*Having Your Baby
by Donor Insemination*

Books by Elizabeth Noble

Having Twins
Essential Exercises for the Childbearing Year
Childbirth with Insight
Marie Osmond's Exercises for Mothers-to-Be
Marie Osmond's Exercises for Mothers and Babies
Having Your Baby by Donor Insemination

Having Your Baby by Donor Insemination

A COMPLETE RESOURCE GUIDE

Elizabeth Noble

1987

Houghton Mifflin Company · Boston

Library of Congress Cataloging-in-Publication Data

Noble, Elizabeth, date.
Having your baby by donor insemination.

Bibliography: p.
Includes index.
1. Artificial insemination, Human.   2. Infertility,
Male.   I. Title.   [DNLM: 1. Infertility, Male—popular
works.   2. Insemination, Artificial—popular works.
WQ 208 N748h]
RG134.N63   1987   362.8'2   87-3372
ISBN 0-395-36897-9
ISBN 0-395-45395-X (pbk.)

Printed in the United States of America

S 10 9 8 7 6 5 4 3 2 1

The quote from *The Prophet* by Kahlil Gibran is reprinted
here by permission of Alfred A. Knopf, Inc. Copyright 1923
by Kahlil Gibran.

TO

Julia, who will always know the truth
Our donor, for his courage and generosity

Your children are not your children.

They are the sons and daughters of Life's longing for itself.

They come through you but not from you,

And though they are with you, yet they belong not to you.

You may give them your love but not your thoughts.

For they have their own thoughts.

You may house their bodies but not their souls,

For their souls dwell in the house of tomorrow, which you cannot visit, not even in your dreams.

Kahlil Gibran
The Prophet

Acknowledgments

The gestation and birth of this book have taken many years, and I am grateful to more people than I can acknowledge in this space.

I would like to mention in particular Pauline Ley and Suzanne Ariel, who met with me many times and shared their literature with me and thus made me so keenly aware of the anguish of genealogical bewilderment. Elinor Hackett's help, especially with arranging interviews with DI couples, is much appreciated. I am also indebted to Rona Achilles for permission to quote her research and insights throughout the book.

I am grateful to Mica Rie and Ingrid Stabins for translating foreign articles, and to Candace Turner, Rita Arditti, Betty Jean Lifton, Joseph Blizzard, and Jan Aitken for additions and corrections to the manuscript.

Several gynecologists helped me with interviews, literature, and criticism of the manuscript, especially Leo Sorger, Christiane Northrup, and Colin Matthews. Psychiatrists David Berger, Philip Parker, and Graham Farrant provided valuable insights. Reuben Pannor, Rona Achilles, and Esther Levine also shared information and support.

George Annas and Lori Andrews gave valuable assistance with the legal issues.

I appreciate my cousin Patrick Bagot's patient proofreading of the manuscript and the support from my husband Geoff and our families. My office manager Ellen Epstein provided much secretarial assistance.

Permission is gratefully acknowledged for quotations from the Australian magazine *Matilda,* Professor Dunstan and the Royal

College of Obstetricians and Gynaecologists in England, Sissela Bok, Mark Karpel, Andrea de Witt and Iowa Resolve, Robert Snowden, Stephen Broder of the Southern California Cryobank, and Michael Leunig of *The Age* in Melbourne, Australia.

The personal quotes in the book have been distilled from phone calls, personal interviews, and letters from couples, women, and practitioners all across the country. By sharing their experiences with me they helped increase the depth and breadth of this enterprise. In most cases the source of the quotation is not identified to protect the privacy of those individuals. Often I did not even know the identity of the interviewee other than a first name, and these names, and locations, have all been changed. Every attempt has thus been made to conceal and protect all the parties involved and any similarity that could be drawn is purely coincidental.

Contents

	Foreword	xiii
	Author's Note	xvii
1	We Did It Our Way	1
2	Coming to Terms with Male Infertility	23
3	Alternatives to Male Biological Parenting	40
4	The Experience of Donor Insemination	49
5	Donor Insemination – Traditions and Techniques	85
6	Semen Freezing and Sperm Banks	106
7	Anonymous Semen Donors	126
8	Known Donors in Collaborative Reproduction	160
9	Ethical Questions and Moral Dilemmas	197
10	Legal Issues and Resolutions	239
11	The Burden of Secrecy	282
12	The Disclosure of Biological Identity	318
	Conclusion	350
	Bill of Rights and Responsibilities	354
	Appendix 1 Causes and Treatment of Male Infertility	358
	Appendix 2 Self-Insemination	366

Contents

Appendix 3
Guidelines for Evaluating a Donor   382
Appendix 4
Sample Sperm Bank Contract and Catalog 396
Resources   402
Bibliography   409
Index   449

Foreword

BY GEORGE J. ANNAS, J.D., M.P.H.

Sam Shepard's Pulitzer Prize–winning play, *Buried Child,* recounts the moral disintegration of a family haunted by a secret they have kept for years: they had intentionally drowned an unwanted infant and buried it in their backyard. During the play, their minister comes to visit the family, but wants to leave as soon as trouble is hinted: "I had no idea there was any trouble. No idea at all." Donor insemination (DI), of course, is concerned with having a wanted child. But it is likely that most people would say the same thing as the minister if asked about keeping anonymous donor insemination a secret: "I had no idea there was any trouble. No idea at all." After reading this book, such a statement is impossible.

It didn't take Alex Haley and *Roots* to convince us that our genetic heritage is part of us, of our identity, and of our birthright. Consciously depriving one's child of the ability ever to know his or her genetic heritage is wrong. As this book so well demonstrates, it is also counterproductive and harmful to family life. As in *Buried Child,* a lifetime of conscious deception can have disastrous consequences. Why does the practice of donor anonymity and secrecy remain almost universal? Why are no standard records kept of donors that can be matched to recipients? Why are parents reluctant to disclose not only the identity of the sperm donor, but even the fact of donor insemination (DI) itself, to their children conceived this way? What can be done to change this practice? These questions, seldom raised in a serious way, are central to this book. And they are relevant to areas well beyond DI.

Donor insemination has become the paradigm for all other forms of noncoital reproduction—from in vitro fertilization (IVF) and embryo transfer to surrogate motherhood, from surrogate embryo transfer to the use of frozen embryos. Unfortunately, as Elizabeth Noble so well demonstrates, it is an unworkable paradigm. The notion that we have solved all the problems with DI is a fantasy. The truth is that we have almost no consistent policies regarding it, and those policies we do have more often than not are harmful to couples and children alike. By exposing the current anarchy of practice and the fetish of secrecy surrounding DI, we are confronted by the issues of donor screening, donor anonymity, legal presumptions regarding rearing parents, commercialism, and control by the medical profession. We need to face these problems as a society if noncoital reproduction is to be responsive to the needs of infertile people, and respectful of the best interests of the resulting children.

Three books have served as useful markers in the brief modern history of donor insemination. The first is Dr. Hermann Rohleder's comprehensive history of DI, *Test Tube Babies: A History of Artificial Impregnation of Human Beings,* which was published in 1934. The book is about artificial insemination with the husband's sperm, and Dr. Rohleder finds DI with "strange sperm" very disreputable. He writes, "What husband or wife, no matter how intense their longing for an heir, will consent to an injection of strange semen? Thank God that most people still have that much tact, decency, and moral feeling." Nonetheless, he believes physicians should be sympathetic to this "outlandish request," at least when made "in desperate, exceptional cases."

The second, much less well known work, is a dissertation by the Rev. William Kevin Glover for his doctorate in Sacred Theology at Catholic University. Entitled *Artificial Insemination among Human Beings: Medical, Legal and Moral Aspects,* it was published in 1948. Drawing heavily on Catholic moral doctrine, Rev. Glover concludes that DI is "obviously and empathically" morally wrong because the marriage union is *exclusive* (and a third party would violate this exclusiveness); the woman has no moral right to receive the sperm of another (and the husband lacks the power to permit it); and the specimen is always obtained by masturbation, a practice unlawful in itself.

The third book is a collection of papers, *Human Artificial Insemination and Semen Preservation,* edited by Georges David and Wendel S. Price, that were presented at an international conference in Paris in 1979. This conference was held years after the IVF birth of Elizabeth Brown, an event that immediately made DI seem technologically trivial. The collection reflects this reaction. Gone are the moralizing and handwringing about DI. Sixty-one of the seventy-eight papers deal with the scientific and medical aspects of semen collection, preservation, and delivery. The remaining seventeen deal with psychological and social issues. The field of DI is described as "young and growing," and having been given great impetus by developments in cryopreservation. One paper, a study at a French clinic, even deals with the issue of secrecy. The authors conclude that "the possibility of sharing the secret could help the couples deal with unavoidable difficulties, and may play a preventive role regarding the secret's potential toxicity."

DI has been written about from scientific, medical, moral, and psychological perspectives. Now we have a book from the couple's perspective. It's about time. Elizabeth Noble and her husband dealt with the issue of the "secret" directly and took steps to insure that both they and their child would know the identity of the genetic father. She tells their story in a compelling manner. But this book is much more. She follows her personal saga with a comprehensive summary of the major ethical, legal, medical, and personal issues any couple contemplating noncoital reproduction should deal with. No doubt some people will find this book disturbing, and will disagree strongly with the notion that truth-telling is appropriate in the DI setting. But this is an extremely useful self-help book for all who must reproduce noncoitally or not at all. Also, because its focus is so clearly on the best interests of the child, it is a helpful book for the future generations of children as well.

The book should also prove eye opening to physicians and legislators, many of whom remain as shortsighted about secrecy as Dr. Rohlelder was about the medical and social aspects of DI, or Rev. Glover was about its morality. With views like theirs common among professionals, is it any wonder that doctors counsel secrecy? I was pleased when Elizabeth Noble asked me for legal advice concerning her wishes for full disclosure to her future child; and equally pleased to write this foreword.

The times *are* changing; not just for medical technology, but also for the protection of the rights of children. Elizabeth Noble takes us beyond protecting the best interests of the sperm donor, to respecting the best interests of the child.

Author's Note

Throughout this book I shall be using the abbreviation DI (donor insemination) rather than the traditional AID (artificial insemination by donor). For consistency I shall also use the initials DI when quoting from references using the term AID.

The terminology for artificial insemination by donor needs to be updated for two reasons. First, it is important that AID not be confused with AIDS (acquired immune deficiency syndrome). The abbreviation AI is also more commonly known as artificial intelligence, and AID also means the (U.S.) Agency for International Development. Second, the term DI indicates that the donor is central to the procedure. (Also, calling the procedure "artificial" insemination is redundant because its artificial nature is already implied in the word "insemination.") "Therapeutic insemination," which has also been tried, is clearly patronizing and misleading, as DI is not a medical "treatment" despite its common presentation as such. I am aware that certain feminists/lesbians use the terms "alternative insemination" or "alternative fertilization" precisely to discount the donor.

I shall also refer to the DI child/adult as "she." In contrast, I shall refer to the adoptee as "he."

As explained in the Acknowledgments, the names and details of those individuals involved with DI who requested anonymity have been changed.

Articles and studies are identified in the text by the authors' last name(s) and date of publication. Complete references can be found in the bibliography at the back of the book.

1

We Did It Our Way

THIS BOOK IS A GUIDE to help others make choices and take responsibility, as we did, in a difficult and controversial area—artificial insemination by donor (DI). Many individuals will not want to engage in such a deep level of personal responsibility, and will prefer to have their physician make the important decisions for them. Others will feel great anguish at reading what I have to say, because they followed their doctor's counsel and now it is too late. For the majority of DI parents, it will be too late to tell the child the truth about her parentage without admitting to years of deception and too late in most cases to retrieve information about the donor. However, guilt is a destructive emotion. Parents generally do the best they can given the circumstances at the time, although later they may look back and feel they would have done things differently. DI parents, like adoptive couples in the past, are victims in a system that is not in their or their child's best interest. I hope that the trend toward open adoption will influence the practice of DI and that the questions I raise in this book will force consideration of the most central concern—the rights of the child.

No one, of course, will ever have all the answers to such a complex issue as donor insemination. Every DI family situation is unique and we are learning as we go along. We also have to realize that learning occurs through mistakes. The information that I gathered for this book is primarily for the benefit of the parties involved in our particular situation, so that we all can be aware of as many dimensions as possible. I also deeply hope that by writing our story and sharing all the information and research I uncovered, the practice of DI will change. As with adoption reform, greater public awareness will enable other parents to make a more informed choice, and provide support for an ethical position that will guarantee the child's right to know her paternal origins.

The Diagnosis of Male Infertility: A Heavy Blow

My husband Geoff and I spent our late twenties studying, traveling, and experimenting with different jobs and life-styles. The thought of children was happily postponed. Indeed, I can even recall casually making the comment that our marriage was so complete it wouldn't matter if one of us were infertile. Feelings certainly change! Reaching our thirties, we decided we were ready for the adventure of parenting. Geoff started running a business by himself, which he hoped would give him the freedom and time to interact with a child. I had my IUD removed to give my uterus at least a year to recover from that foreign body. I remember telling the gynecologist who pulled out the IUD that I didn't need any more contraception—I would play Russian roulette. He talked me into using a diaphragm.

About a year later, we stopped using the diaphragm and actively tried for a pregnancy. I had been keeping records of my basal body temperature for a few months, and was familiar with my most fertile time. I didn't worry too much when the first couple of months went by—we both had a heavy workload. But when no pregnancy resulted after a month's vacation in the Caribbean, I sensed that something was wrong.

We were driving back to Boston from Miami when I got that postvacation menstrual period. My temperature charts showed the expected dips and rises, so we suspected that the problem did not lie with me. We decided to have a semen analysis as soon as we got home. Not all laboratories do a semen analysis, and none of the ones that we contacted wanted to do any investigation without a doctor's order. Lacking any concrete evidence we did not see any need to consult a physician at this stage. It was annoying that a woman can get a pregnancy test without a hassle (finally), but a man cannot have his sperm count checked without medical referral. I put some pressure on one lab—stressing my paramedical background. After much discussion with the supervisor, the lab eventually agreed to do the test.

Several days went by and we heard nothing. So I called the laboratory to see how the semen analysis was proceeding. The test had been completed, but it appeared that we were not going to learn the outcome. A faint voice faltered across the line, "We *must* have the name of a physician to contact with the results. We are not supposed to give out any information to the patient." I knew immediately that something was seriously wrong. Quietly insistent, I pushed for the results. Finally the voice blurted out, "Are you sure your husband hasn't had a vasectomy?" The technician then went on to explain that *no sperm at all* had been detected.

I wanted to believe that a huge mistake had been made. Perhaps I had kept the sperm too warm when I drove to the lab with the sample inside my blouse? But then, at least dead sperm would be visible. *No* sperm? It just seemed incredible; some technician must have mixed up the samples, or the reports. On the other hand, I knew that I had not become pregnant. Still in the denial phase of my grief reaction, I reminded myself that we had tried for only three months, and it is perfectly normal for a couple to take a year to achieve a pregnancy.

As we slowly became accustomed to the truth, I was relieved that we had not waited any longer and that we at least had clearly identified the problem. Geoff took the news very quietly, whereas my emotions always rise quickly to the surface. His feelings were a mixture of dismay and "Well, there must be a cure." We both decided that now it was time to seek medical guidance.

Searching for Medical Care: Consumers' Frustrations

I did not know a single urologist in our area. I called a few friends with medical connections—but they had no one to recommend. Finally, I contacted an infertility organization in Boston and was given the name of a couple of urologists. The first recommended doctor was heavily booked for a few weeks, but his partner had an opening within days. We were anxious to proceed so we made an appointment with the junior physician.

Geoff remembered that when he was about one year old he had spent several months with an aunt while his mother was confined in a sanitarium for tuberculosis. Seriously worried that TB may have been the cause of his sterility, we wrote the news to Geoff's mother in Australia. But she could not remember any childhood incidents or illnesses that might have caused the problem. Also, she told us that her TB diagnosis had been completely mistaken.

Perhaps Geoff's diagnosis would also turn out to be an awful error?

Now that we had the name of a urologist, I called around to check out his qualifications. My colleagues in obstetrics and gynecology, like myself, knew little about male infertility. In order to look into this urologist's reputation, I needed to be open about our problem. This was our first experience with the stigma attached to infertility. People reacted with discomfort, as if we were revealing that one of us had cancer.

Nobody could give us much information about the physician we consulted except that he was known to be keenly interested in infertility. He discovered no obvious abnormalities in Geoff's reproductive system, but a repeat semen test revealed the same result: no sperm. He explained the possible causes and recommended a biopsy of the testicles to determine if there was any kind of sperm production. The presence of sperm in the testicles suggests that there is a blockage of the sperm ducts. The potential solution is to cut and rejoin the sperm duct to another area of the testicle to circumvent the blockage. It was also made clear to us, as I had read in the medical literature, that the chance of success for this surgery was very low—about one case in four regained sperm in the semen. Even in these fortunate cases, the count or quality of the sperm was not necessarily normal nor was there any guarantee that a pregnancy would ever result.

A more experienced surgeon would have presented the option to us of doing both the biopsy and reconstructive surgery together during a single hospital admission and anesthetic. For couples who have decided that they want to try every possibility, this saves time, money, and medical intervention. However, in our ignorance, Geoff only had the biopsy done.

By this time, I was poring over books and articles in medical libraries on the prognosis of this surgery for Geoff. I discussed the biopsy results with physician friends. A urologist out West whom I knew from high school, told us of a urologist who specialized in microsurgery and vasectomy reversals. The infertility counseling group in Boston had never heard of him. However, I checked his credentials and obtained his address and phone number from the *Dictionary of Medical Specialists* in a hospital library.

Doctor Shiller, as we will call him, spent a great deal of time on the telephone with Geoff, explaining his qualifications, procedures, and results. He was very eager to operate, but so was our urologist in Boston, whom we shall call Dr. Kraus. Doctor Shiller had operated on hundreds of men with Geoff's condition, and, he reassured us, "over a thousand rats." Doctor Kraus said he had done only a few. There was also a big price difference—$750 for Dr. Kraus compared with $2500 for Dr. Shiller, plus the travel out of state. Nevertheless, it seemed clear that for such a new and complex type of surgery we should go to the expert. Consequently, we made arrangements to schedule Dr. Shiller and booked Geoff's flight.

Dr. Kraus, however, became incensed when we told him of our decision. He was emphatic that he could do just as good a job, stressing that he had recently completed a course in microsurgery. We felt particularly vulnerable when Kraus added that he would not provide follow-up care if we went to the other surgeon, and that this follow-up was very important.

As we wavered over the decision a contract came from Dr. Shiller: $2,000 to be paid in advance, and in "U.S. currency." The information package was slick and organized. The hospital offered limousine service, gourmet meals, and hotel accommodations for the wife if she wanted to accompany her husband. It almost sounded as if there would also be slippers and a bathrobe embroidered with the patient's name!

We were on the horns of a dilemma. There was the threat of no follow-up from our Boston doctor (although at the time we were never informed as to exactly what this follow-up entailed). Yet we were not comfortable with the super sales pitch of our long-distance microsurgeon.

Finally, we allowed ourselves to be persuaded by Dr. Kraus that he had equivalent expertise.

The First Operation: Inexperienced Hands

After the surgery, Dr. Kraus was quite optimistic to me on the telephone. Geoff's impression was not so positive. The operating room was not well organized, and he lay on the table for nearly an hour waiting for the microscope equipment to be set up. Further delays occurred before the assistant surgeon, Kraus's partner, arrived. (We later realized that he was actually the senior surgeon, who was more experienced and was teaching our physician.) When Geoff awoke and found out that the surgery had taken over four hours, he felt the outlook was bleak. Dr. Shiller had told us that he spent less than two hours on this type of operation so we knew then that Geoff had not been in skilled hands.

A month later, there were still no sperm in the semen.

We knew the results were only 25 percent successful in the best hands. Now we deeply regretted that Geoff had not made the trip to the other surgeon. Kraus dismissed us with, "Well, you have to give it some time—come back with another sample in six months." So much for the follow-up.

In cases of low sperm count it is possible to filter and combine semen samples to obtain a higher concentration of sperm. However, when the surgery is a failure and the absence of sperm persists—then what follow-up is possible? Semen tests we could get ourselves from a laboratory. Our anger was immediate when we realized we had been misled by a beginner aggressively seeking experience in this rare type of surgery. Also, it didn't make sense that time was an issue. If there were no sperm coming through right after the rejoining of the ducts, then why should they be expected to pass through later? This doctor was simply unable to tell us the truth, that the situation was hopeless, unchanged. It made him feel more comfortable to leave us dangling with some false expectations. We were too disillusioned ever to consult Dr. Kraus again. Nowadays, we can even wryly joke that he was "not on the ball"! We organized another semen analysis at a lab six months later. By this time, we were smart enough to put the sample in for a "postvasectomy evaluation," which was done without question. Still the same bad news.

These few months of waiting after Geoff's unsuccessful surgery gave us some psychological space to process our grief. Although we had lost all confidence in Kraus's surgical ability or experience, we fell victim to enough mind games that at moments we let ourselves think that maybe there was still hope.

Neither of us was ready, then, to look into the next round of options. My emotions were a mixture of sorrow and anger. My anger rose when I started to think about the resolution. While the situation was hopeless and final for Geoff, it was just the beginning of a lot of hassles and hard work for me. I was resentful that I could not just fall pregnant in the marital bed like other women. At other times, the sadness was overwhelming. I felt deep sympathy for Geoff's feelings, and I also felt sorry for myself. I grieved for the child with Geoff's honey eyes that we would never create together. (Although I was fully aware that genetically a child could resemble either parent, in those emotional states I only had images of *Geoff's* child.)

Geoff became very quiet and withdrawn. He sold his business, decided not to pursue any employment, and involved himself heavily in yoga, meditation, and philosophy. His father died during this phase as well.

By chance, I noticed in an Australian newsletter we receive that the award for Microsurgeon of the Year had been bestowed on a Sydney surgeon in San Francisco, Dr. Hope. I telephoned the Australian consulate there to find out how I could reach this microsurgeon, but found out that he had returned to Australia. His name rang a bell—it was the same doctor who had taught Dr. Shiller. In fact, Dr. Shiller had told us there were only three good microsurgeons in the world—himself (of course!), one in Australia, and one in Europe. (In retrospect, his judgment was probably quite accurate.) I wrote to Dr. Hope in Australia that we were planning a visit and requested his opinion on the value of a second attempt.

Despite his reluctance to do repeat surgery, Dr. Hope did agree to try it once more. Dr. Hope had never heard of our novice, Dr. Kraus, but he did consider Dr. Shiller very skillful.

The medical fees were most reasonable in Australia and we both wanted to leave no stone unturned. We had learned the hard way that the low chances of success with this difficult surgery need to be maximized with the greatest expertise. If the world's best microsurgeon could not fix things—then no one could. A year after the first surgery, Geoff underwent the second attempt.

Trying Again: Last Chance

Accompanied by the music of Beethoven, Dr. Hope efficiently completed the surgery within a couple of hours. Sperm were flowing freely through the joins he had made on both ducts, but he warned us that "it was like sewing wet blotting paper together." This was evidence of a long-standing chronic problem. The very narrow vas deferens suggested to him that the pathway had probably been inactive since early childhood. By this time, our hope was faint. It was more a case of knowing the worst, knowing when to close this chapter of seeking and hoping.

The repeat surgery also proved unsuccessful. After we returned from Australia I often checked Geoff's semen myself under a friend's microscope. At those times, every air bubble and speck of dust looked like a potential sperm to me and he would have to tell me the hard truth. The lab tests continued to be negative.

What Next? Sorting Out Options

By this time, most of our friends knew of this sequence of events, and from time to time the questions of adoption or artificial insemination came up—both of which I flatly rejected. Geoff reacted noncommittally, realizing how much the decision now rested with me. I was fully aware of the lengthy waiting lists involved with adoption because so few healthy newborn babies were available. We did not want to be bothered with social workers, interviews, home visits—the whole bureaucracy around adoption. There are always children with social or physical problems for adoption, but I had worked with handicapped children and did not want to adopt one, and I did not want any extra parenting challenges with my first child. We also wanted a *baby*, and pregnancy and birth. I especially wanted any child of mine to have the most optimal prenatal environment (physical, nutritional, and psychological), which I did not feel was the case when a mother is planning to relinquish her baby, usually under duress. And I certainly did not approve of the severing of links that occurs with conventional adoption.

Artificial insemination—having a doctor choose some unknown person's sperm for us—was an even worse alternative. I could never trust anyone, and especially a stranger-physician, to make such a decision for me. We felt extremely uncomfortable about the conspiracy of secrecy that surrounds the whole process, especially the belief that the *child* should never be told. Another problem is that even if parents wanted to be honest with the child about the conception, any information on the donor is unavailable or even destroyed to maintain anonymity. The child then loses all genealogical connections with her biological father.

From the very beginning we had always been quite open with friends and family about the tests and surgery. How else would we have obtained the leads that we did which guided our decisions— for better or worse? Although people generally don't know how to react to infertility (it embarrasses them, as they are usually fertile), at least we did not have that heavy burden of secrecy. Nor were we isolated in medical hands like typical infertility patients.

During this whole sequence of events, some of our male friends casually suggested that they would be happy to help out with our conception problems. A few of them had artificial insemination in mind, whereas others seemed to prefer the natural route! We just laughed off these sexual innuendoes. Several friends regretted that they had undergone vasectomies and wished that they had stored some semen that could be used for our benefit. Geoff, my sister, and I would joke about a nose that was too big, or legs that were too short, among our potential donors. One wife volunteered her husband's sperm, and another woman was sure that her lover would oblige. An old friend said she would love to recommend her son—but he suffered from hereditary cataracts. A formerly infertile couple we knew, who now had three children, were initially keen to help. However, they consulted a lawyer and became very anxious about possible birth defects and lawsuits. They moved abroad shortly afterward anyway.

No couple wants to have donor insemination—they want a baby. We wanted a child as much as ever, even more so after putting so much effort into the struggle. Both of us wanted to experience pregnancy and birth, especially since that was the field in which I worked professionally. It looked as if donor insemination was the only possibility left.

However, the medical practice of DI was repugnant to me. I could never contrive to conceive a child knowing that I would deny him or her the essence of his or her roots and history—however ideal the nurturing environment might be. The overwhelming evidence from adoption studies shows how important it is for individuals to know their origins.

We were aware from general reading and television programs that adoptive parents today are strongly advised to disclose the truth to their children, because many traumatic experiences occurred when the child found out about the adoption accidentally. Parental deception is much more shattering than the knowledge of adoption. In fact, Geoff had an adoptee in one of his college psychology classes who personally described such an experience. Geoff never forgot how great an effect that disclosure had on this man's sense of trust. He couldn't even knock on anyone's door without first peeking in the windows. This adoptee searched for several years, and at great expense, before finding his birthparents and thus setting that fundamental curiosity to rest.

Of course we would tell the child the truth about the conception. We saw this as simply our moral duty as sharing and honest parents. On a more immediate and personal level, *I* was the one to become pregnant. Never could I carry a child if I did not know from whom it came. Trusting another to select a donor for me would be worse than an arranged marriage with an unknown spouse. All the potential disasters, such as a technician mixing up semen samples, tormented my mind. And having a child, even under ideal conditions, is such a big commitment. One can be an ex-husband, or an ex-teacher—but never an ex-parent.

Because resolving our problem now lay in my hands, Geoff, in his accommodating way, would have gone along with whatever route I might have chosen. However, he also shared my deep concern about the secrecy that surrounds DI. In our case, it seemed absurd. Everyone else knew our situation, so why shouldn't our child, the person to whom the truth is most significant? Also, for us it was already far too late to be secretive.

Because of the double bind with DI—secrecy about the circumstances of conception and anonymity of the donor—it was clear to us that we had to make the arrangements ourselves for "open DI."

The Big Step: Getting Started on Our Own

Actually, this was the easiest decision of all. True freedom in this case meant no choice. There was no ambivalence, no sitting on the fence, no postponing the issues. We knew in our hearts what we had to do. Our belief that we were following a path of honesty and self-reliance gave us courage. Geoff and I regarded our potential offspring not as our possession, but as a child of the universe. Raising a child is a privilege and an avenue of emotional growth. Blood lineage is not necessary for human attachment. It is a well-known cliché that you choose your friends but you are given your relatives. Spouses are never kin, yet no one questions that bond. Some people even prefer a different species for a companion, as evidenced by their devotion to a dog or cat. The biological act of fatherhood takes but a moment; the psychological and social joys and responsibilities endure for a lifetime.

I now had come to accept the idea of DI, but only if we controlled the whole process so that our highest ideals could be met.

I admit that I had distinct advantages in my knowledge of gynecology and access to medical resources. However, DI never seemed to us to be a medical matter at all. (In fact, the actual procedure of DI is very simple and is explained in Chapter 5 and Appendix 2.) Women attending DI clinics are required to do most of the work anyway, such as taking their daily temperatures and sometimes charting changes in their cervical mucus.

Furthermore, we were both tired of doctors, tests, hospitals, and surgery. During the twelve months of Geoff's biopsy and two unsuccessful operations, I had a breast lump removed (due partly, I believe, to the frustrated desire for childbearing) and both my first ribs (because I was developing muscle weakness in my hands from nerve compression in my neck). It was a year of four general anesthetics and seven surgical incisions for the two of us.

Realizing that the ramifications of DI extend far beyond the basic skills required to perform it, we felt that the next task was to examine the legal position of do-it-yourself DI. I had seen a television program about surrogate motherhood, and I contacted a lawyer in another state who had worked on this type of contract. He was fascinated by our intentions, but we were turned off by his elitism when he said, "Boy, I bet you guys have had a college education to want to do this." He asked us to fly him to Boston so he could discuss the details. Fortunately, before we made that mistake, I suddenly remembered a Boston attorney whom I had heard speak at a birth conference. I was sure he would be sympathetic and knowledgeable. This lawyer was a strong advocate of patients' rights and alternative medicine. When we learned he was counsel to one of the DI clinics in Boston, we felt we had selected someone uniquely qualified to advise us.

At the outset, he pointed out to us that the standard practice was to keep the donor anonymous and not to tell the child. We explained that we had given these questions serious thought and had found this medical practice unethical and unacceptable to us. We were relieved to learn that there was nothing illegal, at least in Massachusetts, about the action we were contemplating. Originally, we had thought we should have things arranged so that Geoff would legally adopt the child, but the attorney pointed out some difficulties with this approach.

Our lawyer had never heard of a couple with a request like ours, but he agreed to research the matter and draw up a contract to be signed by Geoff and the donor we chose. In his legal opinion it was important to keep the donor relationship strictly as a sale of sperm under contract. He also made it clear that the enforceability of the contract, while valid in his eyes, could only be tested in court (see Chapter 10).

At this point we felt a little powerless. We had some doubts about our male friends who had volunteered themselves as donors. Were their offers in jest or for real? Could we afford to be particular? In pessimistic moments we almost would have been glad of any known source of sperm!

Shortly after meeting with the lawyer, Geoff took on a temporary research job in Canada. I wanted to maintain my practice in Boston so we decided that we would take turns commuting. I can still remember all those weekends, sitting around in airports, looking at every man who walked by, considering each one as a potential donor. I never saw one prospect whom I would have chosen!

We wanted to use a donor who was geographically convenient; offers from Australia and the West Coast were obviously not practical. However, for the right donor we would have made any sacrifice. We easily dismissed the notion of asking Geoff's brother. Apart from his location twelve thousand miles away, we agreed that the combined role of uncle and biological father would be too confusing—for us, anyway. Former lovers of mine were not acceptable, as we wanted the whole procedure to be aboveboard and free of sexual implications. Because the donor, for a moment, would be "assisting" Geoff, we agreed that he should be Geoff's choice.

Both of us were extremely happy with a certain friend of Geoff's in Montreal who had offered to donate semen some months before when he first knew of Geoff's sterility. This individual was a relaxed family man with several children of his own. When we raised the question again with him, he said "sure," that he had mentioned it at that time to his wife, and she didn't mind at all. We felt it was important that the offer come straight from his heart. While there were certainly significant questions to consider, the whole idea was basically something with which both parties were completely comfortable from the outset. The issue is similar to deciding on a homebirth, for example. If you need to ask others if you should do it, then you shouldn't. (Further discussion on qualities of a donor can be found in Chapter 8.)

So he and Geoff each signed a release and one dollar was paid to our donor. We parted on a friendly note: "Let me know when the time is ripe!"

Beginning DI: Excitement and Disappointment

The next three months were full of excitement and despair. Each time I was *sure* I was pregnant! It was a great relief to be working positively on achieving a pregnancy—to have everything in *our* hands at last. But the waiting and hoping were a great strain. Despite all the traveling we both did between Canada and home, Geoff and I continually investigated my temperature charts, the changing features of my cervix, and the quality of my cervical mucus. I continued to read up on all the ways to detect ovulation and the different techniques for insemination in medical libraries.

I decided that I would use a rubber cervical cap for the insemination, although they were difficult to find in Boston. There were very few practitioners fitting them, and the waiting lists were long. Finally, when a feminist clinic in New Hampshire offered me a canceled appointment, I drove eighty miles for a fitting. I could have used a syringe, rather than the cap, but then the semen would have to be withdrawn from another receptacle. A diaphragm probably works fine too, but it is more flimsy. I wanted to maximize my chances by avoiding trauma to the sperm and keeping them as close to the cervix as possible.

The donor would collect the specimen in the cervical cap and leave it in the soap dish. I would then go into the bathroom and insert the cap. Next, I would go into a shoulder stand or rest with my hips up on a chair, remaining in that position for about twenty minutes. I wanted everything, even gravity, to help those sperm get to their destination.

Sometimes I went to our friend's office after hours, and sometimes we went to his house. I could make myself useful watering the garden while our donor was busy in the bathroom. One time I went to mail a letter and returned to find him keeping the precious specimen warm on a kettle! Geoff joined me sometimes, depending on our schedules. Once I remember all of us watching the evening news on television; my view was upside down because I was doing a shoulder stand! Another time, we sat around chatting over strawberries and cream. The experience was incomparably more friendly and personal than visiting a medical clinic!

The cervical cap worked well mechanically, but when I first removed it after twenty-four hours there was a foul odor. We figured the smell came from the latex in the rubber, which must not have been healthy for the sperm. Because this cap was designed for contraception, damage to the sperm wouldn't have mattered. Our donor also commented that perhaps the suction with the rubber cap was too powerful for the sperm to migrate uphill against it into the cervix. The suction is certainly very strong. Once, when I was impatient in removing the cap, I didn't break the suction properly and nearly turned myself inside out.

A friend of mine who worked as a nurse for a DI practitioner told me about a plastic cervical cap, actually called a cup as it was designed not to cap off the cervix but to contain semen. I called her in California and she kindly sent me a couple of different cups by return mail. While this cup was rigid and more difficult to insert, it completely solved the odor problem.

I started to become anxious when I was not pregnant after three inseminations, and during one month we actually had two attempts. I decided to have a serum progesterone test to confirm ovulation and check that my hormone levels after ovulation were adequate to maintain a pregnancy if fertilization occurred. By this time a physician friend of mine was kindly writing any prescriptions and giving any orders I needed, and instructing the lab to give me the results. The test results were normal and the encouragement it provided was worth the thirty-five dollars it cost.

Next, I recalled that a tubal blockage often results from using IUDs, which was the form of birth control I'd used for many years. (It made me furious to think I had polluted my body with all kinds of contraception when all the while my husband had a "natural" vasectomy.) I called every gynecologist listed in the Montreal and Boston telephone directories to see if I could arrange for a tubal insufflation (Rubin) test. This simple evaluation of tubal patency involves passing carbon dioxide through the uterus and Fallopian tubes. No one did them any more except for one physician who was away on vacation, but I was in a hurry to move on with my fertility investigation. I soon learned that the hi tech of dyes and x-rays, called a hysterosalpingogram, had taken over. I didn't fancy the radiation, but I allowed myself to be persuaded that the x-ray was more accurate. I also rationalized that even if I'd been able to have the tubal insufflation test and it was fine, if I still did not become pregnant I would have to consider the x-ray evaluation anyway. Precious time would be lost. I was already thirty-five. How long would our donor want to go on contributing his semen—three months, six months, a year? I felt a sense of panic. He was away on a business trip that month and I decided I would go ahead with the x-ray investigation.

It wasn't easy to arrange the x-ray procedure. All the infertility clinics insisted on seeing the *couple* in consultation first. We did not want to backtrack over Geoff's medical history and I particularly did not want to alert anyone, least of all a disapproving physician, to our scheme. (In medical situations, I felt the need to be secret about our openness!) I had studied the procedure for these x-rays and learned that I should shop around for a service that used an organic, water-based dye, and a gentle plastic cannula. I finally found a hospital where the radiology department met my requirements and accepted the story that my supposedly fertile husband was in Canada and unavailable.

The test was unpleasant. A very cooperative physician spent a great amount of time trying to coax the soft rubber tube into my tight cervix. There was a burst of unbelievable pain—I felt like my bowels and bladder would explode on the table—and it was all over. The test showed that both my tubes were open.

Prior to this test, I was obliged to visit the infertility clinic and receive some antibiotics to take as a precaution against infection. The physician I saw was delightful and supportive of the independent way I had organized my fertility evaluation so far. He suggested that I should come in for a postcoital test to check for viable sperm in the cervical secretions. I agreed to this, although I was not sure how I would synchronize the timing of the donor, the flight back to Boston, and the appointment at the clinic!

Somehow, the next month it all worked out, and within five hours of the insemination the sample was being examined. This egalitarian doctor beckoned me to the microscope. I could see for myself; just one poor stray sperm bogged down in a mass of white blood cells. "Cervicitis," announced the physician with satisfied finality.

I was stunned. An infection in my healthy body? Maybe I had gotten this low-grade inflammation from my IUD, the tail of which can act as a bridge whereby germs from the vagina can enter the cervix. I left with a prescription for broad-spectrum antibiotics. Later I felt I should have insisted on a culture and sensitivity test, to identify the particular organism.

I wanted to make sure that the treatment would be completely effective. In addition, in my office I gave myself deep heat treatments with a shortwave diathermy machine to improve the pelvic circulation and to make sure that the antibiotics were carried to the depths of my reproductive organs. Also, I knew that antibiotics altered the vaginal environment and lead to an overgrowth of yeast cells. I douched preventively each day with Betadine, but I was overconfident and stopped the last two days of the course of medication. Sure enough, the itch and the typical cottage cheese discharge appeared. That led next to another course of medication to cure the yeast infection.

I was ready to try again the same ovulation cycle, but we decided that perhaps it was better to wait until the following month and give my body time to settle back to normal. We still regularly plotted my temperature curve and watched how my cervix changed around ovulation. Now that all the apparent problems were behind us, we were back playing the hoping-and-waiting game again. Sometimes it seemed easier to be busy working on a problem instead.

It was now six months since we had signed the papers and had undergone the first attempt. There had been three months during this time when inseminations had to be postponed because of vacations, business trips, and irreconcilable schedules. I was starting to get cold feet. What I would have given to have looked into a crystal ball and *know* how long it was going to take. We watched a David Susskind show on DI, and one woman (interviewed in darkness) had one hundred and fourteen attempts before finally achieving pregnancy. We certainly didn't think we, or our donor, would be able to go on that long!

I was in the habit of giving our donor a few days' notice, as I observed the changes in my cervix and predicted the time of ovulation from my monthly charts. He took his responsibility seriously, and would "put himself out to pasture" for a couple of days beforehand. I called him one evening and we arranged for a breakfast insemination at his house before work the next morning.

I awoke early that day and immediately checked my cervix. It looked dry and closed; no signs at all of imminent ovulation. I telephoned our donor and said I had misjudged the day. About three hours later, I noticed that a bowel movement had dislodged a good amount of perfect mucus—clear and stretchy like egg white. I'd never had such magnificent mucus, probably because of my previous low-grade cervical infection. I phoned our donor at work, hoping that we could somehow get together at lunch time. However, his schedule did not permit this. In fact, he had to attend a meeting after work and would not be home until quite late. I was crestfallen, feeling sure that I was one of those women who had fertile mucus for just a few hours each month and that much precious time would be lost.

I was further delayed by traffic in reaching his house later that evening, which was full of children staying over for a pajama party. Shoulder stands would be out of the question that night! In fact, it was almost impossible to get into the bathroom, with the teenage girls shampooing their hair and fixing their makeup. I began to feel that the long drive to Montreal was a waste of time. Everything seemed to be going wrong—bad luck and bad management.

Eventually the donor and I went out into the garden together to discuss the logistics. I was to stay near the bathroom and listen carefully for when he came out. It was essential that I follow him into the bathroom before anyone else could get in there. I did not have to hover for long and dashed right in as soon as he came out. Although I had given up all hope for this try, I nevertheless felt a bit nervous this time as I squatted down on the floor and inserted the cap, hoping that my shaky hands would not spill any semen. My cervix was very high that night and I did not really feel sure that I had reached it properly.

The next day Geoff came down to Boston and we went camping

on Cape Cod. There was a full moon and I hardly slept. The next morning I took my basal temperature. It had dropped again! How could that be possible? And it rose again the next day. There was my chart, with a W instead of a V in the middle. I tried without success to think of any reason for a false reading, such as a headache, alcoholic drink, or activity prior to taking my temperature. Perhaps it was a double ovulation? Perhaps I would have twins? We joked about this, while knowing in our hearts it was another botched month.

Exactly one week after the insemination, Geoff looked at my naked body in bed and said, "I think you are pregnant." Music to my ears, but I skeptically asked how he got such an idea in his head. "Just an intuition," he said. "Your breasts look different."

On the plane back to Boston I felt my nipples tingling from the cold air jet. Did I feel pregnant, or was I just imagining all of this?

I continued to take my temperature, and it stayed elevated. That was an encouraging sign although my cervix was not yet turning bluish according to the books. Three weeks passed—no period. I started to think I was pregnant after all and that Geoff had sensed the actual implantation, which occurs about seven to ten days after the conception.

Then some blood appeared. Rage and disappointment overwhelmed me. It had been a most unlikely month and in my desperation I had let myself be carried along by a couple of positive signs. Again, my chicken was not going to be hatched. My emotional state was clearly making my cycle irregular. I wondered how *anyone* kept pursuing such a stressful activity as DI.

Then the bleeding suddenly stopped. My temperature stayed high. Maybe it was just a breakthrough bleed that sometimes happens when the fertilized egg implants in the uterus? I called a women's health clinic offering free pregnancy tests. It was the first day since the insemination that the test could be valid.

A Positive Pregnancy Test!

As soon as I received the news that I was indeed pregnant, I telephoned Geoff and our donor. We were all ecstatically excited. All those inconvenient rendezvous were over! We could now go ahead and enjoy our pregnancy like any other couple.

Geoff named our baby "O" (short for embryo) and from the very beginning she lived in our thoughts, feelings, and awareness as if she were already born. It was a great joy when she was born, two weeks early, although I wouldn't have minded being pregnant forever—it was so enjoyable.

When I first saw her I gasped, "She's so pretty." Geoff had the same reaction. She looked just like a china doll and suckled at my breast immediately. I had seen hundreds of newborns, but as the saying goes, your own looks the best of all. In view of our third-party conception, I am sure we would have admitted anything we didn't like about her inherited features. Always a calm and relaxed baby in the uterus, she looked at us with great repose out of her gray-blue eyes. We especially admired her rosebud mouth, one of the contributions from our donor.

We named her Julia Phyllis. Both grandmothers are called Phyllis, and they were thrilled to be honored as her namesakes.

During her first year of life Julia went with me twice to Australia, once for family illness and once for vacation. The family response has been most positive, and Julia would claim love anyway for being so lovable. We have since made three more visits to our Australian relatives and friends, and she is certainly an accepted member of both sides of the family.

Because we had been completely open all along there has never been any secrecy or suspicion surrounding her conception. As often happens with adopted children, people will comment that Julia looks like Geoff, or that she is a nice mixture of both of us. Even people who knew about the DI, will comment on a resemblance to Geoff, and then apologize!

Julia does not look like me at all, but resembles our blue-eyed donor who is tall and thin, with blond curly hair. One great benefit of do-it-yourself DI is that you can choose characteristics you like. In fact, because we planned to be honest from the very beginning, we did not worry about a match of physical features. What mattered more to us was the donor's good health, personality, and the spirit in which he took this courageous and generous step.

DI couples are told that they will forget about the insemination, just like mothers were told that they would forget they ever had a baby if they gave it up for adoption. Nothing could be further from the truth. How could anyone forget an extramarital conception, especially such a planned one? The actual presence of the child with her genetic endowment is a constant reminder of the donor. Because we chose our donor, however, we are happy to see him reflected in Julia's appearance and expressions. She is probably even more special and precious to us because we have not deceived ourselves, or others, about her origins. In fact, once we made the decision to go ahead with our donor, it became a privilege to have such a wonderful donor, and to know that we could even hope to have another child with his help.

Our donor, and his family, have the pleasure of seeing part of himself in a child that he would not have otherwise created. We do not live with mystery, secrecy, lies, or shame. Our donor and his family enjoy their visits with Julia and she is always very excited to see them. I feel she senses a special bond with that family. We have often discussed Julia's conception with her and answer any questions she has when they arise (see Chapter 12).

When I first thought about writing this book, I considered our action only as an alternative, which I felt should be shared with other couples attempting DI, as well as the professionals involved. For us there was no choice and we would not have done it any other way. Although I realize that the last chapter of this experience has yet to be written—and that may be generations away—I have become convinced, in the course of my research, that we did DI in the best way for us all.

DI is an irrevocable step that requires much time, thought, and sharing. Yet these very considerations are prevented by the secrecy that traditionally surrounds this medical practice. It seems so old-fashioned, in today's pluralistic society, that something like DI has to be hidden. I feel that prospective parents who cannot put the DI child's long-term needs ahead of their own needs on this matter, should seriously question their desire to parent in this way. Physicians who cannot meet these standards should not be involved in DI, in my opinion. Every child must be guaranteed knowledge of his or her origins, especially when the conception is premeditated among knowing and consenting adults.

If you have discomfort about telling the child the truth, if you won't be thrilled to share the new way of extending your family, thrilled enough to talk freely about it and secure enough to survive others' judgments . . . if you are trying to utilize this method of procreation to hide infertility or genetic connection, then it is not based in human respect and understanding but rather in fear and selfishness. The child is still primary. Not your needs for a child. Parenting in any fashion is serious business whether it is as a sperm-donor parent, a surrogate parent, an egg-donor parent, a birth, adoptive, foster, custodial or noncustodial parent, or any other type of parent our scientific community may invent.

—*Mary Jo Rillera and Sharon Kaplan,*
Cooperative Adoption

2

Coming to Terms with Male Infertility

ALTHOUGH ONLY ONE PARTNER—in this case the male—is infertile, both individuals form an infertile couple. This additional pressure adds to the solitary pain. Even though a couple may not remain childless—adoption or an assisted conception can circumvent the problem—these resolutions do not cure the heterosexual couple's infertility. While much of the reckoning with infertility is related to the options available, it is very important to distinguish between the infertility itself and the form of resolution.

Couples have usually tried to create a pregnancy for a long time before hearing the final diagnosis. Even then, "infertility" is not an easy word to hear or say when it refers to you. Obviously the verdict is less of a shock if it is given sensitively, in a manner that encourages the couple to ask questions. But often the doctor's evasive attitude signifies such hopelessness that the possibility of further discussion may be discouraged. Such bad news given over the phone or left as a message comes as a dreadful blow. Sometimes a wife is asked by the physician to inform her husband, or even to pretend the infertility lies with her.

My husband just couldn't believe there were no sperm.
It took three semen tests to convince him.

Infertile couples have already felt the injustice of their destiny in a world where millions of women have abortions and great numbers of parents neglect or abuse their children. With the advent of contraception and the women's movement, there has been a trend to postpone childbearing. When a couple already in their late thirties discovers their infertility and realizes time is running out, there is the added pressure of time. It is often on reaching what Erik

Erikson called the "stage of generativity" that couples are most shattered when they cannot automatically share in creating their offspring. Career women who postponed motherhood may feel much anguish at this point.

The pain of infertility is worsened when couples are the butt of "humorous" suggestions and home remedies, such as "eat broccoli," "try putting your legs in the air," "wear a black negligee," or "take a vacation." Some couples suffer value judgments such as "Don't you think you should stop working so hard at the office and start a family?" or "Since your name is on an adoption list, why worry about infertility?" Sometimes there is "reverse jealousy" with quips like, "I wish Jane had your problem. I only have to look at her and she's pregnant." Others may think that a couple is not trying to get pregnant, all of which reinforces society's view that childlessness is abnormal and in some sense even wrong.

The Man's Feelings About His Infertility

Do men have a primary reproductive drive, a paternal instinct akin to the maternal instinct, which sociobiologists would have us believe? It is only very recently that infertility has even begun to be studied and understood, and the focus has been much more on the woman's experience due to her greater losses (of gestation, birth, and breastfeeding). Presenting infertility as a "couple's problem," which it clearly is, nevertheless can cloud or even hide the man's personal experience, not only in the marital relationship, but also in the workplace and the world at large. As Jan Aitken, a social worker with the infertile in Melbourne, Australia, puts it, "The fear—and the task—is whether men who are infertile still have a potency to be fathers and have a place as functioning adult men in the world?" Men in our culture do not feel as sanctioned as women to express deep feelings; instead, most men defend themselves by repressing their emotions. It is very difficult for women to write about the male experience of infertility, and as yet there are few resources written by men for men. A national organization called Resolve offers information and support to the infertile and publishes newsletters that serve as contact sources for men such as Joel Wilcher, who shares his rage and grief over the loss of his "dream child," quoted later in this chapter.

In anthropological history, fatherhood became a social role only when the man's part in procreation was understood. Yet since biblical times it has been assumed that if no progeny issues forth from a marriage then the wife is barren, and that myth still persists today.

Culturally, there are only concepts of male sexual impotence and lack of virility; the concept of male "infertility" does not really exist, although this is starting to change. Margaret Mead wrote that in modern civilizations every normal man wants to beget children, and infertility is experienced as a great loss. The diagnosis of azoospermia (no sperm), in particular, may revive a man's repressed castration anxiety, together with his fear that both the diagnosis and his anxiety over it may be exposed. Studies have shown that the great majority of infertile male partners suffer feelings of inadequacy, inferiority, and guilt that they have frustrated their partner's yearning for a child. With lowered self-esteem the infertile man feels different and incomplete compared with his other male friends. Although the renunciation of children may be personally less traumatic to men than women, a man doesn't expect to experience infertility any more than a woman does, or even less so, thus the news is always perceived as a great shock. Controlling feelings always leads to tension. The loss of fertility may affect a man's mental and physical health, with bouts of anxiety, nightmares, and other sleep disturbances. He feels he has failed his wife, and to atone for his procreative problems he may try to compensate with fulfilling her material demands. Sometimes career and job difficulties arise, or else the man throws himself into his career, which sometimes enables him to evade conflicts and responsibilities.

Solitude and stress within the marriage, problems with communication and future planning, are commonly experienced. Confusion between sexual potency and reproductive capability is frequent. Sexual relations especially may diminish, not only because of the shock and subsequent grieving but the couple may feel that sex is pointless if they cannot create children. Men who associate masculinity or virility with fertility may feel grossly inadequate, with resulting impotence. Other men may become sexually aggressive with their wives and other women to prove they are still potent males. Envy of the fertile partner is another issue, as well.

Psychotherapist Z. Stephen Bohn (1957) contends that men who are infertile and/or impotent already have developed a neurosis as a result of brooding over their inadequacies for a period of years. The implication is that some corner of the mind does know of the body's infertility. He suggests that this process is unconscious and occurs while the infertile man is busy getting an education or developing business concerns to become financially secure. That all of us determine our health, diseases, or accidents is explored by such physicians as Lewis Mehl in *Mind and Matter* and John Harrison in *Love Your Disease: It's Keeping You Healthy*. Such books emphasize the links between mind and body and empower us to effect our own growth and healing. Cabau (1973) in France describes how a woman was able to conceive on the eighth cycle of DI after discussing why she might be preventing the conception with self-induced spasms of her Fallopian tubes. Graham Farrant, a psychiatrist in Melbourne, Australia, has helped many couples to conceive after addressing the psychosomatic components of organic problems.

Karl Ostrom, writing in a 1971 *Hastings Center Report* dealing with DI, outlines how from a Freudian perspective the male identity shifts from the primary identification with the mother to that of the father, so that the little boy denies his early dependence on his mother. This is necessary to develop the kind of independence that will eventually enable him to carry out an adult masculine role and become a husband upon whom a wife and children can depend. The attraction of a dependent relationship, with its comfort and security, although denied, nonetheless remains strong, and normally re-emerges as the male becomes ready to enter into the relationship of marriage. Ostrom concludes that to the degree that a man's sense of independence and competency is securely established, he is once again able to enter into an interdependent and intimate relationship with a woman without fearing that his sense of masculinity will be overwhelmed—as it might have been during earlier stages of his development.

In contrast, Eichenbaum and Orbach, the authors of *What Do*

Women Want?, observe that men are conditioned to expect uninterrupted nurturing of their emotional needs. Boys are trained to expect that a wife will take over from the mother, and girls are trained to provide that kind of mothering. As a result, women are brought up to suppress their needs and to remain emotionally independent. Infertility counselors frequently observe that women assume much of the burden of infertility—which often adds to their partners' guilt.

Parenthood presents special developmental tasks that require personal growth and transformation. Society provides support and assistance because parenting is seen as an important part of the social structure. Social conditioning in a male-dominated world has caused men to be orientated toward self-assertion and independence, and paternity demands that a male balance his self-interest by nurturing a person other than himself (such as an infant). The traditional emphasis on a child as "issue" or "seed" of the male's body, serves to flatter the male and encourage him to enlarge his ego to encompass his children. In this context, the woman is merely an incubator, or the "dirt" (soil) in what is described as the "flower-pot" theory. However, as I will discuss in Chapter 7, the traditional use of anonymous donor semen actually strengthens the opposite position. That is, sperm is merely seed, and the woman-incubator provides the secret shroud to the myth of the male issue so that the patriarchal line apparently continues as usual. This also helps to make it easier for the infertile man in DI to accept another's semen.

The Woman's Feelings About Her Partner's Infertility

The women's movement has long fought against the idea that "biology is destiny." Feminists have struggled for the right to abortion, contraception, better working conditions and wages; and recently they have seen the issues around childbearing and infertility as being political. In a patriarchal society, motherhood is still promoted as the primary goal of women, although many women are resisting this social pressure and remain child-free. Nevertheless, whether the influences are physiological, psychological, or political, the great majority of women certainly have a strong drive to bear children.

The feelings of the female partner of an infertile man may range from compassion to hostility. She may have been originally considered the one "at fault," which might cause deep resentment. On the other hand she may feel guilty that she is *not* the cause and did not share in his failure. She may even need to set up some kind of punishment for herself to relieve her guilt feelings. Some women prefer to spare the husband by "taking the blame" and making up a story about their infertility problems.

The woman may expect compensation for his lack of fertility by his increasing financial and professional success, and it is extremely hard on a marriage if the husband is unemployed or having job difficulties. There are reported cases where the man's emotional reaction to learning about his infertility meant he became unable to work. Dreams about the husband falling ill, becoming assaulted or injured—even committing suicide—and other themes are not uncommon, and suggest the woman's unconscious desire to be rid of him. Rage, vengeance, phobias, and a host of psychiatric symptoms may develop now that her partner's problem becomes her problem, especially if he is her husband. A woman who postponed pregnancy in order to build up a career for herself, or to put her husband through college, has additional pressure and resentment.

Most psychologists agree that usually the wife's first conscious feeling on the discovery of her husband's sterility is "human-bound," to include a feeling of having been "cheated." Then her anger changes to guilt and a need to protect him. Because the male is the one forced to come to terms with the finality of his own situation, the female partner may remain depressed longer than he does. The woman's hostile feelings and revenge are sometimes directed against her husband, who may further annoy her by becoming depressed and withdrawn. While de facto unions may split up over the infertility, temporary separations and counseling can help resolve the anger and helplessness felt by married couples. Berger (1980) stresses the need to distinguish between conflict and psychopathology. Conflict between a couple undergoing DI is inevitable; psychopathology will be the outcome if this conflict is not re-solved.

Infertility is not always primary. It may be secondary due to injury, disease, or vasectomy. Men need to be well informed about treatments that impair fertility as the following story shows. A woman called me one day for information about doing DI with her brother-in-law's semen. Her husband, Greg, was rendered sterile from chemotherapy for a blood cancer. They had experienced a very rough time, first adjusting to the shock of the cancer diagnosis, then the unpleasant medical treatment, and finally, learning—to their great surprise—that the husband was infertile. The oncologist had never informed them of that side effect of chemotherapy. Thus they are grieving the loss of his sperm, which could have been banked, and also an abortion undergone a few years earlier because the time was "not right" for a child. The husband expressed morbid feelings that he "had to trade his fertility for his life."

> After trying unsuccessfully to conceive for about nine months we started to think about what might be the problem. Obviously we thought my husband's illness might have something to do with it. But when we went to the oncologist, neither of us was prepared for her callous, blaming comment "Didn't you know that sterility is a side effect of the treatment?" I felt like lunging out of my chair and strangling her. We accused her of negligence and she further irritated us by backpedaling and saying things like "Well, even if you had banked sperm, you still might not have become pregnant." We realized then that you have to be your own advocate, you have to learn what you can by yourself.
>
> Luckily Greg's brother, who has four children from two marriages, agreed right away. He didn't even consult his wife, so I don't know if she has been told yet. So we are fortunate that we can keep this in the family. I couldn't ever consider DI with an unknown donor; I would have remained childless. This was our only option; we had no other choice.

The Stages of Grieving

The depth of loss that each person feels about infertility varies from frustration to extreme depression. Reactions depend on such factors as the time spent dealing with the medical workup (which can take years), the style of handling by professionals, and the support received from friends and family. The way each couple copes with stress is also significant. For many couples, infertility is the first major life crisis and loss they have had to face.

Although most infertile couples will eventually give birth or adopt a baby, just having this baby will not simply dissolve the loss that a couple may feel about their infertility. Time and healing are essential ingredients. As Patricia Johnston, past president of Indiana Resolve and author of *Understanding: A Guide to Impaired Fertility for Parents and Friends*, points out, infertility doesn't just represent a single potential loss, but rather a number of losses, such as:

1. The loss of individual genetic continuity and an unbroken family blood line.
2. The loss of a jointly conceived child.
3. The loss of the physical satisfaction of the pregnancy/birth experience.
4. The loss of the emotional gratifications of a shared birth/breastfeeding experience and the mystic goal of parent/child bonding at birth.
5. The loss of the possibility of parenting.
6. The loss of control.

As in all losses, the infertile man will need time to mourn, to let go of the hope of giving himself and his mate his biological child. Although in this case it is the loss of something potential rather than something actual, it is nevertheless like the death of a special person.

The stages of grieving have been well defined by Elisabeth Kübler-Ross and others. They include shock, denial, anger, social isolation, guilt, depression, and (hopefully) resolution and acceptance. Let us now look at the emotional sequence in more detail.

Shock

Heterosexual couples usually do not anticipate any difficulty becoming pregnant and are surprised when a pregnancy does not automatically occur. They have usually spent their life since adolescence making sure they will not be "caught" by an unplanned pregnancy. Having used contraception for years, their surprise is intensified as they realize that their fertility is not under their control after all. By the time a couple seeks evaluation and treatment, they generally have experienced increasing anxiety, frustration, and embarrassing questions from family and friends. Yet the diagnosis of infertility, especially if the outlook is bleak, is still a dreadful shock.

Denial ("Not Us!")

Some couples initially deny their infertility. Pretending that this is not really happening buys some time to adjust to the news and muster resources. Denial, which closes off many avenues of feeling and sharing, may also be reinforced by well-meaning advice and suggestions from friends, such as "Just be patient, it took us two years to have Johnny."

There may also be a mutual need to deny wanting a child, and by not admitting how much they really want children, the couple may delay seeking treatment.

Anger ("Why Us?")

Anger is the most powerful and common reaction. It may be directed at each other, at family members, at the physician who fails to treat or cure, or at friends who do not give support (and even worse, get pregnant). Finally, it is directed toward oneself—why me? Infertile couples feel angry about others' ease of pregnancy and the rising incidence of abortions and child abuse. The frustration, inconvenience, and expense which their infertility causes adds to the store of anger.

Isolation

Withdrawal and social isolation are more common with infertility than other forms of loss or death, because infertility is invisible. Infertile couples have a strong fear of criticism and failure. They feel that they will not only be left out of the world of families, but they may even fear social rejection in general. Infertility is not a condition that is readily shared with the fertile world, so coping with the emptiness and loss of control is particularly difficult. Baby showers and christenings are painful events that infertile couples try to avoid. As one woman said, "Infertility is the loneliest way of life I have ever known." In an overpopulated world (although zero population growth is based on two children per couple), there is less sympathy for infertile couples than they deserve.

> People who have had a normal family with no problems can't see our problem. One chap I know said he felt there were enough children in the world anyway without us wasting all this money on producing the odd one or two. I don't think they can comprehend the circumstances, the pressures, that drive people.
>
> —*Infertile husband in Australia*

In addition to the functional loss that infertility represents to their union, the partners may be isolated from one another as they work through the different stages of the crisis. Couples may not want to seek help, for fear that something psychologically wrong with them will be discovered that will affect their eligibility for DI or adoption.

Guilt

Couples may feel guilty because they waited to finish degrees or become financially secure before beginning a pregnancy. The male partner may carry guilt alone, for example, because of a former venereal disease that he may or may not have shared with his mate. The man feels badly that he has frustrated his partner's desire to achieve pregnancy and motherhood, and that the woman may now become the subject of lengthy examinations and treatments because of his inadequacy. Both men and women may feel guilty about not sharing or understanding their partner's feelings. Many husbands offer their wife a divorce at this time, which indicates the deep level of their remorse.

Infertile couples are often anxious to try any procedure that will promise them the slightest hope of conception, and are vulnerable to medical exploitation. Thousands of dollars can be spent on surgery, hormones, office visits, and lab fees, to say nothing of the new reproductive technologies, and many of these procedures are not covered by insurance.

Ada Armstrong, president of Concern for the Infertile, a self-help group in Western Australia, observes that the guilt may lead to a bargaining situation. Some couples with a strong Puritan ethic want to suffer so much that God will give them a baby, somehow. Such couples expose themselves to almost unrealistic treatments, some with a high risk of side effects, in the hope that even if the treatments are not successful, God will see that they are genuine in their efforts and desire for a child. It is easy for the infertile couple to get stuck in this stage, with unproductive infertility therapy. Indeed, it is the social pressure on women to bear children, for their mates as well as for themselves, that fuels today's questionable technology. Ultimately, medical stocktaking must be done and the decision must be made that "enough is enough." On the other hand, some couples can never make this decision, but will readily concede if their doctor does.

Depression

This is an emotional and physical experience of sadness, lethargy, and despair. There may be loss of appetite, motivation, sleeplessness—the whole body feels "battered." Depression is a normal reaction, but if it persists pathologically it may mask suppressed anger.

Mother's Day and Father's Day, Halloween and Christmas, and the "bulging bellies of the fertile world" intensify the depression.

> One day I was looking through a friend's baby cards and one said WELCOME TO YOUR BABY—AT LEAST IT WAS CONCEIVED THE NATURAL WAY and it had a picture of a test tube with another baby in it. I thought that was really sick. I felt like ripping up the card.
>
> —*Infertile woman in Australia*

Grief

Grieving for the invisible infertility is the long, lonely, painful process of burying the dream. The couple grieve for the loss of the biological child for themselves and for other family members. Time is needed for infertile couples to mourn their infertility, and waiting lists for adoption or DI give space for this growth process. Letting the sadness wash out is essential for the next step of resolution.

Joel Wilcher, past president of Resolve, Washington, D.C., wrote about his grieving:

In October 1982, I attended a workshop with Dr. Elisabeth Kübler-Ross on Life, Death, and Transition. One of the issues discussed was unfinished business—those important things in your life that you haven't dealt with—the anger, hurt, pain, unexpressed love, and the tears. Unfinished business can prevent relationships from ending, keeping you from moving on in life.

I went to this workshop with a strong desire to mourn the loss of the child I can never have. I stated this in my introduction on the first day. On the second day while observing a man work out his unfinished business with his murdered daughter, I had a tremendous urge to cry out, "I cannot take it anymore!" I had a strong desire then to see my baby, to touch him, hold him, and to be a parent. This experience triggered my mourning the death of my dream child. I cried, screamed, and generally got angry at the unfairness of the world. I beat the hell out of a telephone book. Later, in a meditation, I visualized my baby boy. He was beautiful. I spent some time holding my baby, whom I named David. I simply loved David, cuddled him, cared for him, feeling proud to be his parent.

On the third day when a woman worked on saying good-by to her stillborn baby, I felt I wanted to say good-by to David. In my work session I took a pillow (David). Crying all the while, I held my baby tight, rocking and loving him I told David how much I loved him, and how good it felt to be his parent. We shared secrets that a parent and child share, loving each other the best we could at the time. Then came the time I was terribly afraid of, the time to say good-by. Good-by can be one of the hardest things to say to someone you love. Yet, to be able to move on, I had to finally finish this relationship, I had to say good-by to David. My baby died, and on October 20, 1982 I buried him. I felt scared, weak, uplifted, revived, and free. I became free to go on with my life because I was able to close my relationship with David. My unfinished business was now finished.

Wilcher concludes that it is important for anyone who experiences the loss of their dream child to find a way to ritualize this loss, and overcome it.

1. Acknowledge that the loss of your dream child is important to you; let yourself mourn the loss.
2. Name the child.
3. Say good-by to your child.
4. Ritualize the burial of the child. Some people have a ceremony for the child.
5. Celebrate the anniversary date.
6. Plant a tree, write or pledge a gift to charity to help emphasize the memory of this very real person in your life.

Acceptance and Resolution

The next step is for the infertile husband to evolve a new concept of parenthood and to redefine himself as a parent and a sexual person. He must seek dimensions in his life to balance the loss of procreation and come to terms with fear of death and loss of immortality through his blood line. However, the use of DI to conceal male infertility is tempting. D'Elicio (1980) et al. write, "It could be argued that the need to deny sterility to other people and to manipulate this undoubted reality expressed a failure to work out the problem personally and consequently a certain emotional immaturity."

As Glezerman and White, in Israel, wrote in a 1981 article on 270 cases of DI: "The belief that sexuality and procreation are irreversibly connected, so deeply embedded in subconscious strata, has to be uprooted by a conscious logical process."

Each person works through the stages of grieving at his or her own pace. Most need much time, sharing, and support, although some can accept the infertility more readily and move on to the next step.

For the couple who have truly come to terms with the male infertility, they can embark on the adventure of assisted conception with a genuine commitment to the rights and welfare of the child.

> My infertility resides in my heart like an old friend. I do not hear from it for weeks at a time, and then, a moment, a thought, a baby announcement or some such thing, and I will feel the tug—maybe even be sad or shed a few tears. And I think "There's my old friend." It will always be part of me.
>
> —*Barbara Eck Menning, founder of Resolve*

Counseling and Support

Infertility is a major life crisis, whether or not a pregnancy results. There is an enormous sense of loss and damage with negative feelings that can either bring the couple closer together or tear them apart. Treatments are stressful, sometimes exacerbated by attitudes and comments by doctors, nurses, and social workers who lack experiential understanding of infertility. The couple are obliged to bring very personal aspects of themselves and their relationship into the open. Feeling very uncertain about the future, withdrawal may seem easier than trying to explain the situation and having to cope with the reactions from family and friends, who rarely guess that infertility is the problem. Yet it is often necessary to tell the truth, perhaps in gradual increments, to family and friends in order to stop jokes and comments. Parents too may feel guilty if the man has had a history of childhood disease, trauma, infection following circumcision, or the like.

When they are all talked out between themselves, it is helpful for couples to start to talk to others in their situation. (Also, group discussions raise issues that help to get a couple communicating at home.) The group process can be helpful as some couples will accept options that others reject. Decisions are made on emotional as well as logical grounds, and the right choices will be made by those in touch with their deepest feelings. Making decisions can be frightening: the Latin root of the word, *decidere,* means "to cut away from." People are reluctant to let go of other options, or the hope for a treatment that they may have been cultivating for a long time. This makes it hard to choose a course of action. Furthermore, each partner may be going through different phases and it may take time before they both are ready to move on to the next step. Taking a break from treatment and even counseling, is often necessary, or perhaps simply saying "we will not discuss anything about our infertility for one day" or a week or a month.

Counseling and support can help the couple not only resolve their feelings about infertility, but also help support the decision-making process as they explore their parenting options. These are two discrete processes, although they are intertwined. Guidance and sharing certainly help the couple move through the transitions more smoothly, as gynecologists don't usually explore the psychological dimensions of infertility. Several men describe their resolutions:

> Somehow it seemed easier to admit that we had an infertility problem, we could not have our own children, that was a fact of life— accept it or not, it was true. There was no reason for it, no way of understanding it, but I was beginning to come to terms with it. It was definitely out of my control. I did not have to try anymore, the responsibility of overcoming our infertility problem had been removed. At last I could relax.

> I feel by finally coping with the crisis in my life that I have gained a better understanding of myself, my wife, and human nature. I now feel better prepared for parenting and much better armed for coping with any future crisis that life will undoubtedly bring.

Isabel Bainbridge, founder of IVF Friends in Melbourne, Australia, says that

> I'm better now at accepting the inevitable, although I shall never feel complete. It's like living in a house with many rooms, but that one room remains closed. I can never enter it.

In 1974 the nonprofit organization called Resolve was founded by Barbara Eck Menning in Boston, and it now has over 50 chapters across the country. Each chapter has a board of directors that includes infertile couples, professionals, and infertility specialists. Resolve offers telephone counseling through their national phone line in Boston. Chapters provide referrals to infertility specialists, therapists, adoption services including international adoption, in vitro clinics, DI practitioners, and other contacts in the medical system. Support groups and educational programs are available, led by trained professionals. Many of these professionals have themselves experienced infertility, which increases their empathy. As one female member said, "Resolve kept me from going insane." The Resolve national newsletter is published five times a year, and is free to all members. Books, articles, and fact sheets on all aspects of tests, treatments, conditions, and options in infertility can be obtained from the national office (see Resources, page 402).

Patricia Johnston, author of *Perspectives of a Grafted Tree,* has provided some helpful guidelines on how family and friends can offer support.

1. Do listen, but don't offer unsolicited advice.
2. Do be sensitive—don't joke about infertility.
3. Do let the couple know that infertility can be a difficult problem and that you care about them.
4. Do be patient.
5. Do be flexible.
6. Do be realistic. Support the decision to take time out from the treatment or to stop it entirely.
7. Do be supportive. Don't put down the couple's chosen treatment or alternative.
8. Do be truthful. Don't try to hide your own pregnancy, but be understanding that your pregnancy may be difficult for them.

9. Do be an advocate. Educate other family members and friends to the pain of infertility.
10. Do tell the couple if you are finding it difficult to know what to say, rather than saying nothing at all if you cannot find the right words.
11. Do remember that infertility is a highly individual condition. Some reactions may be quite severe.
12. Do recommend infertility counseling groups like Resolve. Consider volunteering or donating to such organizations.

3

Alternatives to Male Biological Parenting

WHEN MEDICAL TREATMENT can no longer offer any hope for improving fertility, then other parenting options can be considered. These include DI, adoption, fostering, or remaining childless or "child-free" as some like to express it. Whatever the path of action, making an informed decision requires study, support, and time. It bears repeating that none of the options are a "cure" for infertility, but they are part of a resolution process that has many dimensions. As we saw in the last chapter, the couple must really grapple with the meaning of infertility in their relationship before rushing into one of the parenting options. Success must not be measured only by whether a child is finally obtained, but rather by the quality of the resolution of the crisis and by the return to normal emotional and psychosexual functioning.

> When one door of happiness closes, another opens. But often we look so long at the closed door that we do not see the one that has opened for us. We must find all these open doors and if we believe in ourselves we *will* find them and make ourselves and our lives as beautiful as God intended.
>
> —*Helen Keller*

Who decides, and how, that a person has come to terms with their infertility? Some questions are unanswerable. There are always unknown factors, such as the possibility that unconscious feelings of disappointment and inadequacy may persist in the husband as well as some resentment of any nonbiological child that may be born or adopted. In fact 95 percent of our functioning happens below our conscious awareness. Aspects of the infertility will surely arise and need to be reintegrated with life crises, such as death or divorce.

Examining the Motives for Parenthood

Personal continuity through children is an almost universal expectation of human beings. However, as the infertile pair redirects those dreams, the key question to be asked is, "Why does a person want a child?" In the past, most parents never examined this issue—babies simply arrived. Today, because of reliable forms of birth control, children are usually planned, and with the advances in reproductive technology they can even be engineered.

Some people cannot give thought-out reasons for wanting children. Often it is a case of "give your decision but not your reasons—your decision may be right but your reasons may be wrong." The infertile couple has to decide whether the joy of parenthood depends on having a biological child. They need to review their original decision to have children and see how it has been affected by the knowledge of their inability to do so naturally. Typically they begin to soul search their motivation for parenting, and indeed they may be obliged to explore this in depth in order to be accepted for adoption or donor insemination.

An important first step is to come to terms with one's own parenting experience, before moving on to parent others. It is also necessary for a couple to examine the values and role models that they share, as well as areas of mutual support and conflicts. The Montreal physicians Watters and Sousa-Poza (1966) point out the need to distinguish between wanting to bear children and wanting to parent them (the latter requiring maturity to encourage independent growth within the cultural framework). Wanting children is not the same as having the ability to fulfill the parental role. Many parents want children for selfish reasons—to be loved, to have a love object, to have someone to take care of them in their old age, to save their marriage (divorce is higher among the childless), or for conformity. Often one partner has a deep desire to give the other a child. This individual dimension of the creative act usually remains unconscious when there is no interruption of the flow of reproduction, but becomes highlighted by infertility. Some women have a strong inner drive to experience pregnancy, birth, and breastfeeding, and would rather have a child than a husband, and for such couples it is DI or divorce.

With a second marriage, there is another constellation of factors. Sometimes the man's infertility or vasectomy is known beforehand; other times not. If the man has children from his prior marriage and was sterilized, then the wife may feel that they need a child together, not just for her sake, but to cement the divided loyalties of the marriage due to pre-existing ties.

Books such as *A Baby? . . . Maybe* by Elizabeth Whelan and *Why Children?*, edited by Stephanie Dowrick and Sibyl Grundberg, attempt to define the motivations for parenthood. Such guides are useful for infertile couples to explore, rather than looking for quick solutions. Formerly, children were important economically and socially, but today they are desired more for psychological and metaphysical reasons. This may explain why biological parenting is so sought after today, even if for only one of the partners. Obviously for the male, parenting is more social and psychological than biological. Many parents feel a sense of duty toward society to have children, and are aware of their prestige value.

Ideally, parenting is a road to personal development and certainly a great deal more than just a way to hide male infertility. In the light of these issues, reproductive decision-making takes on a new form. It involves coming to terms with the infertility and becoming highly informed about the options to male biological parenting. Also, one of the benefits to the eventual child is the self-exploration that the parents undertook, which they might never have done had pregnancy occurred naturally.

Adoption or Donor Insemination?

Adoption is the most well-known resolution to infertility. Two out of every hundred individuals in the United States are adopted, and over twenty-nine million American lives are touched by adoption. It is a legal, clearly defined process, with an honorable and responsible status in the community. There is a ready-made child with a partially known history, without the possible complications of pregnancy and birth. Adoption is seen as a good deed because a home is found for a child who needs one. The relationship between each parent and the child is balanced. Some believe that to reject the idea of adoption indicates that the wife is not able to tolerate, along with her husband, their mutual frustration at being unable to create a baby together.

However, fewer infants are available for adoption these days and many couples think there is too much insecurity in raising a total stranger; they worry about the mother's prenatal stress, nutrition, environment, and "bad blood." Adoption is a public acknowledgment of infertility and the need to have a child that some couples feel is "second-best," and who may not resemble them at all.

It is interesting that adopting couples usually request a girl, in contrast with the traditional desire that the first-born or only child be a boy. This shows society's patriarchal pressure: a girl does not carry on the family name and lineage. (Ironically, in DI more males than females tend to be conceived than in natural conception, due to the more accurate timing of insemination with ovulation.)

Handicapped or multiracial infants, and older children, are available for placement, but Caucasian infants can rarely be found. This situation is due to the falling birth rate, earlier access and wider availability of abortion, increased use of contraception, and the improved social and financial support of single mothers. Some couples have adopted babies privately by writing to all the obstetricians listed in their state, or even the whole country.

There are independent agencies and churches that arrange adoption of third world children. While this may take months rather than the years required for an American baby, there is still a lot of paperwork, immigration hassles, transportation and other costs. Fraud and deception are not uncommon in the "baby market." A Taiwanese adoption agency was recently the focus of a scandal when it was determined that babies were being snatched from their mothers in the streets of Taipei, and with false papers "sold" to adoptive parents in Australia.

The criteria for acceptance onto a licensed adoption waiting list may be quite stringent. The list includes age, marital status and length of marriage, employment, accommodation, existing children, medical history, financial history, nationality, race, attitude, sexual communication, emotional stability, acceptance of infertility, and the depth of your desire for children. Older women, lesbians, single mothers (for whom donor insemination is a definite alternative), usually are not accepted for adoption. In 1985, a bill was brought before the Massachusetts legislature to prevent foster children from being placed with homosexual couples. However, for many years in San Francisco and Los Angeles, adoptions have been arranged for single and gay parents. The children involved are usually older, hard-to-place, or suspected/known homosexuals. As one disappointed couple complained:

> They said we couldn't adopt because we hadn't been married long enough. When we had been married long enough, they then told us we were too old.

There are two types of adoption—closed and open. Either may be conducted by state agencies or done independently (often at a very high price) through private attorneys. There are more infants available for private adoption because the pool of surrendering birthparents usually consists of pregnant teenagers. The attorneys doing independent adoptions connect with a wide network of obstetricians who have a steady supply of pregnant teenagers. Obviously, teenagers do not have the resources or the insight to investigate their options, such as open adoption. Thus most adoptions remain closed, that is, the birthparents do not "choose" or even meet the adoptive parents, nor do they have a means of exchanging information concerning the child's life. However, more and more agencies, especially in California, will accommodate a birthmother who wants an open adoption. In this case, the adoptive parents must decide if they are willing to enter into such an arrangement, as is also the case with a private open adoption. Adoptive parents must believe that it is in their child's best interest to forego secrecy, anonymity, and severing ties. The infertile community needs to be convinced of these merits as they form the future adoptive parent pool. It is up to medical practitioners, social workers, and infertility support groups to join the adoption reform activists in this matter.

Open Adoption Resources in Portland, Oregon, is an example of an agency that promotes open communication between both parties. A catalog describing couples and single women wanting to adopt is given to pregnant women planning to relinquish their babies. It is possible to adopt a healthy, white baby within a few months.

While adoption agencies screen parents more on social grounds, DI is typically medical in its orientation. Adoption through agencies is usually arranged by social workers, but in DI, which is controlled by physicians, consultation with social workers and counselors is occasional and arbitrary. Indeed, in DI the lone physician is free to select couples and sperm in a way that would never be allowed by adoption laws. Rarely is a couple turned down for DI—there would have to be convincing evidence of problems such as a passive, immature, inadequate husband having difficulty accepting his infertility, or a hostile, aggressive wife pushing for pregnancy and threatening divorce if she is not accepted.

Adoption agencies are set up to find the best possible home for the child. This inevitably brings about feelings of rejection in the couple if they are overlooked in favor of a better match, even though they could make perfectly suitable parents for a child in another situation.

By contrast, in DI a child is "matched" to the parents. By matching the child, a fraud can be developed that denies her the knowledge of her origins. Couples who prefer DI feel that the child is "more nearly theirs," that there are stronger emotional ties forged through the pregnancy and birth. Another reason given is that DI offers "better scientific planning than the hit and miss of adoption." Parents feel they have control over at least half of the child's genetic history, and they trust their physician that they will have "guaranteed stock." There is also the possibility of planning siblings at regular intervals, using the same donor.

However, the genetic identity of a child does not guarantee responsible parenting, as we know from child abuse statistics. On the other hand, many parents have happily raised adopted and foster children. It is also worth pointing out that no one questions the strength of the husband-and-wife bond, although they are never related by blood.

Some women reject DI because "it is the woman's gain and the husband's loss." As one woman said, "I could never be happy being the mother to a child if my husband was not the father. I would have everything and he would have nothing."

Few couples who choose DI seriously consider adoption, because of the greater wait and cost. Some couples keep two irons in the fire by going on waiting lists for both adoption and DI. Sometimes their decision is made by whichever opportunity presents itself first. However, adopting parents often feel that because there is such a scarce supply of babies, women who are fertile should have DI and leave adoptable babies for women who are infertile. While conception can sometimes occur after a distracting event in a couple's life, it is erroneous to believe that after you adopt a baby, you will conceive naturally. The percentage who do conceive after adoption (5 percent) is the same as for those who do not adopt.

Unfortunately, the majority of infertile couples, lesbians, and single women prefer DI over adoption primarily because the other party involved in the conception is unknown. One single mother said, "The anonymity really appealed to me, the notion that there was no legal recourse, no father to appear eighteen years from now." Some couples, on the other hand, dismiss DI outright because they feel they couldn't possibly keep such a secret or that it is wrong to do so. (The issues of secrecy, anonymity, and sealed records which taint adoption and DI are discussed in Chapter 11.) Poignant books such as Joss Shawyer's *Death by Adoption* and *Dear Birthmother* by Kathleen Silber and Phylis Speedlin argue convincingly for open adoption.

Foster Parenting

Many argue that the primary concern of society should be the welfare of children who already exist and that infertile couples should provide a home for some of these children instead of bringing more into the world.

Foster parenting, which is not intended to be permanent, is easier to achieve than adoption. The child is usually awaiting adoption placement or return to the natural family after resolution of some problem. A temporary parenting experience may be enlightening for an infertile couple. They can try out the role of mother and father without making an irreversible commitment, although of course the child has not been raised by them since infancy. However, it is often very painful for the parents to return the child when the bonds of attachment grow strong. Many foster children end up being adopted by the foster parents.

There are over 100,000 children waiting for homes, but they should not be adopted just because they are readily available or all that is available, or the only recourse to an infertile couple. Such children require special parenting skills, usually developed only with experience.

Child-free Living

Couples need to explore not just the need for having a biological child by the other partner, but whether they really need to have a child at all. Couples without children can also become involved with others' children in many ways.

Theologians will remind infertile couples that the commitment of marriage represents a total acceptance of each other—for better or for worse. The misfortune of an infertile husband is similar to that of an infertile wife and it is only recently that husbands have arranged to have a child by another woman (surrogate motherhood).

Children do not "cure" infertility any more than they will prevent loneliness in old age. (One has only to look at the number of nursing home residents who have neglectful families.) With social change, more couples are choosing not to have children and are comfortable in rejecting society's natal pressure. After the child-bearing years, their lives will converge more easily with other couples. However, there is a huge difference between making a choice not to have children and being infertile. These same couples may later change their mind, only to discover they were infertile all along, and perhaps when it is very late in the woman's reproductive years.

4

The Experience of Donor Insemination

IN THIS CHAPTER we will look at the experience of donor insemination, beginning with how couples make the decision and come to terms with the unknown donor, through the phases of pregnancy, birth, and child-rearing. Some long-term results will also be discussed. This chapter is based on many interviews that I had with women, couples, health practitioners, researchers, and DI offspring over a seven-year period. Teper et al. (1983) observe that "there is a need to delineate, to acknowledge, and to understand the way in which the 'wooden leg' of DI parenthood affects the structure of the family and the relationships within this, the fundamental unit of society."

Rona Achilles, a family and medical sociologist in Toronto, arrived at some profound insights from her extensive study of the participants in DI. In her 1986 thesis, "The Social Meaning of Biological Ties," she points out that

> the defining social features of DI practice—anonymity and secrecy—testify to the social significance attached to biological ties. If biological ties were considered socially irrelevant, anonymity between the sperm donor and recipient, and secrecy about the procedure would not be necessary. Acquiring sperm, in other words, would not require the mediation, distance, and privacy provided by a physician. The seemingly distinct voices of denial and acknowledgment are therefore grounded in the common assumption that biologically linked individuals are bound to each other by legal rights, by responsibilities, and potentially by issues of identity.

Thus she suggests that this "wooden leg" is tied to an understanding of the social meaning of biological ties and has implica-

tions for understanding the social (and psychological) consequences of other forms of collaborative reproduction that employ
donor gametes. The diverse range of family forms today necessi-
tates the "clarification and redefinition of parental roles." Although DI recipients emphasize the social and rearing aspects of
parenting and minimize the biological aspects, there is a "latent
social stigma attached to nonbiological parental roles. They are
seen as less legitimate, less taken-for-granted, with fewer links of
commonality." Yet when couples are asked why they choose DI
over adoption, the importance of the biological connection to the
child is acknowledged because at least one member of the couple
would be the "real" parent of the child. This is the dissonance that
Achilles repeatedly observed in her research. Likewise, DI offspring when wanting to search, refer to their *real* father. This "primacy of an unknown individual over a parent who has reared
them is strong evidence for the cultural strength of biological ties,"
she concludes.

Making the DI Decision

DI presents the opportunity for childbearing and allows the
woman to fulfill her desire to experience the dimensions of pregnancy, birth, and breast-feeding. Likewise the husband can "give"
his wife a child by consenting to her being impregnated by the semen from another man. However, DI brings with it conflicts and
potential emotional problems that need to be recognized and
worked out by husband and wife, especially with regard to his inability to satisfy the wish for his own biological offspring. The
husband yearns for fatherhood and also wishes to conceal his infertility, but the transition through DI brings up understandable
ambivalence and fears. The fear that makes wives hesitate more
than anything is whether their partner will be able to make the
immediate and long-term adjustment to another man's child.
Much more exploration of DI fathers' feelings (unconscious as
well as conscious) are necessary before all dilemmas can be acknowledged.

Alexandre (1980) sums up the situation: "In every case [of
anonymous] DI means for the woman an experience of pleasure

and fertility . . . and of having a child from 'nobody.' For the man, it means accepting being replaced by 'nobody' and certifying with his name the tangible proof of his sterility."

Sokoloff (1987), commenting on the husband's deep feelings about his loss of genetic input, suggests that the husband may consent to DI "either out of a strong need to satisfy his wife's desire for a child or out of fear that she will leave him or have an affair." Langer et al. (1969) warn that "there is no doubt that when looked at from the viewpoint of the psychoanalyst, the diagnosis of infertility in a husband, followed by insemination of his wife by a doctor with semen from another man, would seem to strike a blow at the most fundamental roots of psychosexual development in both sexes and might well give rise to many untoward reactions, either conscious or unconscious."

Couples experience much conflict as they grapple with the DI decision.

> I am afraid to try DI. I'm afraid of how my husband will feel. I'm afraid of how I'll feel too. I'm most afraid of telling or not telling the child. A psychiatrist I talked to said he thought I should tell the child. I worry about that.

> I think the secrecy with DI is scary. With adoption, we don't have to hide anything.

> I am anxious about whether he will harbor any ill feelings toward the child.

> For me, DI is very easy. It allows me to be pregnant like everyone else, to have natural childbirth. The wait for a baby is much shorter and most of all I know I will take care of my body while pregnant. For John it's a lot harder because his ego has been injured by the infertility. There were times when he was depressed, understandably so, but now he has mourned the loss of his body functioning normally like other men. After he got through that he was better able to make a decision about DI. We are definitely going to try it, but not until next year. We feel we need more time to keep talking about it.

> I am feeling *almost* ready to try DI with an unknown donor, but still do not know if I can go through with it because of the "unknown." I am interested in writing to you as I know you used a *known* donor. That is my dream. My husband and I love the idea but have never gotten the courage to ask his brother or a good

friend. I would be happy to adopt a baby from any country, but my husband is afraid of adoption.

The wife may feel pressured to go ahead with DI in order to conceal her husband's infertility.

> At first, when I found that DI might be the only hope for us, I was immediately against it, but my husband was all for it, even though I was not.

> But it sometimes strikes me as being a sin. Then it helps me know that I did not do it for my own sake. I personally would prefer to adopt a child but my husband was absolutely against it. He was scared by the thought that people should know he was no good. I would gladly have taken the blame. On the other hand it was very unpleasant for me to be snubbed by my parents-in-law with whom we live, because they believed I was to blame for our childlessness.

Yet d'Elicio et al. often had the impression that the wife had done everything in her power to persuade the husband to suggest DI, that "DI is looked on as a kind of cement capable of consolidating an existing marital bond that sterility has impaired."

It is interesting how indebted some wives feel for their husband's consent, even concluding that such a decision is a gift that surpasses natural conception in its merit. This is clearly an adult rationalization. In my opinion, a child ideally deserves the best conception possible and it seems bizarre that artificial means could ever be found superior to the natural way (except by lesbians).

> My husband is a Catholic and DI is considered adultery. This was very difficult for him. I was very angry at his church for that attitude. He wrestled with this for a long time and somehow was able to resolve it. His decision was a wonderful gift to me—far greater than the way most husbands give their wife a child.

> To go through DI makes you stronger as a couple than going to the bedroom and conceiving naturally.

> My husband had some difficulty because his religion forbids DI. He thought about it for three years and was finally able to consent.

The infertile husband may feel pressured to agree to DI to assuage his own guilt over his inability to impregnate his wife. Typically he feels that to reject DI would doubly deprive her of her own fertility. As one man put it, "Half a loaf is better than no loaf at all." Another said, "I chose my wife and I love her. I want my child at least to be like her." A husband in England wrote, "I know my wife longs to bear a child and as I am unable to give her one, it is surely better that her maternal instincts should be satisfied in this way."

Dealing with the Unknown Donor

In Chapter 7 we look more closely at the denial and depersonalization of the donor, but here we will review these functions in the decision-making process. Almost all couples deny any personal interest in the unknown donor, which is probably the only way they can accept the anonymity. Likewise, couples readily accept any donor their doctor selects—the less they know about him, they generally feel, the better. The majority of couples want some information on donor selection and medical history, but actively refrain from asking too many questions, not gaining "too much" information which would make him seem "real." They unconsciously deny to themselves that the donor is giving the child exactly half of her genes, and with her genetic unfolding the donor will thus be represented through that child all her life. I believe this is a suppression of their anxiety about the donor and reveals their need to resolve this by making him an abstraction. Women with previous DI babies have confessed their obsessions with the donor and his physical appearance, even while they insist they still would not want to meet him. Some couples admit they would like to see the donor through a one-way mirror, but that meeting him is "not necessary," a curious word that I noticed was commonly used. Some fear disappointment if they meet the donor.

Unfortunately, couples who are too interested in the donor may be turned down (typically told that no matching donor is·available). One husband, quite reasonably, said he wanted to meet a DI father before he agreed to the procedure. Another man wanted to know if the donor had any living normal children.

> If I could see a picture of him and be guaranteed I'd never run into him on the street, I'd like that. But I would never want to recognize

him. Sometimes I want to tell the donor . . . gee, thanks so much. Maybe he wonders, too, where his sperm went. I wonder about that and maybe the donor does, too. But maybe it is just something he brags about and he is a real creep.

The guidance by professionals who deal with infertile couples has a powerful impact. If the powers-that-be are silent, then so are the couples. So many patients feel that "doctor knows best" and when he says, "never tell" they accept it unequivocally. Thus, there is an implicit collusion between DI couples and the physician with regard to communication and discussion.

In Chapter 7, I will discuss anonymous semen donors, and a sample catalog from a sperm bank can be found in the Resources. Usually, very little information about donors is given to DI recipients, except by the Repository for Germinal Choice in California. Usually just the donor's phenotype is described to give reassurance that the donor will be of similar appearance to the husband (or the wife). One couple interviewed by Barbara Eck Menning (1981) related this:

> We live in an area with very few donors. When I asked the doctor how closely the donor would be matched to my husband, he said, "I promise the donor will be male."

Even couples who admit to themselves that they would like more information about the donor are aware that too many questions may threaten their acceptance into the DI program.

Women seem to admit more anxiety about the donor than do their male partners, but generally feel powerless about asserting their needs.

> I'm pretty much resolved about the donor now, I guess. I'm not really interested, I'd just as soon leave it all up to the doctor.

> In years to come I may wonder about leaving such an important decision in the hands of my doctor.

> We don't think about the donor at all—we just believe we are making a baby together.

> I am not interested in the donor's genetic background. That is more important in adoption than DI. It's the way the child is raised that counts.

I didn't feel that they check out the donor enough.

I don't want to know who the donor is, but I do want to know who he *isn't*.

We didn't ask anything about the donor, but we do want to have him the second time.

I would like to have had a photo as well as a medical history. I gave my doctor a photo of my husband, but I didn't like to really ask about how they choose the donor.

Løvset, in a 1951 article, describes patients' attitudes in Norway:

From the wife's point of view it is quite clear that no low motives are bringing her to use DI. She knows very well that there are other ways in which she could have a child. However, she chooses this, which must be unpleasant to her. But so strong is her want for a child in the marriage with this man that she does it. It's a considerable sacrifice she makes to fulfill one of the main purposes of marriage.

D'Elicio found that husbands were more concerned about the donor than the wives were. My interviews did not always confirm this. Rubin (1965) and Berger (1986) found the wives were more interested in the donor's identity. One husband became anxious when he smelled the "terrible odor of semen" in the doctor's office.

The donor was a very big issue. My husband pressured the doctor for about five minutes to get details. For the next appointment we have compiled a long list of requests.

My husband wasn't choosy about the donor—"It's just sperm," he said.

I don't like to think about the donor. It's the child's—not mine. I don't care whose sperm it is.

Some couples have specific requests, such as a Jewish couple who wanted a non-Jewish donor so that the child would not be exposed to anti-Semitism. Others are clearly desperate, such as the women who said:

I would have done anything to get pregnant, I just decided the donor didn't matter. It is the last chance a woman can take if she wants to give birth to a child and can't get pregnant any other way.

I want a baby, and I want it now. I don't care who the donor is.

I know of two obstetricians who were asked by their patients if they would provide the semen! But fear of errors, and racial or genetic "contamination," are common.

We took one year to decide about DI, wondering if the doctor could get the right donor for us. My husband is worried about the child's characteristics, wants to make sure it will be white, and won't have red hair.

I'm scared of that frozen stuff. What if the kid turned out to be Chinese or black?

I couldn't help making cracks about guys walking down the street.

Kremer et al. (1984) observed that as the date of delivery approaches, many DI mothers become preoccupied with fantasies of the donor's looks and personality. Eventually most couples base their decision to go ahead on the importance of nurture rather than nature, despite increasing evidence of the importance of genetic influences.

We feel a lot of the development of a child is environmental. My husband considers what an impact we will have on a baby, that someone else's sperm is not going to raise the child, or be there when the baby cries at night or teach his values.

Psychological Evaluation of DI Couples

Some practitioners have tried to describe the effect of DI on couples who select this alternative way of parenting. Lamson et al. in a 1951 article in the *Journal of the American Medical Association* defined three types of sterile men. The neurotic husband sees DI as adultery, the relaxed man is glad to solve the problem and is proud of the pregnancy, even sending gifts to both the doctor and unknown donor, and the third type of man is ambivalent. He wants to become a father, but he has misgivings about many aspects of the process of DI. Likewise, other authors have tried to categorize women applying for donor insemination. Sometimes DI becomes, in part, an act of revenge and hostility on the part of the wife, and there are many cases where the husband has felt victimized by the DI, or at least pressured into it.

Behrman (1961), one of the early pioneers in DI, initially referred women for psychiatric consultation. However, he met with such resistance that he abandoned this after referring twenty-five women. Rather than focusing on the women's refusal to have a psychological evaluation, he circumvented it by giving them the Cornell Medical Index Health Questionnaire. However, counseling revealed that for two of these women a baby was really the last thing they wanted.

A 1981 Danish study by Rosenkvist found that 23 percent of women and 31 percent of men had psychopathological traits. Twenty-seven percent of the candidates had sought psychotherapy in the past, but this was no different from the population at large. Psychiatrists and psychologists who have written about DI have found it very difficult to gather data, and the documentation is often poor, with impressionistic conclusions. It is very hard to predict which couples will have problems as DI parents, because it is not clear whether eventual problems are solely caused by DI or might have arisen with natural conception too. Some physicians, as well as couples, believe that if a psychological evaluation is required, the implication is that any couple may not be good candidates for DI or parenting, a catch-22 situation. Poyen (1980) reports that 2 percent of couples requesting DI are refused after a psychological interview.

Donor Insemination Counseling

Although DI is considered a transient medical treatment by its practitioners, successful results have an ongoing lifelong impact. The appointment of psychologists and social workers at some DI clinics is a recognition that the implications of DI are much broader than a simple solution to male infertility. In some clinics the infertility team also includes a urologist and a moral philosopher. The experience of social workers suggests that when counseling is available at the time that DI is being considered, the attitudes of the couple are more flexible and a more positive adjustment can occur. It also helps to be counseled by someone other than the physician, who is not in a position to provide or withhold DI.

Most social workers attached to DI programs do not see their role as selecting suitable recipients, but rather as raising the important issues that must be dealt with by DI parents. One of the greatest problems with DI is the lack of information available to couples. While there is more and more information available about infertility in general, a dearth of information exists about DI in particular because the process is so shrouded in secrecy. Many couples are utterly amazed to find out that there is a waiting list, which means there are others in the same situation as themselves. Some women are initially repelled by the idea of men masturbating to provide sperm for them, and one woman, overcome by veterinary associations, exclaimed, "I am not a cow!" Another DI parent complained to Achilles:

> One of the hard things about doing DI is not knowing anybody else in the same situation to talk with and discuss matters that come up with us, because you can't talk to other friends or anybody, really, and I really don't know how to. I don't think I can ask the doctor at the clinic if we could speak to somebody else that he knows because of the confidentiality of the procedure. He doesn't want to put people in touch with each other. I think the attitude is that if you make the decision to do this you should be able to handle it.

A support group would help individuals explore their emotions, especially as some group members may accept options that others reject. A group leader also helps couples articulate their feelings and explains medical procedures to family members. Unfortunately, few DI parents want to expose themselves by being available for questions, and few couples considering DI become actively involved in meetings and counseling—they go underground.

It is a regrettable fact that DI specialists, almost without exception, advise couples to enjoin in a pact of silence, with no understanding or concern for the emotional ramifications. A major women's hospital calls the DI program DELTA. As one DI recipient commented, "I was struck by the symbolism of the logo." A major problem with secrecy is that it clouds *all* of the issues in DI, and as the Toronto psychiatrist David Berger suggests, and I strongly agree, secrecy itself can eventually become the primary problem. The couple tries to keep everything secret and to forget about the mode of conception, but at the detriment of their need for sharing and support. In Chapters 11 and 12 we will see how keeping secrets and lying can harm relationships of trust and hurt people when they learn they have been deceived.

Secrecy about DI can put a wall up between the couple and others. If everyone were more open about DI, then couples would more readily find others with whom to share the experience. In the long run, it is better to keep family and friends discreetly informed, without necessarily telling them *everything*. However, one spouse may be ready to share before the other, so there may be delays before a unified course of action is possible. Also, as one couple pointed out, telling increases the pressure to succeed with a DI conception.

> It appeared difficult to me, if not impossible, to preserve deep, lasting, and developing relationships with people to whom I denied my crucial preoccupation. That loss used to sadden me dreadfully.
>
> — *Joseph Blizzard, DI father,* Blizzard and the Holy Ghost:
> Artificial Insemination — A Personal Account

Not surprisingly, couples who share details with their family and friends have greater confidence as they participate in DI. They don't have to create excuses about leave from work or trips to another town. Neither do they have to live in fear of exposure. Sometimes this fear can become obsessive. I heard from a social worker about a couple who spent the afternoon in the toilets after glimpsing someone they knew in the clinic.

It is easier to share the DI decision with the mother's kin, as the child will be her biological offspring. The husband's mother may feel that the wife influenced him to have a child for her sake, and the wife may feel that his family will view the child as an extramarital conception. Some couples tell the maternal grandparents during the pregnancy and the paternal grandparents after the birth. One father-in-law said, "You never know what you will get," and my mother-in-law said, "You'll wonder why you went to all this trouble when you get morning sickness" (which I never did!). Some couples who confide in friends find that while some feel squeamish about DI, others are very curious.

> The sterility was such an ego loss for my husband, that if he hadn't had surgery, I wouldn't have told anyone on either side of the family.

> We told my mother-in-law—she witnessed the consent form—and she never mentioned it again.

A vital ingredient in coming to terms with DI is just time, which may be involuntarily provided by the length of waiting lists. Some couples intuitively sense that they need more time to process the issues, but others leap right in and get pregnant immediately. It seems that with DI recipients are either rushed right into it or there is the frustration of a long waiting list. Psychiatrist Berger (1986) recommends an interim period of at least three months between the discovery of the infertility and commencing DI.

I cannot emphasize too strongly or too often that all my regrets, resentments, and objections are nailed into the failure to be given or to find enough time. . . . It could be a major tragedy, and it is certainly astonishingly irresponsible to inflict upon two little children, growing into a state of awareness, the ambivalent sentiments which they inevitably elicit, children who through no fault of their own have emerged from an obscure origin of indecision.

— Joseph Blizzard

Glezerman and White (1981) write that the couple must be given sufficient information and enough time to overcome "suspicions about the partner's attitude toward the use of donor sperm."

> The myth of "blood and flesh" has to be uprooted and a state of consciousness has to be achieved in which the donor, from the psy-

chologic point of view, does not exist. Donor semen should then be regarded as a "material" from an anonymous testes, the donor actually being a *"nonperson"* [italics mine]. For this purpose, we restrict information about the donor to an absolute minimum.

Unfortunately, most women and couples going for DI simply want to get pregnant as quickly as possible and resist counsel on the subject of informing the child in those rare clinics where it may be recommended. Often couples are pessimistic about their chance of becoming parents. As Manuel et al. (1980) noted, the attitude is often, "If we can have a child—we'll see later."

Undergoing Donor Insemination

Even though a woman has a history of normal cycles, anxiety and stress—especially with the first insemination—can cause cycles without ovulation, reported as high as 30 percent. This has been interpreted as unconscious resistance to DI. Some physicians encourage the male partner to participate in the DI, to observe the cervix, to see the donor's sperm under a microscope (or even projected on a screen), and sometimes to deposit the semen. As we shall see in Chapter 5, the male accompanying his partner is a significant factor in her being able to become pregnant. Yet husbands often do not take advantage of the opportunity to be present during inseminations, and it can be very lonely for the women, especially if she has to travel long distances.

> I really don't have any feelings. It was just a little vial of semen, that was it. I don't even visualize a donor. I knew it was semen and I knew it came from a man, that was it. I have never even given any thought to the donor, except as I said, I think she's got a bit of wop [*sic*] in her. It was simply a medical solution to a medical problem. It really didn't trouble me and maybe that's because I'm a nurse, I really don't know. I used to work in obstetrics and things like that.

> DI is a clinical treatment, it's just like an allergy shot, there is no personal contact, there is not another person, it is just a treatment. It's just a means to an end.

> DI is a means to an end. You don't want to know about the donor, there is no personal aspect.

> It was a good means to an end. It was the best way to go about it.

> No, as far as I'm concerned, it's not a stranger's child. It's our child. Gosh, that never occurred to me. I mean, it's not a stranger, it's semen. I don't even conceive that there was sort of a person on the other end before it got to be semen. No, that didn't even occur to me. It's certainly not giving me nightmares.

Achilles (1986), together with Carole Anderson and Gena Corea, suggests that the emphasis of ends over means represents an attitude to reproduction that perceives it like the production of goods and manufacture of commodities. "Reproduction is viewed as an instrumental project where the means to achieve a desired end (a child) is of no significance other than its instrumental value."

Many women comment on the lack of privacy and impersonality of some of the DI clinics, sometimes concluding that the staff have to keep their emotional distance so as not to become personally involved.

> It's a matter of either you put up with it because you have greater motives, or else you get very upset. And there were times when I got very upset and I would go home and think, I know I could not possibly conceive today because I'm just all uptight and that doesn't help. Especially when you think how costly it is. That's another thing. Each time you go there you think, God, it's so expensive. I hope it works this time. It's difficult, I find it is so difficult to deal with people over such an intimate thing and they are so rude, matter of fact and cold, and you are just shunted in and out. . . . It doesn't cost anything to be a bit more supportive and they are not supportive at all. . . . If you can think of the worst sort of circumstances to conceive then that would be it. It tells you something about how badly somebody wants it. It's just that when you are trying and the whole focus of your life revolves around periods and temperatures and that . . . it just becomes so difficult. I became quite obsessed with it to be honest. I couldn't think of anything else to the point where I realized myself that it was unhealthy and I thought I'd give the idea up for a while. It didn't work for that so I don't know if I would have been able to give it up.

They didn't even talk to me beyond the initial interview with the doctor where things were sort of laid out. Beyond that, he didn't even talk to me again . . . half the time he didn't even say hello. I was there and ready, he would come and do his thing and leave. I tell you, it couldn't have been more impersonal. It was awful. It took a lot of getting used to. I remember when I got pregnant with Danny—mind you, that was after two or three tries—I was ready to send him a letter saying what an awful environment it is. You know why I didn't? I thought, I may have to go back there someday for another child. So, I don't think I'll send this letter.

Many women continue to experience doubts, especially about their husband's feelings and attitudes.

My husband came with me once but he wouldn't go into the examining room.

A mother in Løvset's 1951 Norwegian study said:

I believe (my husband) is a bit jealous of me. Coming home after having had DI, he seemed somewhat strange. The idea occurred to me that he regretted it and I therefore told him there would be no child if he did not take part in it. He is not unintelligent, but I persuaded him to have intercourse with me. Maybe that is why I succeeded in being pregnant after DI only once. Anyway, I made myself believe that as a kind of consolation.

I've been feeling rather miserable over deciding to give DI a trial, since not only does the identity of the donor concern me more than I thought it would, but the reception of my husband of a failure to "deliver the goods" was not quite as sweet as might have been thought had it occurred to me previously.

Achilles saw that couples who favored secrecy made an effort to deny the process to themselves and each other. The lack of discussion about DI—before, during, and after—is a way of denying that the DI has occurred and consequently denying the significance of the nonbiological tie to the social father and the biological tie to the donor. Achilles also observed that this silence on the part of the wife was central to the denial that the child is genetically linked to another man and was conceived during their marriage, the only precedent for which is adultery.

Conceptions can occur after the first attempt, which results in less reflection about the whole process.

It was just like more tests and surgery, just another procedure.

I thought the insemination was exciting. All the way home I kept saying, "Swim, little sperm, swim." I was overjoyed when I found out that it worked.

However, for many women the process goes on month after month with increasing frustration.

I wish I had a dime for every day I took my temperature.

I would get just furious when I got my period.

I wish they would give you more information, something to give you *hope*. All I knew was what I had read in a magazine article.

The money was the worst thing. Twenty-six months at $130 a month—but it's still cheaper than adoption.

Chevret reports anxiety expressed in such comments as: "Will I be able to conceive even though I feel depressed and am still undecided?" or "After failure of the first few cycles, could I be sterile?"

Cases of infection from contaminated semen have been reported in the literature, but are probably underreported for the understandable reason that practitioners are unwilling to expose their negligence. One woman I interviewed had to have hepatitis shots after it was discovered (in Australia) that her donor had that disease. AIDS had also been contracted through DI prior to the development of the AIDS screening test. However, I was told by the American Association of Tissue Banks that there had not been one case of AIDS transmitted by donor semen as yet (1987).

Karl Ostrom (1971) reviewed the effects of DI in relation to the Freudian psychodynamics that underlie the usual way of procreation. A young girl's envy of Mother, who can produce a child for Father, is compensated for when she creates a child for her own husband. In turn, the husband's part in this creation strengthens her feelings of love. But pregnancy by DI means that the residue of the little girl's desires for her father tends to be separated from her feelings toward her husband, instead of being integrated. The unknown donor acts like a "blank screen whereupon unconscious

"Barren Rhythm"
by Andrea DeWitt
(Courtesy of Resolve, Iowa)

Dot . . .

Dot . . .

Dot . . .

My life pours

out

dot after dot

in

an unending row

on a

basal graph

of

Dot . . .

```
Dot . . .                      nd
                            i   a   r
Dot . . .               m  f   pe io
a                          to        d.
  n                    ee
  d t             s
      h     s
        e ot a    s
        d  l  y
           wa
```

fantasies are projected. This factor, together with the atmosphere of secrecy within which DI is shrouded, evokes and intensifies the incestual quality of such childhood desires and fears, thereby creating conflict about the pregnancy." To get around this, Ostrom explains, many women will regard the child as the doctor's responsibility (as indeed do many of the doctors themselves). This helps the women to alleviate fantasies about the donor.

Berger (1986) postulates that for the wife, the stranger who impregnates her may represent the oedipal father, and for the husband, this stranger may represent the hated oedipal father who has stolen the wife/mother from him.

Not all couples wanting DI are childless. They may already have adopted children or stepchildren or the man might have children from a former marriage prior to his vasectomy. In cases of voluntary sterilization, the DI is seen as a practical solution, easier than surgery, without all of the emotional ramifications of primary male infertility. Of course, sometimes the vasectomy reversal is not successful; I have interviewed DI couples who have had even two rounds of surgery with no success.

Another category of couples who seek DI are those with incompatible blood groups or hereditary diseases they wish to avoid. Twenty percent of DI is done to prevent the transmission of genetic disease. Chevret quotes one man: "In my dreams, I populate the earth with monsters." While there are still major issues with DI for such couples, they are less oppressive than where male infertility is concerned. Nevertheless, they are actively circumventing a genetic problem of their own by substituting unknown genes.

Why Couples Drop Out of DI Programs

Couples undergoing DI should be advised at the outset that it takes twelve months for about 80 percent of women to conceive. Put another way, about 20 percent of natural conceptions fail. Therefore, it is reasonable to give the DI program at least a year.

Sometimes couples decide that their desire for a child is not that strong anymore, or they are dissatisfied with the DI procedures that produce a high level of strain. Hurried, impersonal staff, with different personnel at each visit who have little understanding of the emotional experience of DI, are typical complaints.

> I was treated in an infantile way. The people at the clinic just don't listen to you. We are lined up there like birds on a fence. There is no privacy; they call out your name and everyone else can hear. We all know why we are there, especially on a Sunday morning.

> After six months of DI, I was utterly exhausted, mentally and physically. We've applied for a private adoption now. It may take two

years, but that is better than going to the clinic every month six days in a row.

There was no information, no handouts, no support groups. I had to *keep asking* the doctor so many questions, and I felt he didn't want to answer them at all.

My physician didn't recommend self-insemination, so I brought in sperm from a friend, keeping it warm in my crotch. The doctor was very busy. I would wait for ages for him to come and do it, lying on the table with a plastic straw coming out of me. I preferred it when he used the cup, otherwise I would feel the semen running out of me. One day, the doctor was so late, I was crying, convinced that all the sperm were dead, and I would have to pay forty-five dollars . . . forty-five dollars for dead sperm. After three visits like this, I decided to do it at home with a flashlight, speculum, and a seventy-nine-cent eyedropper. I felt so out of control with the doctor calling the shots, wasting my time, and charging me all that money.

It is not uncommon for some women to try to become pregnant extramaritally, sometimes gratifying their need for mothering at a high cost to the relationship. Separations and divorce occur among those who discontinue DI (as with those who achieve a child this way), and one woman even developed endometriosis and had a hysterectomy. Unfortunately, women and couples who drop out are considered lost to follow-up, and they may need counseling even more than those who remain in the program. Support groups are necessary not just to help with making the DI decision but throughout the stress of inseminations and after the arrival of the child.

I know of several cases where a woman has conceived with DI but felt that she could not go through with the pregnancy and birth and subsequently chose to abort the child. This has also happened with IVF conceptions, which are achieved at even greater personal and social cost.

In summary, DI can be time-consuming, tedious, inconvenient, repetitive, expensive, and emotionally draining. The process is punctuated by disappointment and there is no guarantee of success. The strain is increased in some clinics where couples know that if conception has not been achieved after six months, the woman will go back to the bottom of the waiting list again. While a great number drop out of DI programs, some eventually conceive after dozens of inseminations, such as one woman in England who conceived four children after a total of 210 inseminations.

Glezerman and White's survey of 270 couples found that significantly more patients from the higher age group and lower socioeconomic class dropped out. Other contributing factors were long duration of infertility, especially primary infertility, and ovulatory disturbances. The large number of dropouts in DI programs indicates the need for more investigation and counseling. While many DI clinics are unaware of the reasons, a common one is fear—of the donor, secrecy, incest, even adultery. Women have made comments as follows:

> I feel something sacred is being violated in accepting another man's semen.

> I cannot tolerate the thought of another man's sperm in my wife's vagina.

> To go into this room and here is this little vial of stuff that is going to become a child. I think it is rather cold-blooded, it does just make my blood turn cold.

> I just couldn't stand it, physically and psychologically, to go into that treatment room.

> The thought of several donors' semen being used over time is like having intercourse with many men.

> I felt dirty after DI and rejected my husband when I came home.

> I was totally brokendown and impossible to live with for a week after the treatment.

> I feel wrong, like I'm doing something wrong.

The Experience of Pregnancy from DI

Achieving pregnancy can be a mixed blessing. There is tremendous relief in being able to stop taking your temperature and going to the clinic and begin enjoying a pregnancy like any other couple. On the other hand, it is now a fait accompli. Just as the couple had to come to terms with the diagnosis of infertility, and then chose DI as a parenting option, now they have to reckon with the pregnancy, which is a catalyst for growth and change under any circumstances.

As we have seen, DI poses a threat to the man's masculinity. The diagnosis of sterility was a blow to his ego, and now his partner is successfully pregnant with the sperm of another man. This brings the man back to the time when he was unequal to the competition of his father in the struggle for his mother's affection. As a substitute for the child he cannot produce, the man may throw himself into his work and try to increase his earnings.

Thus, DI can evoke deep-seated feelings of helpless dependency in relation to the wife and also feelings of inadequacy in relation to other men. Even homosexual panic has been reported in some men. A man experiencing such an emotional crisis over the pregnancy and birth perhaps can tolerate a passive infant, but will surely have difficulties with the assertiveness of a toddler or a teenager.

One DI father described the loss of his genetic continuity to Menning (1981):

> After considering DI, I had hoped that my wife would deliver a girl, whereas before I had expressed no preference. Somehow in my mind a son would highlight my loss because he wouldn't be a small version of me.

Rather than being wonderful news, the pregnancy may be an anticlimax, especially if the couple lies about the DI and says it was a successful insemination with the husband's semen or that some other form of treatment was undergone. The lie becomes concrete with the achievement of pregnancy, as one of Achilles's respondents expressed.

> We felt more relief than excitement with the pregnancy. It was sort of deflating, an anticlimax. Everyone around us was so happy because they thought it had happened naturally. Actually, I was joyous to be pregnant, but as the pregnancy went on, at about seven months, all of a sudden, I got very very scared, as I realized how out of control of your life and body you are. I thought, what if I have a half-caste baby? I don't know what has been put inside my body. You've given yourself completely in trust to a doctor to do

this to you, and I thought how devastating that could be on your whole life. And just the whole thing hit me as to what we were doing, then, and until the baby was born I was very uneasy a lot of the time. If you asked me if I would do it again the answer would be "no." And certainly not while we are still trying to resolve our feelings with what we've got. I don't think we could have another one this way. The emotional trauma has been too much for one thing. . . . It's such a major thing, you know, having a baby is such a major thing in your life. . . . I don't want to live a lie. [deep breath] I don't want us to lie to ourselves, to each other . . . to anybody, and this is what this makes you do.

Berger (1986) describes a woman who, despite the success of DI, was "unable to overcome the feeling that her husband had somehow cheated her out of a 'normal' pregnancy."

The burden of secrecy is so great that couples, like donors, are eager to be interviewed and share their feelings and experience. Many find it easier to confide in a stranger and some hope to learn what others have to say about the DI experience.

Your request for information satisfies a great longing on my part. Ever since I became pregnant I've wanted to advise other infertile couples to try DI, but my husband insisted that I not do so openly in order that our son be protected from suffering any stigma.

Basically we are both honest and direct people and you cannot make a decision in your life like DI and pretend it has not happened . . . and this is one of the things that I feel we have to get out into the open because it can produce all kinds of problems in a couple's relationship later . . . your relationship to the child . . . everything. I just don't see how it can be done. I just think because it has been such a closed subject, I just think, if we believe in it enough to do this, then let's believe in it enough to say we did it.

One woman felt "survivor guilt" (as Carol Frost terms it) about her gain in experiencing the pregnancy and birth, but this was alleviated when she saw how much her husband enjoyed those phases too.

There was a lot of pain and grieving initially and we went through some rough times. That was all lifted from my shoulders when the insemination "took." Perhaps my husband grieved longer through the pregnancy, but I honestly believed that the joy of parenting has kept us too busy to grieve.

Joseph Blizzard (1977), in a chapter called "Getting Stuffed — Inlaws and Outlaws," writes:

> We really needed help during that pregnancy. The inseminator had conducted his affairs with decorum and with dignity but he had defined the limits of his professional brief pretty clearly. He had solved some problems but he couldn't solve the problems which he had created by solving the problem. My problems were now the problem he had solved. . . . If DI only produced children then the apparent complacency of its advocates would be in order. Pregnancy is, however, a more pernicious consequence. It is a condition which must be survived by the man and the woman despite the statement and restatement of unforgivable things. It is a period of helplessness beyond help, a commitment to fraud, an exposure to hazard as told in myths and lived in nightmares. . . . When she finally became pregnant it was a very matter-of-fact business . . . no celebratory drinks or a party. Many of our friends and acquaintances who found out, inadvertently, must have thought it very odd that we didn't consider that they might be interested to know. These experiences and the anesthesia which they have created around the affairs of childbirth have made it difficult for me to feel, express, and display pleasure in other people's pregnancies and children, as freely as I might.

> My husband accompanied me to the doctor's office for most of my inseminations. He was with me the day I conceived. While it was not exactly a romantic experience, the whole process and its miraculous product have made me love him much much more. I deeply admire this man who set aside his personal feelings about machismo, etc., to enable us to achieve our parenthood via pregnancy rather than adoption.

> I had nightmares all through my pregnancy. The child looked different each time. Last night he was Chinese and cross-eyed.

> I wanted to discuss names for the baby with my husband. He said, "You choose the baby's name, it's really your baby and not mine."

The issues of DI re-emerge when a second DI child is considered. The desire for a second DI child, according to various studies, ranges from 10 to 42 percent. Not all husbands agree, as one woman confessed to Levie:

> I had many feelings of guilt toward the child, and although this seems contradictory, of resentment toward my husband for denying us another child, as you know.

Thus we see that DI evokes mixed feelings among recipients, especially married women. Until DI is done openly and people share their feelings as they do with abortion, divorce, euthanasia, and other controversial psychosocial problems, we will never know much more.

The Arrival of the DI Child

Medically, DI children appear to be as healthy as those conceived naturally, even DI offspring from frozen semen. A Japanese study found DI children to be 77.5 percent longer and with a 26 percent greater birth weight. The major issues, then, are emotional rather than biological.

The secrecy surrounding DI is so great that rarely is the obstetrician (if different from the DI practitioner) informed about the DI. Those who do know treat the unborn as a "premium baby" with inevitably more Caesarean sections.

> I was so worried through the pregnancy that a mistake had been made, that I had gotten the wrong specimen. Well, it all ended beautifully. The delivery was a great relief in more ways than one. I wonder if next time I'll have the same worries.

> I never went into labor. When the baby was three weeks overdue I had a Caesarean. I feel that because my body was so separated from the act of conception, because it did not participate then, I could not participate in giving birth later. I didn't see my son taken from me and it took a long time for me to bond with him. . . . I didn't feel he came from me at all. I wonder if I was also afraid to enter the next stage . . . of meeting the baby. What I had really wanted to achieve was a pregnancy. While I was pregnant, everything was fine. But I remember breast-feeding him in a rocking chair at the hospital and thinking, "I wish this could all go away

and he could be a regular child." However, my husband commented happily, "I knew you wanted to get pregnant and I did this for you. But I never realized what this [the new baby] has done for me."

After the birth, women have fantasies about who the child resembles. Compared with mothers of naturally conceived children, twice as many DI mothers think their child resembles kin members. However, they generally protest that the child does not look like any male members of the mother's parental family. Ostrom (1971) writes, "One may safely infer that their 'incestual strivings' had been likewise stimulated and were threateningly close to conciousness." All forty-three of the DI mothers in his survey studiously avoided naming their child after anyone on either side of the family, whereas thirty-two of the naturally conceived babies were freely named after family members.

Achilles notes that physical resemblances among family members is important for blood-tied family members. When the blood tie is not there, physical resemblance serves to "normalize" the DI family relationships. One DI mother hoped to have the same donor for a second child, "in case there is an identity crisis they can comfort each other."

> The child does not look like either of us. This puts a question in people's minds because they know how long we have been married.

I have found a very strong need in DI mothers to dismiss any thoughts or concerns about the donor. DI children, like adoptees, consciously and unconsciously pick up the mannerisms of their nonbiological parent, so that likenesses occur that may be commented upon by unknowing family members and outsiders. As one couple said, "We have the last laugh when people say he looks like Peter." DI, as one mother wrote, is only for strong marriages because babies create more stress, and added that "I'm careful never to say *my* kids." Another woman recommended that

> the mother should try to see the husband's or grandfather's characteristics in her child for the in-laws' sake.

As the child gets older, and more and more characteristics emerge, this must get harder for the DI parents with an unknown donor. It is so natural to point out family likenesses, as our donor does, linking the child with those who have gone before her, and putting her in her correct genealogical context. In the new mothers' groups that I teach at the Maternal and Child Health Center in Cambridge, I observe much sharing as to which qualities come from each parent. This, I believe, is a natural parenting instinct to "place" each feature of the child. Certainly, I found it fascinating to see that my daughter has my fingers and toes (from my mother) and my body build (from my father), yet her facial structure, coloring, and broad nails come from our donor. I find it hard to believe, as the gynecologist Finegold claims in his 1964 edition of *Artificial Insemination* that a couple with four DI children, all with different donors, successfully concealed the DI from their family and neighbors. How can Finegold possibly know that? He doesn't live in their neighborhood from day to day and no one can know the final outcome.

> I feel that the members of my husband's family looked for resemblances to him at the birth of both my children, and they can't see it. I just have the feeling that my mother-in-law is really disappointed that the children don't look like him, but I could never explain.

DI parents do harbor fears and fantasies about the unknown genes, although most of these fears are suppressed and such comments as "You raise it—it is your child" and "The donor only surfaces when I consciously think about him" are typical. Some parents develop a "bad seed" theory about the origins of the child. There is always the temptation to blame any of the child's difficulties on her genetic heritage.

> I wonder what characteristics might be showing up in the kids. Both boys play with their hair.

> My in-laws were very distant during the pregnancy and first year. Now that the baby is walking around they are showing more interest.

Glamour magazine featured an article on DI in November 1980.

> When the baby was a few months old, Diane began speculating about which of the child's personality traits might have come from

the donor. "The baby would throw a temper tantrum and I would say, my God, no one in my family does that," she says. "He must have gotten it from that strange person." Now she says she has overcome these feelings, largely by talking them out with her husband. "Let's face it, all babies are new and different people," she says. "As far as I'm concerned, my husband is the father in every way."

Fred reacted to the newborn quite differently. "I was just so happy," he says. "I had a tremendous feeling that we had overcome something, that we had beaten out the storm. We had our sanity intact, and a baby."

Manuel and Czyba did a 1973 follow-up study on children born by DI in France that concluded there was a deep emotional investment by both parents for the DI child. They observed an "overinvolvement" of all the DI fathers, and described their behavior as "very maternal." This corresponds to a Swedish study by Milsom (1982), which noted that DI fathers avail themselves of paternity leave at a higher rate (30 percent) than other fathers in the population (12 percent). Manuel and Czyba found that the fathers took a large share in the physical care of the child from the beginning, and were often even more responsive than the mothers to signs of frustration by the child. They also found that seven of the sixty children had psychosomatic disturbances clearly related to the mother's anxiety. Problems such as the waiting period prior to conception, risk of conception, and difficulties at childbirth were highly correlated with this anxiety, which continued during the first month of the infant's life.

Long-Term Outcome

It is hard to believe that there is so little information available regarding the outcome of a procedure that has been practiced for a century. *The Artificial Family,* written by Snowden and Mitchell in England, as recently as 1981, admitted that it was not possible for them to interview a single DI child who is now an adult!

Most physicians don't do follow-up because they prefer not to remind their patients of a procedure that everyone wants to forget. The questions are thus unasked, as well as unanswered. How much of a DI child's problems, if any, are behavioral in origin rather than genetic, and in response to the big family secret that is sensed? What fantasies of the donor are experienced by the husband, mother, and child? Does the mother feel guilt at the child, who daily confirms her husband's infertility? How does the husband respond to this constant reminder that his wife conceived with another man's sperm? Does she compound his inferiority by turning all her affections to the child? How does the mother's husband relate to an adolescent daughter, lacking the usual incest taboo, or the emerging sexuality of an adolescent son who might threaten his virility? Are DI children angry—if they find out—that they were conceived unconventionally? Are they afraid that they may mate with an unknown relative? Are they furious that they have no recourse to their paternal genetic origins? Some light will be shed on these matters in Chapter 11.

Positive Results

With regard to the physical and mental parameters, the few studies of DI offspring report a favorable outcome: two Japanese studies (Mochimaru, 1980; Iizuka, 1969) found DI offspring to be superior to controls.

Practitioners often exaggerate their claims about positive outcome, relying on Christmas cards, notes of appreciation, and requests for another DI child. Nationally, only 10 percent of couples request a second child by DI. A study of the psychological results of DI in Holland by Levie (1967) found that 96 percent of couples expressed a positive outcome and no problems were reported. Rubin (1965) reports a similar optimistic outcome, however only 50 percent of DI mothers he contacted did respond. Strickler (1975) claimed an 81 percent success rate, and 46 percent of the respondents said that their marriage had been strengthened by the experience of DI. The experiences of the other 19 percent apparently were not known.

Negative outcomes tend to be dismissed by enthusiastic DI practitioners. For example, Warner, reviewing thirty-two years of experience of DI in a 1974 article, mentioned that only one husband had had a "bad reaction" to the DI (it would be interesting to know more about that reaction). He found that only five couples divorced after the birth of a DI child (but we were not informed as to whether the divorce had anything to do with the DI). In only three cases did a wife wish a second series but was unable to get her husband's consent (but we are not told why).

Sandler, writing in a 1965 issue of *Mental Health*, denoted that

> there is no evidence whatsoever that the use of DI disturbs the family or produces psychological problems, and I am sure that this is because candidate couples are selected with care, as of course, are the donors. Indeed we may say that DI brings about the fulfillment of marriage.

Simmons interviewed 125 couples in 1957 and concluded that he could state "unequivocally that DI is successful." But how could anyone find unequivocal marital success among 125 couples!

One of the amazing results of the surveys and studies is the low divorce rate—about one percent (compared with a national average of 50 percent). It almost seems too good to be true—is the secret that the couple hides so powerful that they will tolerate any marital situation rather than risk exposure? (Candace Turner, founder of a support group called *Donors' Offspring*, says she has yet to meet any adult DI offspring whose parents did *not* divorce.) The two divorced DI mothers whom I interviewed said (as did Baran and Pannor) that the separations had nothing to do with the DI. One mother had conceived twins, because her husband had a vasectomy, which she had known about prior to marriage. One husband left the marriage when the baby was six months old. The wife felt that her spouse had no "natural feelings" toward the child. She reasoned that it was the idea of having a family—which meant giving up time spent on his boat—not the DI itself. It was her hope that the huge developmental changes that occur in the second half of the child's first year may help to recharge her partner's interest, that this more interactive time "helps to grow love."

Negative Results

It is important to balance the "positive vacuum" claimed by physicians who practice DI. The amount of psychological research about DI is scant, and usually based on the Freudian model. Gerda Gerstel, a New York psychiatrist, published the first paper on negative outcome in 1963. While that paper is over twenty years old, it is concrete evidence that the outcome of the DI is not always so rosy. She describes five cases in which severe emotional disturbances were triggered off in both parties by the husband's azoospermia and the DI. The DI aroused varying degrees of hostile feelings in the wife toward the husband. Gerstel feels that on a deeper level, the wife's feeling that she had been cheated stimulated a revival of the oedipal rejection. The revival and reinforcement of that oedipal rejection, she continues, may be said to lie at the source of the wife's feelings of hostility and revenge, which were now directed toward her husband. All the women attempted to deny their pregnancy and avoided wearing maternity clothes. Gerstel also speculated that revival of that rejection may also stimulate the wish to look for another father, and the unknown donor symbolizes the fulfillment of this wish. However, the patients felt guilty over this desire and punished themselves with anxiety that the child would be born deformed or with some genetic disease.

The women had fantasies about the identity of the unknown donor that began before the DI and continued through the process. Sometimes these were transferred to the physician or other males in his office or waiting room. Some women saw their unborn child as having superior qualities and others thought the child would be defective in some way. Gerstel claims (and this is backed up by recent research on prenatal psychology) that such attitudes adversely affect the child.

Donor fantasies led to guilt feelings toward their husbands and impaired their sexual relationships. As well, all the women were tormented by the fear that the DI would be exposed, and four of the five refused any anesthetic during labor in case they lost control and revealed their secret. Severe and prolonged depression was observed after birth in all of the women and the babies were all cared for by substitutes. All the women refused to nurse. Some did not look at the baby for days and one mother did not relate to her child for almost four months. Gerstel judged that all the children were subsequently overprotected by their mothers and rejected by their fathers. Separation anxiety was a problem, especially for the boys who could not establish a positive relationship with the father who had withdrawn. All of the children were aware of a big family secret and knew that this secret somehow involved their father. One of the boys took on the same fantasies as his mother, that his real father was a famous person. Persistent denial of his legal father was revealed in psychological tests and play therapy.

Any problems that the children developed, and they all had problems with feeding, colic, and vomiting, were thought by the couples to be hereditary, rather than stemming from the marital difficulties and emotional climate in the home.

Becoming a parent is usually an opportunity for a husband and wife to resolve conflicts from childhood through maturation. Gerstel notes that

> the fact that neither the prospective donor nor the marital pair are investigated to any extent in DI, in contrast to the thorough adoptive study of both the prospective and the natural parents, is particularly striking. Again the psychological advantages of informing the child of the circumstances that surround his birth, so strongly advocated by adoption agencies, is in distinction to the unfavorable effects that are an inevitable concomitant of the secrecy which surrounds DI.

Gerstel concludes that the psychological issues in DI are taxing to most normal couples, and that the "decision to participate in DI is in itself indicative of an emotional disturbance." (Dr. Finegold thought that a request by an *unmarried* woman for DI was an indication of "psychological disturbance.")

Schellen (1957), in one of the early texts on DI, also discussed the manifestations of psychic trauma. For the husband, they include:

1. pathological jealousy of the wife and donor
2. grave reactions of hatred toward and aversion from the child, which may result in his repelling and repudiating the child

3. feelings of hatred toward the doctor
4. exacerbation of his sense of inferiority, which is accentuated by the presence of the child
5. the mental strain of secrecy, which may be discharged in neurotic projections such as ardent longing, hope, fear, and suspicion
6. estrangement from the wife, fostered by the husband's sense of being pushed into the background by his alien child.

For the wife, problems arise from:

1. yearning to know the donor who has completed her happiness
2. estrangement from her husband brought about precisely by this yearning toward the donor and by the presence of the child which is wholly hers, but in which her husband has no share at all
3. as with the husband, the mental burden of secrecy.

Adverse psychological reactions among DI parents have also been reported by Peyser (1965) and Kremer (1982).

A French group of DI parents observed by Manuel and Czyba expressed their gratification in terms of having a child who is "loving" and "without grudges." These were the two most frequently cited qualities for children of the ages of eighteen months and three years. The researchers felt this was related to their general refusal to reveal to the child its origin. The parents' fear of traumatizing was associated with a fear that their child might "bear a grudge against them for not being like the others," upon learning of his or her origin. Manuel and Czyba commented that:

> "The truth is that it is *our child*" is the attitude most commonly expressed by the parents: the truth of the desire is truer than the reality.

David Berger (1986), associate professor of psychiatry at the University of Toronto, notes that DI can generate significant psychopathology.

Psychiatrist Herbert Peyser in 1965 described a disturbing array of "untoward effects" of DI experienced by two couples. One woman ended up having electric shock therapy, but the other couple—despite extramarital affairs and other problems—agreed to return to the same gynecologist for another child!

Alexandre reports four adverse outcomes to DI in France, yet two of the couples sought a second child.

Achilles interviewed five adult DI offspring, and all were informed of their origins due to a family crisis. In two of the five cases, a parent had even committed suicide.

Annette Baran and Reuben Pannor, coauthors of *The Adoption Triangle,* are currently working on a book called *The Secret Seed.* They interviewed over 170 members of DI families, including 19 offspring. Ranging in age from 16 to 68, most were in their mid-twenties at the time, and all but one had learned of their DI status under "punitive circumstances," generally during a divorce. While most of their parents had divorced, Baran and Pannor felt that the DI was not the reason in any case. After years of research, they are "absolutely convinced that secrecy and anonymity have to end in the interests of everyone."

There was a custody battle over a DI child in Melbourne, Australia, in 1983. The wife claimed that she and her husband didn't know what to expect when they joined the program and that there was little counseling available. "It's astronomical, the amount of information we didn't have," she said. "Without counseling and help, it was perhaps inevitable that we would split." (Her mother was the only other person who knew about the DI.) Apparently, her husband had always been very affectionate toward her but after the birth "he hardly spoke to me and tried to dodge me and Brian as much as he could. . . . I think Brian was virtually a reminder to David that he was sterile."

The American Academy of Pediatrics has defined risk factors in the adoptive family that stress the parents and subsequently the child:

1. Unresolved feelings of infertility.
2. Concern over biological identity.
3. Attempts to try harder because of the perceived biological inadequacy.

These issues are all present in the DI family.

The Significance of Secrecy in DI

Two separate issues need to be distinguished when evaluating the outcome of DI. First, the issue of *having a child* per se, which is a life crisis for most parents. What aspects, then, are related to bearing and raising a DI child compared with simply bearing and raising any child? An overwhelming number of respondents to an Ann Landers' survey admitted that parenthood had been a great disappointment to them. However, it does seem clear from the above examples that the unknown donor was a major source of the problems. The second issue to be examined is that of the *secrecy around DI,* rather than the DI itself. Secrecy brings up the taboo of incest in all of us, which resonates much more primally than other sexual taboos such as adultery.

Theologians, such as W. R. Matthews, the Dean of St. Paul's Cathedral in London, writing in the Royal College of Obstetricians and Gynaecologists' report on DI, expressed his concern about the secrecy.

> The integrity of the wife is even more profoundly injured since in order to satisfy her personal desire for a child, she had admitted an unknown person to do for her what no one but her husband has a right to do, and will deprive the resultant child of that which it is his right to receive from her, a *known father.*

The most in-depth account of the experience of DI can be found in J. Blizzard's book, *Blizzard and the Holy Ghost,* the appendix to which is subtitled "One Man's Hell." His pain and regret are undisguised.

> The personal and spiritual impact cannot be circumvented and we are compelled, with all this evidence, to recognize that we have committed a deeply asocial act, whilst pursuing our own, independent biological objectives.

> To run, in solitude, into the teeth of social attitudes, religion and law, requires some courage and a lot of conviction. DI is not momentous as it might appear to its practitioners; it may turn out to be a life's experience or even a life's struggle, voyaging through strange seas of thought, alone.

Although Blizzard takes issue with all aspects of DI, many couples, single women, and lesbians have spoken to me of the great joy brought to them by their DI offspring. We know that the proportion of adoptees is greater in reform institutions and psychotherapy clinics than in that of the general population. What about the phantom DI child? Why has society not learned the painful lessons of secrecy, concealment, and sealed records in adoption? Do we have to spend another fifty years making the same mistakes with DI? Can we not open the records, and our hearts, so that DI families can share their experiences and provide mutual support as they deal with their special circumstances? If fathering really is social, then why hide the biological details?

Children today grow up in a different world with different social rules from those that worked for us, and they will deal with different problems. Already some children have more than two parents, and many more have less. Reproductive technology has increased these "odd numbers" so that a child can now have as many as three "mothers" and two "fathers."

How have open DI arrangements worked out, when donors and offspring know each other and socially interact? I would certainly like to hear from others who share this situation. (Please write to me at the Maternal and Child Health Center, 2464 Mass. Ave., Cambridge, Mass. 02140.) The Adoption Awareness Center in San Antonio reports that five years of experience of open adoption (any form of communication between birth parents and adoptive parents, either directly or through an intermediary) have been *without exception* positive and loving.

Perhaps as our society grows less nuclear (in both senses) and more caring, bonds that extend families and unite people will be valued for their mutual benefits instead of seen as threats to our tenuous notions of "security." Godparents are a socially sanctioned form of this kind of extension, and if a role has been created for them, then a role can also be created for donors to share their gift of life.

There will always be consequences to DI and they will be different in each case. We have seen that the positive experiences are glossed over by DI practitioners, but the negative ramifications have been described in detail by concerned psychotherapists.

Clearly, couple adjustment to DI is complex and poorly understood, not only regarding the conception but the long-term adjustment as well. The ethical and legal issues also create a need to hear more from the counselors, psychiatrists, attorneys, philosophers, and others with an interest in the field of DI, not just from biased gynecologists who either strongly promote or prohibit DI. Only when the subject becomes more open, and follow-up is done, will we hear from the now silent majority—the couples who undergo this experience and the children who result.

5

Donor Insemination – Traditions and Techniques

IN THIS CHAPTER we will review the circumstances under which DI is recommended, the history and different techniques of insemination, and other procedures that a woman may undergo in the process of trying to conceive. Here we will be examining the typical medical practice of DI. The ethical, legal, and moral issues will be explored in later chapters.

Indications for Donor Insemination

It has been pointed out that the ease of DI has directed attention and research away from understanding and treating male infertility. This is in contrast to the aggressive and prolific treatment of female infertility, which is much more interventionist because of the internal placement of the female reproductive organs.

Yet it is precisely the untreatable nature of male infertility, as Achilles observed, that makes it an indication for DI. Although euphemistically termed a "treatment," it does not alter the infertility of the male, and the female is, of course, presumed to be fertile.

One cynic commented that "there are no indications for DI, only requests." We will now look at the reasons why DI is performed.

1. *Primary infertility*. Any of the causes of male infertility that are discussed in Appendix 1, if not medically resolved, become indications for DI.
2. *Eugenics*. In these cases sperm production may be normal, but there is a hereditary or familial disease, which the male does

not want to reproduce. Twenty percent of DI nationwide is done for genetic factors. For example, genetic diseases such as Huntington's disease, Klinefelter's syndrome, Hoffmann's disease, and muscular dystrophy. Some diseases, like von Recklinghausen's disease and Huntington's chorea, have variable expressions and do not show up until midlife. Donor insemination, of course, does not eliminate genetic risk, it simply reduces it. For example, with Werdnig-Hoffmann disease or cystic disease of the pancreas, the risk is still one percent, but that is much better than 25 percent. Also, prenatal screening can be done, such as amniocentesis, and alphafetoprotein blood tests.

3. *Immunological reasons.* The most common situation is when there is incompatibility between a woman and her male partner's Rh factor. Sometimes a woman's cervical mucus becomes "hostile" and causes an immune response to her partner's sperm. (Donor cervical mucus can be tried too and mucus can be successfully stored for a few weeks at four degrees centigrade.)

4. *Vasectomy and remarriage.* This is an increasingly common indication for DI, and accounted for 12 percent of inseminations nationwide when surveyed by Curie-Cohen, et al., in 1980. In California, vasectomy is now more often the reason for DI than primary infertility.

History of Donor Insemination

Donor insemination was the first step of a whole range of reproductive assistance that is available today. Its history goes back centuries. As early as 220 A.D., the Talmud questioned the paternity of a child who was born after a woman was accidentally fertilized in bath water. In the thirteenth century there is documentation of a rabbi's concern about the fertilization of a woman sleeping on bed linen where a man had ejaculated.

The history of donor insemination in animals is more documented than human donor insemination. Arabs in the fourteenth century used techniques of artificial insemination in breeding horses. A wad of wool was first placed in a mare's vagina and then under the nose of a stallion, who ejaculated in response. The wad of wool, which caught the semen, was then placed in the mare, who became with foal. The story goes that a sheik even inseminated his enemy's pure mares with semen from diseased inferior stallions. Varasotto in the same century artificially inseminated sheep. Don Ponchom, a monk in the abbey of Reame, wrote about experimental fertilization with fish eggs. The existence of spermatozoa was discovered under the microscope by the Dutchman Anton van Leeuwenhoek in 1677, but he did not know their function.

Bartholomeus Eustachius in 1550 advised using a finger to guide semen toward the opening of the uterus after intercourse, and in 1779 the Italian priest and physiologist Lazaro Spallanzani artificially inseminated reptiles and dogs, and observed the effects of freezing on human sperm. Around 1790 John Hunter of London first recorded a pregnancy and delivery of a child conceived by artificial insemination with a husband's semen. In 1838, the Frenchman Girault blew sperm into the vagina via a hollow tube. In 1865, a pamphlet on artificial insemination was published by De Haut in France, but he discontinued his experimentation due to great public outcry. In the late nineteenth century Marion Sims, an American gynecologist, reported fifty-five artificial inseminations that he performed on six women. The success rate of his "ethereal copulation" (he used ether on the women) was only 4 percent because he thought that menstruation indicated ovulation. The first reported successful artificial insemination (with husband's semen) in the United States occurred in 1866. That same year the concept of sperm banks was originated by Mantagazzi. De Lajotre, in 1876, claimed a success rate of 88 percent with 567 women by using their husbands' semen. He was later condemned by the Tribunal of Bordeaux for doubtful practices.

In 1884 Dr. William Pancoast, of Jefferson Medical College in Philadelphia, first documented a successful donor insemination. (The accuracy of this well-known story has been questioned.) Dr. Pancoast anesthetized the wife of an infertile man and used semen from the most handsome man in his class of medical students. He did not inform either the husband or wife of his action, which, as

Gena Corea points out in *The Mother Machine,* makes his act a rape. After the birth of the child the doctor did confess his secret to the husband, who reportedly received the news with great enthusiasm.

One must also wonder about the nature of the prior physical examination which Hard (1909), one of Pancoast's medical students, described as "very complete, almost as perfect as any army examination." The author continues, "As a matter of possible public interest, I will say that during this examination was discovered for the first time, as far as I know, the suction function of the uterus which takes place during orgasm." Hard subsequently visited the world's first recorded artificially conceived offspring, by then a businessman in New York.

Clearly, the potential of DI loomed large in Hard's vision at the beginning of the century, as he expressed in the following amazing diatribe:

> From a nature point of view, the idea of artificial impregnation offers valuable advantages. The mating of human beings must, from the nature of things, be a matter of sentiment alone. Persons of the worst possible promise of good and healthy offspring are being lawfully united in marriage every day. Marriage is a proposition which is not submitted to good judgment or even common sense, as a rule. No Burbank methods are possible, even tho [sic] they be ideal. Artificial impregnation by carefully selected seed, alone will solve the problem. It may at first shock the delicate sensibilities of the sentimental who consider that the source of the seed indicates the true father, but when the scientific fact becomes known that the origin of the spermatozoa which generates the ovum is of no more importance than the personality of the finger which pulls the trigger of a gun, then objections will lose their forcefulness and artificial impregnation become recognized as a race-uplifting procedure.

> It is gradually becoming well establisht [sic] that the mother is the complete builder of the child. It is her blood that gives it material for its body and her nerve energy which is divided to supply its vital force. It is her mental ideals which go to influence, to some extent at least, the features, the tendencies, and the mental caliber of the child. "Many a man rocks another man's child and thinks he is rocking his own" for it looks like him. And often two children by the same parents have features entirely dissimilar. It is the predomi-

nating mental ideals prevailing with the mother that shapes the destiny of the child. The man who thrusts his nose into a beautiful blossom to surfeit his sense of smell on the sweet perfume, is merely breathing the lustful odor from the sexual organ of the plant; and if his nose displaces some of the pollen, he may be the father of the next flower. If a honey bee does the work, it might be called the father.

A scientific study of sex selection without regard to marriage conditions, might result in giving some men children of wonderful mental endowments, in place of half-witted, evil-inclined, disease-disposed offspring which they are ashamed to call their own. The mechanical method of impregnation, whether it be the orthodox way or the aseptic surgeon's skillful fingers, counts but little, except sentiment, and sentiment is fast becoming a servant instead of a master in the affairs of the human race. Few are the children that are brought intentionally into this world. As a rule they are but the incidental result of a journey in search of selfish pleasure. They are seldom sought, and often unwelcome when they put in their first appearance. The subsequent mother's love is largely a matter of growth, for affection is but an attribute of selfishness.

The man who may think this idea shocking, probably has millions of gonnococci swarming in his seminal ducts, and probably his wife has had a laparotomy which nearly cost her life itself, as a result of his infecting her with the crop reaped from his last planting of "wild oats."

Hard closes with an indictment of the prevalence of venereal disease at the time.

In 1907 Ivanoff, a physiologist, wrote that there were real advantages in using artificial insemination on a large scale in animal husbandry. In fact, techniques, protocols, and legal lineage (the donor is always the sire) of DI in animals have been much more highly developed than for humans.

By the early 1900s, the practice of DI was well under way. Twenty-four articles had been written on the subject of DI in the United States by 1938, and a 1941 survey estimated that almost 3,700 inseminations had occurred in the United States. In the 1980s, estimates range from 10,000 to 100,000 DI children per year; the state of California alone may have 20,000 annually (Sokoloff, 1987). The numbers are vague because of the secrecy around the procedure. It is estimated that there are over one million DI offspring in the United States, with thousands around the world as well. Yugoslavia, for example, has an estimated 5,000 a year, England and Australia over 2,000, Switzerland and Denmark over 1,000, and over 300 and rising in Sweden despite that country's recent legislation, which protects the child's right to know her paternal origin.

The development of frozen semen and the establishment of sperm banks have given a big impetus to DI. This will be discussed in the following chapter.

Definitions

Artificial insemination is a technique whereby semen is placed in the vagina, cervical canal, or uterus by means other than sexual intercourse, for the purpose of inducing a pregnancy. Because of the association with animal husbandry and to avoid acknowledging the donor, other terms have been suggested such as alternative, therapeutic, or even abnormal fertilization.

Husband Insemination

AIH is artificial insemination with the husband's semen, in contrast to AID—artificial insemination by donor, or DI as we now call it. It is also known as "endogenous" or "homologous" insemination. This is done when some mechanical difficulty prevents the husband from depositing the semen in his wife's vagina—such as impotence, hypospadias (semen lost through a congenital opening on the underside of the penis), or retrograde ejaculation (semen enters the bladder). There may be physical deformities, paralysis, or psychological conditions that also prevent natural insemination.

When oligospermia (less than 30 million sperm) is present, several semen samples may be taken and pooled to increase the concentration of sperm. A centrifuge technique spins the sperm for a couple of minutes. The first portion of an ejaculate ("split ejaculate") is used as it contains less prostatic fluid and thus a higher concentration of sperm. The concentration of sperm seems to be more important than the total number of sperm. Laboratory screening to eliminate abnormal sperm and other debris in the semen by passing it through a nylon membrane may also increase the possibility of conception.

Cervical mucus that is "hostile" to a partner's sperm may be receptive to the sperm from a donor. In such cases, there is a definite body-mind link to be explored. Psychological aids, such as visualization, can help, but it is probably necessary to understand the "hostility" of the mucus first. It is interesting that when the mucus and semen are mixed together prior to AIH, the success rate is doubled (from 21 to 42 percent).

Shapiro (1981) cites a case where a woman was allergic to her husband's semen, developing shortness of breath and hives if a condom were not used or if it leaked. She also had positive skin tests to semen from vasectomized men (who have no sperm in their semen). After seven cycles of AIH, with sperm only, she successfully conceived and delivered twins. There is another case of a woman who developed an allergic reaction to her husband's semen during pregnancy. The authors observe the "immunologic potential of human coitus," which is clearly psychosomatic.

Donor Insemination

DI is artificial insemination with semen from a donor, and is also known as "exogamous" or "heterologous," "therapeutic" or "aided" insemination. Some prefer the more technical names because AID stresses the major drawbacks of the procedure—the artificiality and the presence of a donor. I stated the reasons why I use the term DI—donor insemination—in the Author's Note.

Semen obtained from one donor may be used for many impregnations and can be kept indefinitely through freezing and storage in sperm banks. When two or more inseminations are done in one cycle, different donors may be used for each attempt. However, Langer et al. (1969) in Israel refused subsequent DI unless the same donor was used.

Although the procedure may be helpful, safe, and painless, concern is rarely expressed for the consequences of the procedure, which occupy the major part of this book.

In a couple relationship with male infertility, DI (in contrast with AIH) introduces a third party. Traditionally the donor's identity is highly guarded, in order to protect the donor and physician. Single or lesbian women may also place secrecy at a premium for their own protection against a possible paternity suit.

Mixed Insemination

AIM refers to the practice of mixing the husband's and donor's semen. It is also known as AIHD or CAI, confused artificial insemination; BAI, biseminal artificial insemination; the "French firing squad" technique; or, in German, the "pathfinders' action." Although the Curie-Cohen survey found that 15 percent of physicians mixed semen, only ignorant physicians would recommend it today. Even Guttmacher (1962) protested:

> I feel that if the couple cannot face the reality of the fact that this will be a child of the seed of an unrelated man, then I think they are not intellectually and emotionally ripe for the procedure. Therefore I have not been tempted to lull them into a kind of feeling that this might still be the husband's child.

Before the days of blood tests, Finegold suggested that AIM could provide the means for a court to presume in favor of the husband's paternity.

The rationale that practitioners give for AIM is that the husband may then let himself believe that by a remote chance he might be the biological father. It could be argued that this procedure would make it even harder for the husband to accept DI under these circumstances, where his own chances of biological fathering were not ruled out. Also, the use of AIM implies that the husband's infertility is marginal, if such a conception is at all possible. Therefore, one might ask, why is donor semen being used?

Some physicians mix the sperm from different donors, again to confuse the issue of paternity. Any mixing of sperm offers no advantage for improving the chances of conception and, in fact, may have an adverse effect on the semen. More important, AIM for the purpose of confusing the records to preserve donor anonymity is ethically unacceptable but often practiced by lesbians and single women to avoid future paternity suits.

Techniques of Insemination

As Stephen Steigrad, a Sydney gynecologist, puts it, "The actual technique of artificial insemination is one of life's great non-events." This is why self-insemination, discussed in Appendix 2, is so simple.

Masturbation is the usual way of obtaining a semen specimen for artificial insemination, and sperm obtained this way remain mobile longer. However, semen can be collected in a number of other ways.

1. *Coitus.* Retrieval of semen from a condom or even from the vagina after coitus interruptus.
2. *Surgical biopsy* of the testicle or epididymis.
3. *Postmortem* because sperm production is the last body function to cease.

The semen must be used within two hours, and it can be introduced by several different techniques.

1. *Intravaginal.* The semen is simply deposited in the vagina with a syringe, straw in an applicator, test tube, the lower blade of a plastic speculum, or even a turkey baster. Metal is not used because it has a spermicidal effect.

2. *Applied to the cervix,* in a rubber contraceptive cervical cap, plastic insemination cup, diaphragm, or sponge.

3. *Intracervical application* with a cannula if the opening to the cervix is narrowed (stenosis of the external os). It is important that only a small amount of semen be used, a quarter of a ml or less, and that it be introduced very slowly into the cervix so that it does not enter the uterus. Otherwise, cramps can occur from the prostaglandins in the semen. Also many more abnormal sperm (if not screened) reach the uterus than normally would if they had to make their way through the acidic vaginal secretions. This can

lead to infections such as an abscess, endometritis (inflammation of the lining of the uterus), or even peritonitis (inflammation within the abdominal cavity). However, some practitioners, such as Neil Barwin in Ottawa, Canada, routinely do intracervical inseminations, and report only rare side effects, three cases in four hundred requiring transient hospitalization.

Selection of Women

In the overwhelming majority of inseminations in the United States, the gynecologist simply uses his own judgment in treating couples or single women with DI. In other countries, a team approach—combining physician, social worker or psychologist—is more usual. The role is not always selection, but rather presenting information and alternatives so that individuals can drop out themselves, if they so choose. Sometimes such teams are recommended, not to supply objective advice about the unknown outcome of DI, but merely as a means of reducing any possible criticism of the selection process. In fact, I personally know social workers who have left such teams because of conflicts with other members over the issues of secrecy and disclosure to the child.

Each clinic and physician will have their policies of exclusion— no single women, no women over forty, or whatever—which have made sperm banks that market directly to the consumer a popular alternative. The larger the institution, generally, the longer the waiting list and the more structured the routine.

Determining Ovulation

The most important aspect of donor insemination is timing. The egg is viable for less than twenty-four hours, although sperm survival is longer—up to days. It is crucial, then, to determine the time of ovulation. Usually women are required to take their basal body temperature (BBT) on waking for three months to observe their ovulation pattern.

If conception has not occurred within six months of DI, then

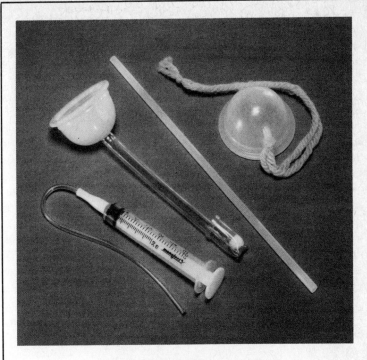

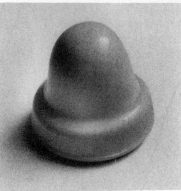

Top: Plastic insemination cervical cups with frozen semen straw and syringe *(Courtesy of Milex Products, Inc.). Bottom:* Rubber contraceptive cervical cap (Courtesy of Lambert/Dalston. *Photograph by Artemis/Harriette Hartigan)*

clinical investigations of ovulation may be begun, which might include systemic tests, such as thyroid function. There are also other unrecognized and poorly defined conditions that affect the success of insemination.

Ovulation can be estimated by radioimmune assay blood tests (which are slow) or rapid LH estimates (which are not always sufficiently sensitive) to check for that hormone peak. Ultrasound scans of the ovaries reveal the status of the ripening egg follicle and reliably can predict or observe ovulation. However, ultrasound scans are expensive, and one to five of them may be necessary until the main follicle ruptures. Other assessments of ovulation include examining the cervical mucus under the microscope (between days eleven and thirteen) for certain qualities found at the time of ovulation such as a "ferning" pattern of crystallization, stretchiness ("Spinnbarkheit"), and the absence of cells. Sometimes estrogen is prescribed for seven to ten days of the cycle to improve the quality and quantity of the cervical mucus because it is very important for conception. Levels of plasma progesterone can be estimated between days twenty-one and twenty-four and confirm whether ovulation has occurred.

However, many practitioners find that it is "more effective" to induce ovulation rather than to predict it. It is not uncommon for the many women undergoing DI to have treatment with clomiphene citrate, (known as Clomid or Serophene) which induces ovulation. It is thus used to produce a predictable ovulation, even though a 1981 study found that the use of clomiphene meant less than a one-day shift of the predicted day of ovulation. This medication is prescribed for failure to ovulate as well as poor function in the luteal, or postovulation phase, of the cycle. It can also stabilize irregular cycles. The decreased function in previously ovulating women is a reaction to the stress of DI. So many women (30 to 67 percent of reported studies) fail to ovulate at some time while undergoing DI that the term "DI-induced anovulation" has arisen. The menstrual clock of the hypothalamus in the brain can be affected by stress due to time off work, travel, expense, or ambivalence about being impregnated with a stranger's sperm. This drug is actually an antiestrogen and it may decrease the amount of ovulation mucus, so that estrogen is often prescribed as well. Clomid is given in doses of 50 to 150 mg a day for five days beginning on the fifth day of the cycle. This will cause ovulation about six days after the last pill, i.e., on day sixteen. There are also side effects from Clomid, such as swelling and possible cysts of the ovaries. Also, the chance of multiple pregnancy is increased when more than one egg is stimulated for release at ovulation. Some doctors, tired of a guessing game each month, will give 5,000 to 10,000 units of HCG (human chorionic gonadotropin, a potent "fertility drug") at midcycle, which will produce ovulation within forty-eight hours. However, Federation CECOS in France (1983) cites a study that implicates inducers of ovulation as a cause of chromosomal abnormalities.

Female Infertility Workup

Many clinics will do six months of DI on the basis of a woman's BBT charts, which show evidence of ovulation. However, some physicians insist on a comprehensive workup, or fertility examination, from the outset. While this may be cost-effective for the physician, it usually isn't for the patient. However, if a woman has not conceived after a few months, it may make sense to undergo some investigations, including psychological counseling. Of course, the woman must also be in good general health and not suffer from such conditions as diabetes or heart disease.

One of the simplest tests is the postcoital test (PCT) to check for survival and motility of the sperm in the cervical mucus. Around days twelve to fourteen, not later than ovulation, and within two to six hours after insemination, some mucus is aspirated from the cervix and examined under the microscope. Prior to insemination, a drop of semen can be placed on a microscope with some cervical mucus to check for compatibility too. Any infection (cervicitis) will be indicated by the presence of white blood cells and can be observed at this time and treated.

A hysterosalpingogram (HSG) is an x-ray to check if the Fallopian tubes are open. A dye is injected into the uterus so that any blockages in the tubes can be observed (and occasionally cleared by the procedure). The HSG has virtually replaced the Rubin or insufflation test, which checked patency of the tubes with carbon dioxide. If the patient felt shoulder pain then this was an indication that the gas had passed into the abdominal cavity and that the tubes were open. Broekhuizen (1980) observed that where routine HSGs were done on women undergoing DI, 80 percent were unnecessary.

A diagnostic laparoscopy is an investigation of the reproductive organs through the abdomen, under anesthesia. It requires an incision so small that this operation has been dubbed "Band-Aid surgery." The abdomen is distended with gas, usually carbon dioxide, to make the organs easier to see through a lighted telescope. Using the laparoscope, the physician can determine whether the tubes are open or closed, whether scar tissue is interfering with the movement and function of the tubes, and whether tubal surgery is necessary. The ovary can be viewed directly to determine whether it is functioning normally. If necessary, a biopsy of the ovary can be taken for examination, or eggs can be collected for examination, testing, or for in vitro fertilization. The HSG and diagnostic laparoscopy are performed during days five to thirteen of the menstrual cycle, after bleeding has stopped and before ovulation.

An endometrial biopsy involves scraping a small piece of the lining of the uterus, prior to menstruation, to examine it for hormone changes that would indicate ovulation. This procedure also proves that the cervical canal is sufficiently open.

Number of Inseminations Per Cycle

The Curie-Cohen survey found that 17 percent of practitioners did one insemination per cycle, 61.4 percent did two, and 20.5 percent did three inseminations per cycle. More inseminations are done with frozen than fresh semen because sperm vigor is reduced by freezing. Interestingly, the success rates were independent of the number of times women were inseminated in a single cycle or the timing with which inseminations were spaced. The only significant factor was the size of the doctor's practice, the larger practices having higher success rates.

Multiple inseminations are typically done on the day before, the day of, and the day after ovulation (-1, day 0 and $+1$). Day 0 is the last day of the lowest point of the temperature (nadir) before the rise. Some say this is the best day, other practitioners found it better either the day before or the day after. DI is sometimes done every other day. Another opinion is that a single insemination per cycle means better timing, with less expense ($75 to $100 per insemination) and wastage of sperm, and has equivalent or better results. A 1980 study by Propping, in West Germany, showed multiple inseminations to be only half as effective as single ones. The explanation put forth is that a second insemination may disturb a pregnancy that has already resulted.

Fifty-one percent of Curie-Cohen's respondents used the same donor for each insemination of a single cycle, but different donors for each cycle, whereas 31.8 percent used different donors within a single cycle.

Results of Donor Insemination

The success of DI is calculated in many different ways. Fecundability means the probability of conception in a menstrual cycle, and fertility refers to the actual conception. Higher rates of success are usually reported with fresh rather than frozen semen. However, patient selection, insemination techniques, number of cycles, and the follow-up of the results of DI are not uniform. Some writers calculate the successful pregnancies according to the incidence of pregnancies per cycle and others total the overall pregnancy rate (the ratio of conceptions to patients receiving DI). This latter rate varies with the number of women who do not complete the advised regimen (losses to follow-up) either because they dropped out or were still hoping to conceive on the program when the data were analyzed. The rate of conception usually refers to the frequency or percentage of conceptions achieved in a certain cycle. The cumulative rate shows the distribution of conceptions by the number of cycles required for conception. This proportion uses as its denominator only those women who conceived and ignores women who did not conceive. Such a proportion does not represent the probability that a woman will conceive by a certain cycle, because it is conditional on a pregnancy being actually achieved.

The cumulative rate of conception obtained by life-table analysis takes into consideration the experience of all the women on the DI program. The life-table method corrects for variable periods of follow-up and losses to follow-up, as it has been argued that drop-outs should be classified as failures. The life-table analysis estimates what conception rates would have been had all patients completed a specific number of DI cycles, and thus provides a true measure of the chance of conception.

Nowhere has the success of DI been 100 percent, and the national average according to Curie-Cohen's survey (1979) was 57 percent. Worldwide rates range from 40 to 80 percent. Guttmacher reported an average of 69 percent in 1962. The highest success rates are in the first three or four cycles, by which time about one-third have conceived. Some practitioners claim that the pregnancy rates fall off after the first few months and then about two thirds of women drop out of the program. Successful clinics have cumulative pregnancy rates of up to 85 percent of those women who persist for a year or longer, using life-table analysis. Glezerman reported that 98 percent of women conceived within thirteen cycles. A study by Bergquist et al. at Johns Hopkins Hospital in Baltimore, published in 1982, concluded that "patients can be advised that their chance of conception with DI should approach that of normal fertile couples." They studied 226 women, using fresh semen, usually two inseminations per cycle with the cervical cup technique. Using a mathematical model of cumulative pregnancy rates, their rate was 62.5 percent after six months and for those who continued to undergo DI beyond six months the monthly probability of pregnancy did not decline. By ten months, 82.4 percent of patients had conceived. (With natural insemination about 30 percent conceive within the first three months, 50 percent by six months, and 80 percent by the end of a year.)

Glezerman and White (1981) describe the ideal DI patient as a woman who is younger than thirty-five, belongs to a higher socio-economic class, has suffered less than seven years of infertility, has no ovulatory disturbance, and has sufficient emotional support from her male partner. In fact, his study found that only 28.6 percent of women whose partners did not accompany them for the inseminations achieved pregnancy, compared with 98.6 percent of those whose partners did. There was a higher abortion rate also in the unaccompanied women, and more than 70 percent of them discontinued DI with or without notification. The absence of the male partner at inseminations was interpreted as resistance, despite his formal acceptance of DI as evidenced by the signed agreement.

An interesting comment on the female factor in fertility was reported by Emperaire, et al. (1980), in the British medical journal *Lancet.* If the male partner's sperm count was zero, 96 percent of the women undergoing DI became pregnant within six months. However, if he had a count of zero to twenty million, only 70 percent of the women did. Likewise, Albrecht (1982) in Boston found a 20 percent fecundability in women with azoospermic partners compared with 10 percent for those whose men were merely oligospermic. They interpreted this to mean that women married to men with low sperm counts are a selected population with subnormal fertility and are unable to compensate for the deficient sperm counts of their husbands. One could also postulate that DI is more acceptable when there is absolutely no hope of conception with one's husband and that this has a psychological effect on the woman's fertility.

Levie (1967) found that four previously infertile husbands showed a "spontaneous remission" of their infertility after their wives had already delivered DI offspring. Each of these men were apparently able to "beget" a child.

Age

Most practitioners find that fertility drops when the woman reaches thirty or thirty-five. Decreased fertility over age thirty-five is often due to the pathology of the pelvic organs. Peak fecundability has been estimated at age twenty-four. Others, like Chong and Taymor, reported (1975) that there was no age effect on fertility. Cesarean rates, which are higher in births resulting from reproductive technologies ("the premium baby") are further elevated in older women.

Fresh or Frozen Semen

Frozen semen was used by 31.4 percent of the Curie-Cohen respondents but accounted for only 12.7 percent of total donor semen. Of those who used frozen semen, 43.7 percent used it in less than 10 percent of their inseminations, and 41.2 percent used it in an average of 90 percent of them. The use of frozen semen was independent of the size of the practice and the size of the population served. Even more striking was the fact that the use of frozen semen was independent of whether the physician treated a woman with the same donor for every cycle or different donors within a single cycle.

Of those physicians who used frozen semen, 87 percent never stored it over two years and 68 percent obtained outside donors. Of those who never or rarely used frozen semen, only 8 percent used donors from outside their own geographic area.

Usually twice as many inseminations are required for frozen as fresh semen, but some practitioners feel the advantages (see Chapter 6) outweigh its lower pregnancy rate. A study done by Kovacs and Lording in Melbourne, Australia in 1980 involved 252 patients who used frozen semen and with at least two inseminations per cycle had less successful results. The life-table pregnancy rates were 47.6 percent after six months and 62.8 percent after twelve months. However, another Melbourne study by Clayton in 1980 showed that 50 percent conceived within three cycles and 85 percent by six months.

As a result of AIDS, frozen semen only is recommended by the American Association of Tissue Banks, the Center for Disease Control, and the Food and Drug Administration. In Australia guidelines require the use of fresh semen. Freezing semen allows it to be quarantined (currently for 90 days, but some banks follow the Australian standard of six months), pending a blood test of the donor to clear him of AIDS antibodies. With such guidelines, a physician who uses fresh semen may be at increased risk for malpractice by not adhering to "standards of practice." Thus sperm banks report increased demand; as one said, "Cleared semen is like liquid gold," and customers are reserving it several months in advance.

When a test for the AIDS *antigen* is developed, quarantining, which allows time for the *antibody* response to the antigen, will no longer be necessary. The American Fertility Society guidelines (October 1986) indicate that fresh semen is safe if their screening procedures are followed (although some AFS members disagree). The majority of physicians are continuing to use fresh semen, according to most sources.

Spontaneous Abortion (Miscarriage) Rate

The rate of miscarriage following DI is no different from natural conception. Numbers range from 8.9 percent in an Australian study to 10.7 percent in a report from Baltimore. Chong and Taymor found the miscarriage rate higher among women aged thirty to thirty-nine compared with those aged twenty to twenty-nine.

Congenital Malformations

Reports of congenital anomalies among DI offspring are less than those naturally conceived, which is 2 to 3 percent. This may be a result of underreporting, although one study looked out for this and concluded that DI parents are more likely to report evident malformations. While the overall incidence of malformations may be lower in DI offspring, the incidence of chromosomal abnormalities may be increased (Fraser and Forse, 1981, Chong and Taymor, 1975, King and Magenis, 1978). Possibly these abnormalities result from stimulating ovulation.

The Sex Ratio of DI Offspring

Although there are reports in the literature that state no statistical difference in the genders of DI offspring, certainly the majority of studies show a much higher number of males than occurs naturally. Kleegman (1954) found that 70 percent were males when the DI occurred within twenty-four hours of ovulation and 70 per-

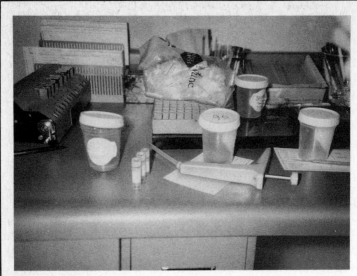

Preparing semen for freezing at a sperm bank

cent were females if the DI was done more than thirty-six hours after ovulation. Edvinsson (1983) in Sweden reported fifty males to thirty-six females.

Hazards for the DI Consumer

Often infertile couples or single women, unless they contact a sperm bank directly, are obliged to place their trust in the physician they consult. Indeed, Lauerson and Ukane, in the November 1982 issue of *Cosmopolitan*, go so far as to say that "your knowledge and trust in your doctor are often essential for a successful conception." Belief surely does play a vital role in health and illness. However, couples are mostly unaware that their physician, if using frozen semen, has no control over the selection and screening of donors or the process of sperm preservation. For example, one of the substances used in cryobanking of semen is Tris, which is used to fireproof fabrics and has been found to be carcinogenic.

The problem with semen brokers, be they your gynecologist or an out-of-state sperm bank, is that the recipient is never 100 percent sure of the semen. Slome, writing in 1973 in the *British Medical Journal* said that his personal experience with DI makes it difficult to suggest a sperm bank because the sperm can't be confirmed. The more parties involved, the more chance of confusion and error. Mail-order sperm can suffer a number of calamities en route. Although I have seen how they prepare, divide, and code the semen, like any bookkeeping system, there are bound to be mistakes. Straws will be misplaced, erroneously labeled, or broken. I have watched technicians in small crowded rooms, chatting away, with the radio blaring, dropping items on the floor, as they casually perform the freezing regimen.

Obviously, elaborate coding systems have been devised to minimize error, with different containers for different sperm. Some clinics have the patient fill in the records for matching the donor so that at least secretarial errors in transcription are avoided. Such doubts never arise when working with a donor friend, and the sperm comes fresh and pure. Discussion of anonymous donor selection can be found in Chapter 7, and Chapter 8 explores the choosing of known donors of semen and other forms of assisted reproduction.

The demand for DI can be expected to continually increase with media publicity, the rising incidence of male infertility, fewer infants available for adoption, more women (single, lesbian) wanting to bear a child without a male partner, and progress in genetic screening.

6

Semen Freezing and Sperm Banks

THE WIDER AVAILABILITY and commercialization of DI has resulted from technical developments that have enabled semen to remain viable after freezing (cryopreservation) and thawing. Cryopreservation for ova first became available in Australia in late 1985, which bypasses all the ethical problems of freezing, storing, and discarding human embryos. The world's first baby from a previously frozen embryo was born in Melbourne, Australia, in 1985, two hundred years after Spallanzani first observed the effects of freezing on human sperm.

In 1866, Manteganazzi originated the concept of sperm banks. In 1938, Jahnels observed the survival of frozen sperm after thawing. British scientist A. S. Parkes and his colleagues developed in 1949 the use of glycerol to protect sperm during the freezing process. In 1953, Bunge and Sherman, using dry ice for freezing and storing semen, reported the first successful human pregnancy resulting from frozen semen.

The Advantages of Frozen Semen

Freezing sperm makes it easier to use the same donor from month to month, or even for subsequent pregnancies. It allows for both a more accurate matching of characteristics and, with a seven-days-a-week service in many clinics or even at home, more precisely timed inseminations. There is not the wastage that might occur if fresh semen is donated, but the timing is not right for the recipient or she cancels her appointment. Specimens can be more readily cultured and screened in a laboratory setting, and the number of progeny by a donor can sometimes be more easily determined. Many practitioners prefer to use frozen semen because the donor is truly anonymous, whereas with fresh semen the physician knows both the donor and recipient and there is always the possibility for information on either party to slip out.

The major advantage cited for sperm banking is the availability of a greater range of specimens at any time or place. Multiple donations from a donor can be dispensed to geographically distant locations. Cooperation among the government sperm banks in Australia facilitates the shipping of semen to different states when

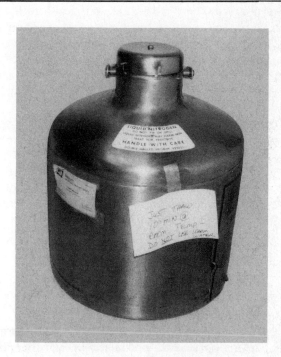

Liquid nitrogen shipping tank

a donor has fulfilled his limit of ten pregnancies in a given area. Dispersing the semen samples in this way helps to diminish the likelihood of inbreeding in a certain location. The development of a wide choice of donors makes it possible to offer a range of characteristics, so that donors can be matched to husbands. This is often very important to DI consumers and may lead them to select frozen semen over fresh. Single women may seek a specific characteristic such as tallness or curly hair. Sperm banks also claim that the couple have the option of a future sibling, i.e., true brother or sister for the child they conceive. However, the sperm bank may have used all the semen from that donor or gone bankrupt.

Computerization enables rapid matching of the legal father's characteristics with those of the donor, particularly race, blood type, and Rh factor. Additional features that sperm banks usually record, and recipients may request, are physical—such as ethnic group, eye color, hair color and texture, height, weight, complexion, build/bone size. Occupation and hobbies are included in some cases. (See Appendix 4 for a sample donor catalog.)

Dr. J. K. Sherman, chairman of the Reproductive Council of the AATB, points out that semen cryobanking is not synonymous with DI. Semen banking also offers opportunities for storage, pooling, and concentration of a husband's sperm if the count is low. Sperm banks are also used by men planning testicular or prostate surgery, chemotherapy, and those who are physically disabled or at risk for occupational hazards. A recent development is the banking of sperm for surrogate mothers and absentee husbands or commuting couples! Some sperm banks are now offering sex selection techniques; these are discussed in Appendix 2. However, donor semen is about 85 percent of the cryopreservation.

Commercial Sperm Banks

The improved methods of freezing and storing semen in liquid nitrogen have led to the establishment of commercial sperm banks as well as banking for research and development in human reproduction, such as sperm antibody research. Sperm banks in the United States are usually businesses for profit, although some are attached to universities or government hospitals (as in Australia). They may be small, a single physician with his own storage facilities, or a major enterprise with branch offices. By 1973 there were sixteen semen banks across the country, and today there are over two dozen whose directors or technicians are members of the American Association of Tissue Banks (AATB). Membership is not required in the AATB, and only six states have laws pertaining to tissue banks, so it is not known how many other sperm banks exist in the country and what their standards are. The AATB has drawn up a protocol for bank inspection certification by peer review, so that soon banks themselves will have the status of membership. However, in the meantime, those individuals who are members of AATB adhere to the guidelines in their facilities. Mascola (1986) writes that artificial insemination should be "at least as safe as a blood transfusion, but its safety is compromised until all practitioners and semen banks adhere to the guidelines."

This association, together with such banks as Idant in New York, California Cyrobank in Los Angeles, and Xytex in Augusta, Georgia, have been in existence for over a decade. Most of the sperm banks offer various reproductive diagnostic tests, and some like Idant (which is the largest sperm bank in the world, with over 20,000 specimens) are blood banks as well. Although the price of frozen donor sperm has increased (with shipping costs it adds up to about $130 a straw), it has not kept pace with other rising medical costs. Yet semen banks have been obliged to do many more tests to screen the semen, and malpractice insurance premiums have soared. A spokeswoman at the AATB said that it would be extremely difficult for a sperm bank to start up today, as insurance companies would not want to take a risk on a bank without a track record.

Donor screening standards established by the Reproductive Council of AATB include: independent screening by two physicians for fertility, health, intelligence, and the absence of infectious disease. Each donor is required to have a physical examination, and a medical and genetic history is taken of the donor for three generations. Educational level and occupation are noted. Because of the AIDS scare, donors are questioned very thoroughly about their life-styles, and most banks refuse the semen of gay and bisexual men. Roxanne Feldschuh, M.D., director of Idant, says that they did not take such donors even before the AIDS problem, because their semen invariably showed high rates of infection.

Reputable sperm banks today screen the semen for HIV (AIDS), CMV (cytomegalovirus), RPR (syphilis), herpes, plus chlamydia, Mycoplasma, and ureaplasma—sexually transmitted organisms that have been identified in recent years. Semen is also tested for candida (yeast), hepatitis type B, gonorrhea, and trichomonas. Urine drug screening is done, plus a blood chemistry profile and CBC (complete blood count). When indicated, donors are tested for Tay-Sachs and sickle cell trait. Karyotyping (chromosome analysis) is done on every donor by some banks, such as Xytex and Biogenetics. Others, such as California Cryobank and Idant, do not do this routinely.

The AATB recommends that donor semen meet the following standards, which some practitioners regard as unrealistic: 75 million sperm per ml, 50 percent or greater initial motility, above average forward progression, less than 30 percent structural abnormalities of the head and neck, and at least 50 percent postthaw recovery rate after freezing.

The guidelines established by the AATB, including the maintenance of records, can be enforced in only the six states that have laws regulating the practice of sperm banks. At least such guidelines serve to establish "standards of practice" that influence the conduct of the member banks. The AATB stipulates that records be maintained for the "life history of the semen sample"—its processing, storage, and destination. It is also stipulated that records should maintain the anonymity of the donor, although each bank is free to set up its own system. Nevertheless, there is nothing to prevent banks from destroying records after the donor ceases participation. Some banks I interviewed said that they would always keep the medical information and genetic profile, but planned to destroy the code that linked that information with a certain donor; thus, if the bank were ever ordered to produce the records, it could "honestly" say that there were none. The link between the semen and physician/recipient is also often destroyed in the interests of preserving anonymity. Other banks, such as Biogenetics and California Cryobank, were committed to permanent records and reported that there were instances when physicians reported genetic conditions (which were not necessarily found to be connected with the donor).

Donors who have a large quantity of semen are profitable for sperm banks, as some ejaculates yield up to forty specimens. Ejaculates range in volume from 2 to 4 cc, but only .25 cc of semen (plus preservatives) is required for an insemination. The donor is paid from $10 to $75, and each specimen is sold for at least $60 to $125, making a profit of over $2,500 with a productive donor!

Most sperm banks maintain at least fifty current donors; some have over a hundred. Several hundred specimens a month are shipped, interstate as well as overseas, at a price ranging from $50 to $75 per specimen, plus shipping costs. Most frozen donor semen in Canada is imported from the United States. Although there are sperm banks all over the world—in Australia, Belgium, Brazil, England, France, Germany, Israel, Norway, and Denmark, to name a few countries—U.S. sperm banks also ship semen to these and other nations. Perhaps some of the requests are made for fear of inbreeding.

There was a satirical article in the German journal *Aus der Medizinischen Welt,* expressing concern about quality control with semen exported to Europe. The author, Wimmer, found some comfort in the thought that surely the Americans would not send over the semen of gangsters, as it is in their interest to build a strong and safe Europe!

Freezing, Inventory, and Shipping of Semen

The sperm are usually preserved with glycerol, plus egg yolk sometimes, as is customary in Europe. Fructose, sodium citrate, or Tris may also be added to prevent the formation of ice crystals. The semen is then placed in sterile paillettes, ampules, or straws (which may hold from .25 to 1 cc., half of which is preservative mixture). After the vials are sealed and identified, they are quickly cooled to -70 or $-80°$ centigrade in liquid nitrogen vapor for forty-five minutes and then placed in a permanent tank, where the temperature of the liquid nitrogen is $-196°$ centigrade ($-321°F$). The storage tanks operate independently of any electrical power source, and the levels of liquid nitrogen are monitored carefully.

Tanks can accommodate up to five thousand vials, making the labeling and coding of specimens very important. Usually the semen is coded by donor number and matched with a color as well. Clearly marked sections of the tanks or even different color-coded tanks may house semen from different ethnic and racial groups. Each stored vial has the donor code, date of the specimen, and number of semen units. Wall chart systems are sometimes used to record the use of specimens on a daily basis, although computers are now more commonly used for semen inventory.

In the United Kingdom, it has been suggested that sperm banks be organized on a national basis, with a series of ten to twelve strategically located regional centers (each able to serve about 5 million people). This Huxleyan scheme recommends that the main centers recruit and select the donors, screen the semen, do all the freezing, and provide the major storage facilities. The proponent, Dr. W. Richardson, suggests that a second tier of the system would incorporate an arrangement of subsidiary satellite storage tanks, holding semen from at least six donors, situated in towns where there were DI centers. The third tier in the system would be individual clinics, and the semen would be sent in a returnable tank that could store the sperm for a week.

The U.S. Postal Service does not accept frozen consignments; they are sent by United Parcel Service, Federal Express, or courier. Some banks have their own free delivery service within a certain mileage. Samples are requested by a physician upon authorization of the recipient, and in some cases they are shipped directly to her. If the specimens are packed and shipped in dry ice, they can be kept frozen for three to six days, and there is no container to return. Some ampules are transported in portable biological dry shippers, made of durable lightweight aluminum, which contain enough liquid nitrogen for a week. Specimens should never be stored in a regular freezer. Insemination equipment and instructions for thawing the semen are usually included. Cryobanks report that physicians are often casual about the thawing procedure, which can affect the recovery of the sperm. Physicians and recipients need to follow the thawing instructions carefully; also, many banks do not demand payment if the sample is less than a promised quality. This sperm count guaranteed may range from 20 to 50 million sperm, with 50 to 60 percent motility, depending on the standards of the various banks.

All banks have informed consent/release forms, such as the one in Appendix 4. Some make clear that the same donor cannot be guaranteed for subsequent orders and that in some states, by law, the physician may be required to file this consent with the Registrar of Vital Statistics if a pregnancy results from the procedure. However, few physicians have the time or the motivation to give results and other feedback to the sperm banks, and many of them, like the banks, ultimately destroy the identifying components, or all, of the records.

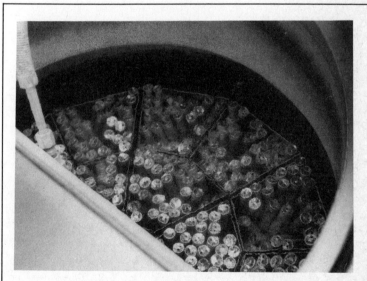

Straws of frozen semen in liquid nitrogen *(Photograph by Artemis/Harriette Hartigan)*

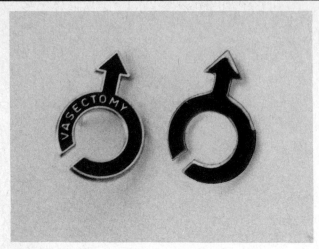

Vasectomy pins *(Courtesy of the Association for Voluntary Surgical Contraception. Photograph by Artemis/Harriette Hartigan)*

"Vasectomy Insurance"

The popularity of vasectomy in the early seventies was another factor in the creation of sperm banking. Many men viewed sperm banks as a way of safeguarding future fertility, if they were going to war, undergoing surgery or radiation therapy, or might be exposed to hazardous materials. "Fertility insurance" was designed to encourage men to submit to vasectomy, without much thought of future consequences. However, when vasectomies were a fashionable new trend and free sperm storage was offered, only one percent of the men requested this, according to Tyler in a 1973 report. A decade or so later, great numbers of those sterilized men have remarried and are now customers of the banks—this time as recipients of donor sperm.

The Disadvantages of Sperm Banks

The major drawbacks with semen banking concern the use of anonymous semen donors, who are often poorly screened. There are no regulations in the United States at present, although since the AIDS scare a screening test has been developed. In December 1985, the American Association of Tissue Banks task force on the role of semen in transmitting AIDS recommended the use of frozen semen as the optimal and safest means of testing for AIDS in semen donors. Frozen semen permits a quarantine period (at least three months was advised) in storage for retesting the donor's blood before the semen is released for insemination. This permits detection of the specific antibodies that may not have been in high enough concentration to be detected at the time of donation. Prior to the development of an AIDS screening procedure, the Australian government closed down all sperm banks in the country.

Frozen semen is more costly than fresh, as commercial sperm banks operate for profit, plus there are shipping costs for the heavy freezing chambers. The process of freezing limits the capability of the sperm, and there is no guarantee that semen specimens will be usable at a later date. The correlation between prefreeze and postthaw motility is controversial. Higher rates of motility are found when the semen is thawed at an environmental temperature of 22 degrees centigrade rather than at 4 degrees centigrade.

In actual practice, about one third more inseminations are required using frozen semen because it is about two thirds as viable as fresh sperm. About 65 percent of sperm survive the freezing technique and 70 percent of potential donors are typically rejected because their sperm does not freeze well and thus cannot meet this criterion. Ice crystallization and respiratory shock are the main problems for the sperm with cryopreservation. (However, a donor may still be adequate for DI with fresh semen.) Conception rates with frozen semen are about 50 percent although some practitioners report greater success, especially in the United States.

Sherman published a study in 1973 of 571 DI conceptions with semen stored at least ten years, noting fewer abnormalities and abortions than in the general population. However, a 1985 study by Forse et al. in Quebec found three cases of Turner's syndrome and a case of Trisomy 21 in a group of 398 babies born by DI. The researchers cautioned against the possibility of genetic damage from freezing sperm.

Some people are worried about potential eugenic (often racist and sexist) manipulations and whether the commercialization of semen may come to mean the most desirable semen goes for the highest price.

Long-Term Outcome

Nobody knows the eventual genetic effects of using frozen sperm, although in thirty years no negative results have been observed. The American Public Health Association warns that "the biologic potency and genetic adequacy of human sperm which has been frozen and stored over a protracted period of time and then thawed remains to be established." Frankel, writing in *Connecticut Medicine* in 1975, points out that as a medical procedure human semen banking should be considered an experimental technique. There is no licensing or protocol—sperm banks are not even obliged to screen donors at all. This warning is not communicated to prospective parents. In fact, there are no standard procedures among semen cryobanks for obtaining informed consent and some provide no consent forms at all. As secrecy is a tenet of DI, records are rarely kept and if so, often destroyed, which means follow-up is impossible. Under these circumstances, how will we ever know if any freezing is ultimately safe, or if it may be safe only for a certain amount of time, or what the long-term effects of semen preservation might be?

Lauerson, a gynecologist in New York, in an extract from "New Ways of Making Babies: How Science Can Help," published in *Cosmopolitan*, November 1982, advises couples to quiz doctors about their sperm source: "Which sperm bank is your doctor using? Is it reputable?" He mentions that a rural doctor with a smaller practice might use frozen sperm obtained from an "authorized sperm bank," although, as we have seen, very few banks are regulated.

What are the liabilities of the sperm bank if the sperm causes a problem? Sperm banks could be held negligent under an implied warrant of mercantility (i.e., a product that would pass under ordinary circumstances of trade), or product liability (if the child is defective or has unexpected characteristics) or misrepresentation (if sperm testing was fraudulent).

The state of the American Male's bodily fluids isn't what it used to be, and though the Commies are not to blame, a lot of other factors are—everything from environmental pollution to tight shorts to excessive use of the hot tub. So serious is the problem of declining male virility that a whole new industry has grown up with a vocabulary—deposits, assets, and liquid withdrawals—that has nothing to do with hard cash but is rather the currency of another form of banking. There, sperm is the legal tender.

—*Los Angeles, December 1982*

Following are profiles of two sperm banks that keep permanent records and market directly to consumers. Other sperm banks are listed in Appendix 4.

Repository for Germinal Choice

This sperm bank in Escondido, California, was founded and funded by millionaire Robert Graham in 1979. Graham, a father of eight who made his fortune inventing plastic optical lenses, set up the sperm bank as part of his Foundation for the Advancement of Man. His aim is to breed higher intelligence by using the genes of men of proven genius. He prefers sperm from Nobel laureates in the hard sciences, but he is now accepting other academics and even top leaders in business. The idea of influencing the genetic quality of a species by choice is unpalatable to most people and Graham's strongest critics find his eugenic illusions reminiscent of Hitler's genetic engineering, or at least "biological nonsense." Others find his assumptions about the inheritance of intelligence to be very simplistic, as IQ scores of children tend toward the mean of the statistical curve, whatever the intelligence of their parents. Graham was quoted in the *San Francisco Examiner,* February 8, 1984, as ßaying, "I have been so concerned getting the sperm bank launched that I haven't looked at the ultimate outcome, especially since I won't be here. . . . I haven't really thought through to the outer limits of this project." However, much of the press hysteria over the Repository can be dispelled by the actual practice: by 1986 there had been only sixty applicants and twenty-four conceptions, hardly an influence in humanity's gene pool!

Graham claims that the program is based on "compassion, scientific study of genetics, and voluntary participation." He sees his role as simply servicing intelligent married women by supplying the finest sperm possible to make that woman a mother. Also, this way he hopes to increase the number of creative scientists (although the children may develop other ideas for their careers!).

Dr. Graham is assisted by his wife, Dr. Marta Everton (an ophthalmologist), and the donor-recruiter Paul Smith. The sperm bank, which originated in an underground chamber beneath Graham's home, now occupies a spacious suite in a modern building in Escondido. It is listed in the yellow pages under "sperm banks." According to the December 1982 issue of *Los Angeles,* the budget was expected to increase from $100,000 to $300,000 to cope with the flood of applicants. Dr. Graham would eventually like to handle about 800 inseminations a month, but there have been fewer than 100 applications in total since the bank opened in 1976. The Repository typically has only about a dozen donors on hand, all unpaid, providing 2–700 specimens in all. An ejaculate from the most popular donor yields 65 inseminations. At present, no donors are Nobel laureates.

The repository only stores and ships sperm—it is not a clinic. By dealing directly with the consumer, physician's medical bills and the long waiting lists typical of hospitals are avoided. The sperm is free. A refundable fee is charged for the containers of liquid nitrogen, which keep the sperm frozen. The deposit for three months is five hundred dollars, less fifteen dollars per month depreciation and ten dollars per month liquid nitrogen. The application fee is fifty dollars plus shipping costs for the tank, which holds enough liquid nitrogen for three months and weighs fifty-eight pounds when full.

I met with the bank director, Juliana McKillop, in early 1985. A dedicated and open-minded woman, Juliana provides emotional support as well as advice on how to do self-insemination. She felt that the public mistakenly believed that women had to be on the same intelligence level as the donors, and that this misunderstanding explains why so few consumers had availed themselves of their top quality sperm. She emphasized that sperm would be shipped anywhere to any woman meeting the requirements of the sperm bank. Although officially only married women are acceptable and they must be less than 40 years of age, several single women have had DI offspring from this bank.

Sir Martin Pyle, a physics laureate in 1974, commenting on the sperm bank said, "The way the human race develops, if it develops at all, cannot be fiddled with." However, as we have seen, there are many sperm banks, and thousands of inseminating physicians who are "fiddling" with the genetic lottery in a much bigger way. Graham's sperm bank happens to be the smallest, and the most famous, but it is also the most thorough and provides the most complete information about the donors.

Consumers may select a donor, identified by number and color, from a catalog, which provides the following kind of details:

Donor **Turquoise #36**

SUMMARY: (e.g. A prominent science professor at a major university, well published in his field, distinguished ancestry, very musical)
ANCESTRY: Swedish
EYE COLOR: Hazel
SKIN: Medium
HAIR: Blond, thick, wavy, no thinning
HEIGHT: 6′ 2″
WEIGHT: 170
GEN. APPEARANCE: Clean-cut features, athletic build, pleasing good looks
PERSONALITY: Good sense of humor, happy, even-tempered
BORN: 1940s
IQ: 160 at age nine
MANUAL DEXTERITY: Excellent
ATHLETICS: Long-distance runner
HOBBIES: Classical music, languages, chess.

BLOOD TYPE: O+
GENERAL HEALTH: Excellent. Grandparents still alive. This person has two children with PhDs.

This is an example that I compiled from the 1985 catalog of seven donors. One had "no time" for athletics, but that wouldn't disturb some people as much as the donor who had coronary bypass surgery at age fifty! Five of the seven donors had "O" type blood group, which is the most common type. These donors almost sound too good to be true—perhaps there should be a slot for their faults! Nevertheless, this information is much more than provided by any other sperm bank in the world.

Donor screening is very thorough—right down to hemorrhoids and myopia. The donor Personal History Form has eighteen pages and can be found in Appendix 3. Donors undergo a physical examination and blood tests. Unlike the recipients of the sperm, no age limit for donors has been set. Indeed Dr. Graham feels that by the time a man has shown he is a "high achiever" or become "world class in his field," he has reached middle age or even advancing years. Graham feels that while the volume of sperm may decline with age, the quality does not.

The aim of the sperm bank is to provide the best genes, not the best sperm, and some of the donors actually have below-average fertility. On the other hand, the most potentially fertile donor in the bank was one of the oldest, in his sixties. In contrast, commercial sperm banks select sperm on the basis of numbers and motility more than genes.

To date, all the donors have chosen to remain anonymous, with the exception of William Shockley, winner of the 1956 Nobel Prize in physics and notorious for his views of racial superiority. However, some of the donors have agreed to have their identity disclosed if the child later desires this. One donor even offered to pay for the education of offspring conceived with his sperm, with the parents' permission. (One wonders how many children he would educate!)

The first child to be conceived from a Repository donor was born in April 1982 to Joyce and Jack Kowalski of Phoenix, Arizona. However, in July it was discovered that in 1976 Mrs. Kowalski had lost custody of her two other children by a previous marriage when Jack was accused of child abuse. During 1978 both Kowalskis had served time in a federal prison on fraud charges. Paul Smith, the recruiter for the bank, admitted that the bank's standards are less exacting for recipients of the sperm than for donors. "We're not the CIA," he told *Los Angeles*. "We don't go in and run a life check on these women." Mr. Smith said they sounded like a perfectly normal couple over the phone. However, he added that the application form has since been increased from one to twenty pages.

Graham's comment was that Mrs. Kowalski produced a "superb infant." (All the men involved in DI seem primarily interested in producing a perfect product, and the life that follows is of less importance to them. However, Graham does make time to regularly visit the offspring from the Repository, I was told.) Despite the negative publicity, Paul Smith claims that the number of prospective mothers jumped from five per month to three hundred.

The second successful recipient was a single mother, Afton Blake. A successful professional woman, she appeared on television shows with her son Doron, which is the Greek word for "gift" and coincidentally an anagram for donor. Picking the donor for the third child to be conceived from the Repository was a mutual decision of the parents: they chose a man who was an athlete and a musician.

> We considered the list separately and compared our reactions to the various profiles. We discovered they were identical. From my wife's point of view, which was the most important, she felt on the basis of the information available that this was someone she might even have married. This may sound arrogant, but the person she chose is closer to me than the average medical student, which was the only thing offered by the other banks. And quite frankly, that attribute wasn't too attractive to us.

I was surprised that the number of conceptions through the Repository was so low. Perhaps the original notoriety of this "Nobel Prize winners sperm bank" has put off people. Surely some couples would prefer to use donors whose motivation has not been money, from a bank which is not set up for profit, without having to go on a waiting list. And most important of all, a bank where detailed records are kept and could be available to the DI child.

Feminist Women's Health Center

In October 1982, the Feminist Women's Health Center in Oakland, California, opened its doors, offering donor insemination with semen from its own bank, the Sperm Bank of Northern California. The brochure lists as its first feature "donor insemination for single women and couples." The philosophy of the clinic is unique.

> We believe that women have the right to control our own reproduction and in doing so, determine if, when, and how to achieve pregnancy. The donor insemination program at our clinic is for all women, regardless of their race, marital status, or sexual orientation. Lesbians, single women, and women with infertile partners are encouraged to participate.... Our program is an important resource for women who have not had access to alternative fertilization.

There is also no age limit for women applying for DI. The average age of the women on the DI program is thirty-four, and thirty-two is the average age of those who successfully conceive. About half of the women had never been pregnant before. Most recipients are college-educated Caucasians. According to the sperm bank's 1984 report, 64 percent were unmarried, 27 percent married, 8 percent divorced, and one percent widowed. The ratio of lesbian and bisexual women to heterosexual women was about one third to two thirds, with pregnancy achieved at a higher rate in the former group. The facts counteract the image of "a bunch of women who want to have babies without men" which caused one fertility counselor to resign. He felt that DI was a "pretty intense decision and that [the clinic's] policy was that basically any woman who wanted it was going to get it." However, the director commented that

> since we've opened up the sperm bank, our respect for the other half of the world has increased tremendously. We think men are doing a wonderful thing by giving us their sperm.

My impression after visiting the Health Center and Sperm Bank was that it was a very professional, organized, democratic, and comfortable self-help clinic.

Usually frozen semen is used, except when women bring in their own donors. As the sperm bank is part of a comprehensive health-care center, a unique program has been developed for clients seeking DI. There are regular orientation meetings that discuss the clinic's overall philosophy, services, donor-screening criteria, and legal information. Orientations are done with either women only or with couples. In addition to a complete physical exam, including blood tests and cultures, there is a fertility-awareness class. Participants learn how to chart and interpret the menstrual cycle, with basal body temperatures, cervical mucus evaluation, and self-examination of the cervix with a plastic speculum. Selection of a donor is done in consultation with a review of medical compatibility. Assistance is provided to women who want to inseminate at the clinic, or at home, or who have their own donor. If the DI is done at the Center, champagne and chilled glasses are available so that the event may be celebrated during the "boring" thirty minutes that the woman rests with her hips elevated! I was told of one couple who held a fertility party the first time they did a home insemination, and invited all their friends. (And they did conceive!) The clinic also offers comprehensive infertility counseling, testing, and treatment for both women and men.

Although the sperm bank was originally set up as a service to women in northern California, at least a hundred calls a month come from all across the United States. Over 150 physicians, clinics, hospitals, and nurses are registered with the sperm bank and order semen. Semen has also been shipped as far away as India, Japan, and a few South and Central American countries. More than 250 men have stored their sperm for future use. The largest group are facing possible sterility due to some type of cancer or its treatment. Prevasectomy storage services are also requested, as well as private donors storing their sperm for a known recipient (in twenty-one cases). Men usually store a minimum of three ejaculates of semen for up to seven years, at fifty dollars a year. The brochure clearly states that "after thawing a percentage of the sperm return to the prefreeze state." There is a twenty-five-dollar semen analysis fee and a thirty-dollar retrieval and preparation fee. A freeze tolerance test is performed to determine initial sperm survival.

Female clients are charged on a sliding scale ranging from sixty-five dollars to two hundred and fifty dollars, based on what they can afford to pay. Local doctors, hospitals, and clinics are charged fifty dollars per semen specimen, as are recipients at the clinic for the first three inseminations.

The sperm bank imposes no limitations on women, and one of the motivations for setting up the service was to offer an alternative to the degrading experiences women often have in going to male fertility specialists who usually charge several thousands of dollars and may be antilesbian. Probably the only woman-controlled sperm bank in the world, the directors feel that nothing could be more natural than "making babies," which is a major reason for their using the term "donor insemination" and dropping the pejorative label "artificial." As founder Laura Brown puts it, DI frees women from the feeling of using men sexually to achieve a pregnancy, from "ripping a man off for his sperm."

About 35 percent of the inquiries come from women whose husbands are infertile for one reason or another. Records are kept, but the current philosophy advises anonymity and confidentiality. The majority of unmarried and lesbian women planned to tell the child about the DI, but only 12 percent of the married couples did. The staff felt that about a quarter of the heterosexual couples might agree to the child's learning donor identity at the age of majority. Donors are informed of the health, sex of offspring, and any multiple births.

Donors, who must be less than thirty-five years of age, receive only a small "honorarium" (from one dollar to twenty-five dollars toward the cost of time and travel), which most of them do not accept. In the first five months of operation about five hundred men called the Center volunteering to be donors. One benefit to the donors is an extensive workup including semen analysis, blood tests, and medical history. Since the inception of the sperm bank, 188 donors were screened, but only 25 percent were approved, 46 percent of these being discontinued at some point. The most common reason for rejection was if the semen had a low sperm count or poor motility. Five births per donor are allowed within any one state and five anywhere outside that state. When I visited the bank in 1985, they had about twenty donors available, but since opening they have used over two hundred donors. From October 1982 until April 1984 there had been eighty-nine births.

There is no standard type of donor, according to the staff who handles the semen. Some donors said they wanted to help women make babies; one man (who was rejected) felt he wanted to "spread his perfect Aryan seed." Gay men wanted to be donors because they felt they had a reserve of potential babies that should be tapped. However, since the advent of AIDS, the sperm bank no longer accepts gay or bisexual men as donors. Unlike the commercial sperm banks, if there is any suspicion that the donors view sperm banking as a source of income, they are not accepted.

In 1984 16 percent of the women achieved pregnancy, 69 percent dropped out, and 16 percent were still trying. This is a very high drop-out rate, despite the supportive environment. Seventy-seven percent of the pregnancies are achieved (with almost all frozen semen) within the first three cycles. Forty-seven percent who do not drop out achieve pregnancy within a year. The sperm bank encourages women to do home-inseminations, which are more effective in achieving pregnancy. Sixteen of the twenty-two pregnancies that year were boys. Also, fresh semen was much more effective than frozen.

7

Anonymous Semen Donors

IN THIS CHAPTER we will look at the information available about that mysterious cocreator of life—the anonymous donor of semen. Theologians, philosophers, and social scientists are much more interested than physicians and couples in examining this major dimension of DI, and the unique ethical dilemmas that arise from anonymity.

Although sperm are liberally provided by nature, the ramifications of what a man does with them can be of profound consequence. As men become more aware, they will see what a pawn the unknown donor has been in the game of artificially making babies. W. R. Matthews, the Dean of St. Paul's Cathedral in London wrote:

> The donor shows lack of respect for his own integrity. He alienates himself from the semen to be treated as an independent physical object, altogether detached from him and his life purpose. But the semen is in a profound sense himself, it is a summary vehicle of his own character and characteristics, physical and spiritual, bequeathed to him by his own parents and ancestors. In a large and deep sense, his seed is his life.

The donor is supposedly selected for his "good character," "responsible attitude," and "morality." He is seen as performing his public service in an apparently nonchalant way with little responsibility for his actions. Dunstan (1975) describes how the donor

> consents to become a donor by masturbation and to be paid for doing so, foregoing all knowledge, not only of who will bring up the child of his loins, but even whether his semen has been used at

all, lest later in life he should "become bothered by the fact that somewhere a child of him lives." The more one reflects upon the DI transaction, the stronger the conviction grows that it is about the donor that the most searching ethical questions must be asked; and then about the doctor's use of him as an accomplice in this deed.

The further the act of insemination is removed, for instance, from the personal union and common life of the donor and recipient of the seed, the further from the human, and therefore the more suspect morally the practice would be.

Yet it is precisely because DI removes the personal relationship that it makes it "easier" for everyone involved to pretend that the donor doesn't matter. In fact, the French word for donor is *l'étranger* (stranger), and we have seen how great the need is for both the recipients and the brokers of sperm to depersonalize the donors who provide it.

As we will see in Chapter 10, United States case law, as well as legislation in many states, has established that the anonymous donor cannot be considered the father because he was not responsible for the use made of his sperm. If he didn't intend to become a parent, then he is absolved of parental obligations. Of course, donors need protection from the possible financial claims of a multitude of offspring. At the same time, it is an insult to both the donor and the recipients that the biological connection through the male is not regarded as having any importance. This is an amazing situation in a patriarchal society, where the language and social and legal systems are based on biological ties.

Sources of Semen Donors

Curie-Cohen found that 62 percent of DI practitioners used medical students, 10 percent used other university graduates, 18 percent used both, and 10 percent used other sources. If the physician is using a sperm bank, he will receive a catalog with donor characteristics. A comprehensive range would include blood type, height, weight, hair color and type, complexion, eye color, ethnic origin, race, religion, years of college, occupation, nationality, interests

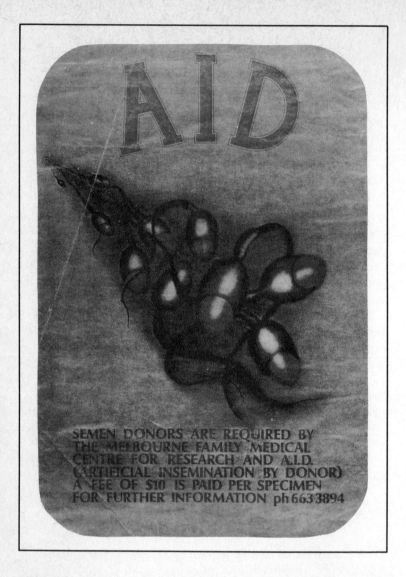

AID

SEMEN DONORS ARE REQUIRED BY
THE MELBOURNE FAMILY MEDICAL
CENTRE FOR RESEARCH AND A.I.D.
(ARTIFICIAL INSEMINATION BY DONOR)
A FEE OF $10 IS PAID PER SPECIMEN
FOR FURTHER INFORMATION ph 663 3894

and hobbies. More commonly, just the first eight items are noted. (See Appendix 4.)

Where fresh semen is used, local donors will be recruited—students, sympathetic husbands of infertile women, grateful husbands of new mothers, or anyone who comes forth from newspaper ads or media requests. At least your doctor or his staff will personally select the donor and you can ask him about his criteria. Physicians using fresh semen match only a couple of characteristics, or some pronounced physical feature, and these may be matched either to the wife or the husband. Eight percent of Curie-Cohen's respondents did not attempt *any* donor matching at all. Regrettably, blood group matching is one of the priorities and its sole purpose is to deceive the child.

Niels Lauerson, who is a DI practitioner, fancifully writes:

> [Your doctor] is searching for a facsimile of an existing husband, and his judgment and sensitivity are crucial. Does your woman's intuition tell you to trust your doctor? You must, because he is helping you to create a human being who will be in your life forever.

Once Lauerson had a patient who requested that the donor be a tall, red-haired, orthopedic surgeon, and he finally was able to meet her request. Lauerson likes to lighten the heavy discussion with such comments as "there are no artificial ingredients used for DI, just like test-tube babies are not born in test tubes." He continues:

> Naturally, every profession has its horror stories, and I can remember hearing about one prominent physician who mixed up semen specimens he was using for artificial inseminations. He gave a white woman the semen from a black man and the black woman the semen from a white man. However, his patients should have noticed that he was a particularly disorganized person even though he had a far-reaching infertility practice. Never ignore personal impressions. The doctor who performs a couple's artificial insemination is a pivotal person in their lives.

Notice, however, in the above statement how Lauerson blames the victim, even though he has been insisting that the patient-victim trust the doctor! Interestingly, he uses an example of racial mixing, one of the very common fears of DI couples. I also find it curious that a DI practitioner would relate such a story, and particularly one that he admits was hearsay.

Le Lannou (1980) reports that sperm banks in France require that all sperm donations be given without remuneration and from a couple with one or more children.

Fertility has been declining in the whole population in recent

years, which is one of the many problems with finding suitable donors. A 1950 Cornell study found that 44 percent of male college
students had over 100 million sperm per ml and only 12 percent
had between 20–40 million. At the University of Texas in 1977,
it was found that the number of men with a high sperm count had
dropped to 22 percent, and twice as many men now had below
normal counts as in the Cornell study two decades before. In
1978, Beck and Marina (1980) found that 50 percent of the men
who qualified on other accounts to be donors, had deficient semen. The Reproductive Council of the American Association of
Tissue Banks developed the following guidelines for donor semen:
75 million sperm per ml, 50 percent or greater initial motility,
above average forward progression, less than 30 percent structural
abnormalities of the head and neck, and at least 50 percent postthaw recovery rate if the semen is frozen.

Medical Students

Medical students are the most common source of semen in the
United States, although donors may come from all walks of life.
Medical students are expedient because they are captive, yet transient, which means that there will be fewer progeny in a given area
for future unknown inbreeding. One practitioner said, "Nowadays
you take what you can get and that means medical students. Of
course, we assume that if they've come that far, they are intelligent." Physicians naturally consider their junior colleagues to be
"ideal, healthy, intelligent donors," as probably would any other
professional group selecting members from its own ranks.

It is assumed that medical students are well informed about genetics and familiar with their family health history. However,
Curie-Cohen found that not even the graduate specialist practitioners of DI had a reliable understanding of basic genetics! Also,
the incidence of disease among medical students is more than
stated, especially Mycoplasma infections, which one physician felt
were responsible for a number of miscarriages in his successful DI
pregnancies.

A 1983 *Journal of Urology* article by Gerber and Bresau reported that thirty-four (79 percent) of forty-three medical students applying to be donors, had inadequate semen analyses by one or more criteria. Problems with the semen quality were more common than insufficient numbers of sperm, even with several collections. Because medical students are the primary donors it is a surprising revelation that they are even less fertile than men in the average population. Is this caused by special environmental factors (e.g., radiation, anesthetic gases, and so forth in the hospitals) or is it the stress of medical education? Searching hard for an explanation, the researchers even wondered if psychological difficulties affected the semen quality because the specimens were produced by masturbation! Are medical students a dependable source if only 21 percent of the potential donors were acceptable? As J. Walter Smyth of Johns Hopkins Hospital comments on the Gerber and Bresau research:

> If that is so of the general population, the woman is truly the determining factor in occurrence of pregnancy, since 85 percent of couples have little or no trouble achieving pregnancy, whereas only one in five husbands has a normal sperm count. If that is so, either the normals for sperm count must be revised or all (semen) tests must, as the authors suggest, be accompanied by an egg penetration test.

Or, we must assume that medical students averaging twenty-five years old are not a good source of donor sperm. Sorry, men.

Medical students become less willing to donate as they progress in their studies. This may be due to their growing maturity and ethical awareness of what paternity implies or perhaps they need the money less as they earn more from their profession.

Finegold, writing in *Artificial Insemination,* assumes that emotional and neurotic young men "probably eliminate themselves." He reassured himself that:

> We have evidence that psychiatrists do not regard donor participation with undue perturbation. At one time our most desirable suppliers of spermatozoa were the fledglings from the house staff of the Western State Psychiatric Hospital in Pittsburgh.

Homosexual Donors

Homosexual men in the past responded to requests for sperm donation, however. Even lesbians are reluctant to have donations from homosexual men, because "street sperm" (which is sperm from donors who come in off the street) is more likely to be contaminated by infection, herpes, or AIDS. Sperm banks and clinics avoid semen from gay or bisexual men. Of course, they are relying on the integrity of the applicants to honestly state their sexual preference, and since the AIDS scare, banks are questioning their donors very thoroughly.

Heterosexual couples are usually not told if their semen donor is gay. I believe they have the right to know such information about the origin of the sperm or to specify that the donor be married or of proven fertility. The idea that homosexuality could be an inherited predisposition seems preposterous, but it has certainly been suggested. Dunstan (1976) quotes a medical doctor in England:

> One young student gave thirty specimens over his four years; all were successful. Payment was nine pounds each time. He is a homosexual. Morality apart, one hopes that in years to come homosexuality will not be found to be genetically transmitted.

In fact, in 1960 the Feversham Committee of the Home Office in the United Kingdom thought that even the questionable "morals and sense of responsibility" of donors might be genetically transmitted! In their report the committee wrote that "the role of the donor is of such a kind that it is liable to appeal to the abnormal and unbalanced."

Perhaps homosexual men become donors in large numbers because they feel they are an untapped reservoir of paternal genes. Huerre (1980), a physician in France, suggested that

> it appears at times that a donation may be related to a latent homosexuality. Since certain donors are recruited by a sterile male friend ("my friend asks me") who comes in each time. The donor explains that he donated "for him" after having come up against the hesitations of his wife who felt dispossessed of "something which belongs to her."

Considering that this particular clinic requires infertile couples to do their own recruiting, it seems unfair to view the recruitment so pejoratively. It is apparent that the subject of DI brings up many racist, sexist, or paranoid fears and fantasies that may be just under the surface.

Criteria for Selecting Donors

In the 1940s, Dr. Abner Weisman drew up a credo for selecting "proper donors." This kind of "*we* shall judge and select" mentality is still very much in operation in DI clinics today.

1. The donor must remain *unknown*. [italics mine]
2. The donor should be in fine health mentally and physically.
3. The donor should be of fine physical stock.
4. The donor should be of high fertility.
5. The donor should be between thirty and thirty-five years of age.
6. The donor should be of excellent character.
7. The donor must be cooperative. He should be willing to persist with each case.

8. The donor's characteristics must match those of the patient's husband.
9. The donor's temperament should closely resemble that of the husband.
10. The donor's religion must be the same as that of the husband.
11. The donor should protect himself legally by ascertaining that the physician has the usual signed documents.
12. The donor should be from men of the science of medicine.
13. The donor's Rh must be suitable. It is best that his blood grouping be identical with that of the husband.
14. Multiple donors should be utilized if possible.

Items that are significant, in my opinion, are numbers 2, 3, 6, 7, and 13. I quite disagree with Weisman on the first point. *I would put as the number one priority that the donor must be known,* or knowable to the child at some time.

In general, there is a remarkable lack of standardization for the selection of donors. The busy gynecologist certainly has not the time or opportunity to complete Dr. Weisman's tall order. Today, the two most important aspects of using unknown donors are genetic and laboratory screening (especially testing for AIDS).

Although in-depth interviews of donors are rare, some practitioners feel that, as physicians, they are able to evaluate and disqualify donors on certain grounds. One writer admitted that the contraindications of "pronounced obsession and hypochondriacal character" are easier to discern than "masked depression"! Apparently, donors should be excluded if they present themselves in compensation for a failed relationship, are "hypersexual," have fears of a possible consanguinous marriage, or might become involved in an imaginary emotional relationship with the recipient. "Financial need as the primary motive" or an "inappropriate curiosity for modern scientific procedures" have also been cause for rejection.

Donor Screening

Because there are no uniform national standards for donor selection and screening, donor screening is usually very inadequate. The AATB has attempted to remedy this in the case of frozen semen, and their guidelines were discussed in the previous chapter. The paucity of donor screening is also not consistent, for example, with other ob-gyn practices such as the pressure on pregnant women today to undergo more and more genetic screening.

As we have seen, donors are asked to disclose any history of physical or mental illness. However, payment for semen tends to discourage truthfulness in such matters, and if the donor lies or withholds pertinent information there are no sanctions that can be used against him.

The Curie-Cohen survey revealed the lack of knowledge that medical practitioners have of genetics, which means that the majority of gynecologists are unable to make sound decisions with regard to donor screening. For example, 71 percent of the DI practitioners reported that they would reject a donor if he had a family history of hemophilia, although it is impossible for a donor to transmit that gene unless he personally has the disease. Although 95 percent of the practitioners said they would reject a donor who carried Tay-Sachs disease, less than one percent specifically tested for it. Likewise, while 92 percent would reject a donor with a translocation or trisomy genetic defect, only 12 percent actually examined donors' karyotypes (chromosome configuration) to determine if the condition were present.

There are over 2,300 Mendelian abnormal phenotypes, and about half of these could be transmitted by a donor with a 50 percent chance of affecting the child. There have been attempts to assess human chromosomal abnormalities in human sperm, for example, the extra Y chromosome that occurs in one to two percent of anomalies. The incidence of chromosomal abnormalities in aborted fetuses is about 30 percent. Therefore if abnormal sperm account for this, genetic techniques may help reduce the number of abnormal sperm used for DI. If donor screening is to be regulated, then screening for the dozen or more common genetic conditions should be mandatory.

Sample of a Donor Consent Form

Date _____

To _____ M.D.

I offer my services as a donor of semen for artificial insemination with the understanding that the identity of any recipient shall not be disclosed to me nor shall you voluntarily reveal my identity to any recipient. For the purpose of determining whether I am acceptable as a donor of semen, I consent to a physical examination, including the taking of blood and other body fluids, by you or any assistants whom you may designate.

To the best of my knowledge:

(a) I am in good health; I have no communicable disease, and am free from any physical or mental impairment or disability, whether inherited or as a result of any disease or ailment, except as follows:

_____

(b) I never have been afflicted with any venereal disease, except as follows: _____

(c) None of my grandparents, parents, brothers, sisters, or children, if any, nor their lineal descendants, have ever been afflicted with emotional illness or any inherited mental or physical disabilities or disease, except as follows:

_____

Signed _____

The foregoing was read, discussed, and signed in my presence, and in my opinion the person signing did so freely, and with full knowledge and understanding.

Witness _____

Of course, there is no way of knowing for sure if the donor has answered the questions honestly, or if he indeed has the knowledge and understanding to give the correct answers.

Payment and Motivation of Donors

One of the benefits of being a sperm donor is the investigation of his health and fertility, a screening that varies from superficial to thorough—depending on the facility. Semen analysis is always done, and it is possible to screen for at least sixty genetic diseases.

Some donors give very personal reasons for donating, such as "my sister is infertile and I know what a tragedy it is" or "I'm an unusual person" or even that there is a "spiritual connection." Men may feel guilty about not having more children, especially if pressured by their wife, or may simply like to think of having more offspring without being directly responsible for them. Even in the most altruistic cases, where no money is involved or the money is unimportant, it is not unreasonable to think that there must be some personal gratification or ego reinforcement in donating.

> I wanted to get my lineage out . . . to have my genes carry on.

One donor, when asked by Rona Achilles if he would donate again, said, "Yup, every week. God, I could start my own country."

Achilles found that donor motivation could not be reduced to either financial gain or altruism, although both play a role. One physician she interviewed said that he now used only "single interns who seem to want to propagate the universe."

> I think the financial thing may have . . . like . . . sweetened the thing . . . but I wasn't looking for financial gain.

> It's great that people think of me highly enough to want me as part of their . . . uh, family history. . . . It's mind boggling to me.

However, the deeper motives, rights, and responsibilities of semen donors also need to be examined. It has long been a principle of Western sexual morality that persons should be responsible for the offspring of their body. Donor insemination has traditionally involved men receiving payment for their reproductive material and forfeiting any moral, legal, or social responsibility for what is done with it. For this reason, George Annas (1980) prefers the term "vendor," and indeed it is the payment (even one dollar) that makes the contract legal. In a recent California court case, a donor sued for visitation rights to the child of a lesbian couple. As he was never paid for his semen, the court found that he was not a "donor," but rather the "father."

There is never any obligation to become a donor, so why do men bother? Are they just in it, as has been suggested, "for the bucks"? Although some semen brokers state that the financial compensation is usually considered secondary when compared with the consequences of the semen use, for some "it is the concrete motivation to take the first step or to continue." Curie-Cohen found that about 88 percent of donors were paid between $20 and $30, although nearly 7 percent were paid more than $35, or up to $100 per specimen. Today the average reimbursement is $50 to $75. Some medical students can donate enough semen to achieve minimum annual earnings for taxation purposes, and others at least can bring in handsome pocket money.

Donors in Rowland's (1983) Australian study felt that they should be paid for the loss of time, for travel, and "to compensate for the embarrassment involved in donating" (this was a question on the form; such a reason may not have been volunteered). Fifty-seven percent, however, would still donate if no payment were involved. Twenty-four percent donated for the money alone. The majority wanted to help infertile couples, although only 7 percent had direct knowledge of such couples.

Most practitioners complain that "in spite of the remuneration, or *perhaps because of it,* [italics mine] we have experienced difficulties getting suitable donors."

Schoysman (1975), defending the payment of donors, uses the analogy that a physician who did not charge would be seen as a saint, but this doesn't mean that medical fees are unethical if they are proportionate to the service rendered. He argues that the donor, especially if providing fresh semen for a physician, has to be willing to be available at unforeseen times. The ovulation of a given woman may be postponed for a while, causing inconvenience to both doctor and donor. Schoysman also feels that if the donor is willing to refrain from intercourse for several days and occasionally sacrifices a weekend to bring a semen sample to the clinic or the gynecologist's consulting room, he should be rewarded.

The CECOS center in Lyon, France, asks infertile couples to recruit donors for the program (not for their own personal use). Donors must have at least one child and have their wife's consent. Twenty-eight of forty-five donors were obtained this way; others were procured through appeals via the media.

We have seen that by paying the donors, couples feel that they have simply purchased sperm, like a bottle of wine, and that any deeper questions or further obligations are thus canceled. Likewise, donors are simply vendors of an expendable body fluid. Nijs and his colleagues (1973) themselves stated that even though a socially open helping attitude toward couples with fertility problems is a positive attribute, "this helping attitude must not keep one from accepting financial compensation which is a means of *neutralizing* the DI" [italics mine]. It is incredible to think a few dollars can take care of the existential questions involved in the creation of life!

Huerre (1980) found that the donors maintained a "watertight" distinction between their actions and the birth that will follow from it, which they do not feel concerns them. They merely "sometimes fantasize about the chances of their children later meeting those conceived through their donation." In some instances, he reports, "donation serves to efface a personal tragedy or serve as balm for a wounded ego."

No Parallel Between Blood and Semen Donors

In the United States, donors of blood and semen have traditionally been remunerated. Abroad, semen donors are paid but blood donors usually receive neither payment nor reimbursement for travel costs. Reimbursing expenses can simply be a euphemism for payment, and is open to the same exploitation.

Not everything is sold in our society. For example, love is not, and under most social codes neither are human beings nor bodies. It is no wonder that some donors feel that any payment, especially under the table, is sinister and smacks of prostitution. To accept money, they feel, would be a slur on their character.

Practitioners of DI see it as a classic physician service (like supplying blood) "to achieve a pregnancy," rather than the "purchase of semen." An analogy is often drawn between semen donation and blood or organ donation, but the two must be seen as completely different. In the latter, an existing life is being sustained (although this may be interpreted as the gift of life in some cases), while in DI a new life is created. Furthermore, this new life is contrived outside of any procreative or even personal relationship between the biological parents.

The donor has no control over the use of his semen. The ultimate legal and ethical responsibility rests with the physician. Achilles observed that "medicalization of DI from the perspective of the donor reassures him that his sperm will be used responsibly, similar to the trust expressed by DI mothers that the physician would choose a suitable donor for them." Aldous Huxley, in his book *Island,* was one of the first to see the overlap between family planning and biological and social engineering.

In his documentary *The Gift Relationship,* Richard M. Titmuss reveals how payment for blood in the United States led to the suppression or falsification of medical history and thus contamination of the gift, through infection or genetic damage. In the United States blood may be sold to support habits of drug or alcohol abuse, whereas in countries such as Britain and Australia it is always donated for free.

Dunstan (1976) argues that "what is so freely given by nature ought not to be sold." One donor, interviewed by phone on the *Phil Donahue Show,* said that he had given between seventy-five and one hundred specimens for forty dollars each. Each specimen, especially if frozen, can yield many straws for inseminations. It has been estimated that a fertile donor, donating twice a week, could father twenty thousand children in a year.

Nijs found that although more than half of the donors compared semen and blood donation (but less than half were blood donors), all confirmed that "the distinction between these donations is so great that it had occupied them very seriously." In Rowland's study (1983) about half were regular blood donors.

They saw sperm donation as being connected to them as individuals, in contrast with blood donation, where they felt they were just one of a crowd.

Donors often perceive the husband's infertility as a failure of manhood. Despite the separation of sexual intercourse from DI, sexual connotations surround the procedure. One donor commented to Achilles that DI was a kind of "institutionalized cuckoldry," and another said, "It is like getting your wife fucked by proxy."

Masturbation

Achilles noted that sometimes there is a sexual motive for donating and that payment proves to be a legitimating cover for what the donors regarded primarily as sexual activity.

> As a student I was really short of money. It seemed like such a funny thing, almost a joke, a kick ... getting paid to jerk off. It was one of those things that I'd heard about that medical students get paid to jerk off.

> My girlfriend wanted to know how they got the sperm. Everybody wants to know that ... and when I told her, she couldn't believe it. She said, "My God." You know, she thought, like I did, that they stuck a needle somewhere and withdrew it ... but I told her that it was the old-fashioned way and she just couldn't believe it.

Robert

Robert and Nelsen were donors interviewed by Achilles. Robert had heard about sperm donation from his "buddy at work." He relates the sexual experience of sperm donation.

> I thought the first time I went down that the nurses would help (nervous laughter). I was disappointed, but I thought what the hell ... you still get the money. I was so embarrassed at first ... I didn't know, if I was doing the right thing or not. ... Well, the first time I couldn't do it ... because it was a male doctor there and I was sort of inhibited to do it knowing that he would be, well,

I couldn't do anything with him waiting. . . . They gave me another chance, well, I came back and I explained the problem and so instead of the doctor they had a nurse wait for me, which solved the problem. Well, I've been dying to ask them if (nervous laughter) the nurse would help me, but I don't want to jeopardize my position at the clinic either.

When asked if he wanted to keep donating, Robert replied, "It's the money and the power trip too." As to whether he would donate if he were not paid, he said:

That's an interesting question . . . probably, yeah . . . I would probably anyway. I make good money at my job. I probably would . . . but don't tell them that. At the first interview the physician asked me why I was interested in this . . . that took me back because I wasn't sure myself. I told him that I knew I was . . . that I wasn't going to get married for a while . . . and I thought if I could help people out who were having trouble . . . I wouldn't mind, but that was what I thought he wanted to hear. . . . Which it was . . . he thought that was ideal. . . . I think the real reason was . . . like my buddy . . . that of being paid for doing what I did (nervous laughter) . . . and to think that it's going into some strange woman (laughter) and I don't know . . . it was some sort of power trip . . . I don't know . . . thinking of myself like Tom Selleck or something.

Later he describes how the sexual nature of the donations wore off as he experienced the impersonal clinical nature of the procedure.

To go into a room and to see men's magazines lying on a sofa . . . it's sort of degrading sometimes. You feel like a little teenager sometimes going in there . . . like your mother sent you, like you've been a bad boy, and you have to go in your room now. . . . It feels real, you know, being alone, closing the door and being in there by yourself. And you know what you do which is sort of like an immature act really. I used to do it for the fun of it, but it has taken the fun out of it in my personal life, really. Like before the whole program I used to masturbate for my own enjoyment, but after going through the DI program it struck me that there was a purpose for that and to do it just for enjoyment . . . well, I feel guilty now.

Nelsen

I just walked into this room not knowing what to expect . . . and the room was filled with syringes on shelves and I thought, Oh my God . . . and the nurse she just handed me this brown paper bag. It was all really clinical and like you'd never talk about what exactly was happening. . . . "Come this way" to the door that said MEN on it. "We would like one sample please." It was just this tiny cubicle like bathrooms in hospitals. Because of the bizarreness of the situation, I just felt supreme alienation. My first reaction was, well, I thought I better get going on this and the funniest thing happened. I felt the same thing I felt, I guess when I was twelve or whenever I was first masturbating . . . was I doing this right? It was totally incongruous. It was the same feeling as eighteen years earlier . . . I felt thrown into this bizarre world. This whole thing had been a sexual thing until then when it was suddenly a medical procedure. . . . So, it was very strange. After that, that was the routine. I'd never see anyone, like "Mission Impossible." . . . "Go to Room Thirty-three." It was a small office or procedures room and they would assume that I knew what to do and I did. No one would be there. No one would talk to me, it was all very uptight. I would just leave this sample and leave. It wasn't like this nice place to masturbate, it wasn't sexual at all. That was one thing, it was like a job. The other thing was that the sense of doing it for someone wasn't really there . . . it was really removed, particularly because I was getting paid. A grand income of one hundred dollars made me feel creepy, it became incredibly alienating . . . a lot of it was getting paid for it. . . . If you give blood you know you're doing it for someone, but this was so different. Part of it was the money, but I would never do it for a friend . . . the anonymity is very important.

Donors in the study by Nijs considered the masturbation an indispensable step to help others, regretting that the sacred state of parenthood had to begin with conception in a cold, clinical climate.

Finegold (1975) writes that donors "rarely ask leading questions or display any interest in the procedure after they hand over the receptacle. Schoysman (1975), anxious to negate the view of donors reading lascivious periodicals to get into the right mood, assures us that the semen samples are always obtained in a "discreet

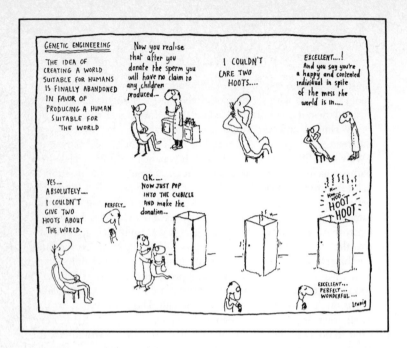

and matter-of-fact way"—whatever that means. Nijs (1973) found that giving sperm was seen as a neutral physical act, that once done is "over forever."

Guttmacher (1962), one of the pioneer gynecologists in DI, advised:

> Never select donors who volunteer. Perhaps such men wish medical benediction for masturbation which otherwise arouses in them feelings of guilt.

Huerre (1973) wrote:

> The fantasies attached, when not forcefully repressed ("I think only of the donation") are directed away from the woman and an ill-advised eroticism; they are nothing if not noble. It is as if masturbation, a forbidden pleasure, is made possible or even categorized by the semen it engenders and the consent of the woman is normally excluded.

Some donors have reported painful feelings after ejaculation, and one commented:

And sometimes you get an empty feeling afterwards, the first few times. I thought is this all there is to it? You know, I thought it was *supposed to change my life,* but it is no big thing. [The italics are mine. What an interesting reaction from the "disinterested donor"!]

I think the last word on the subject belongs to Blizzard:

Masturbation is a disquieting activity, which [the Feversham Report] claim(s) most people would find more objectionable than, for instance, giving a pint of blood. Well, I freely confess that I have done both without making a habit of either, and in my view there is no comparison.

Number of Pregnancies

DI offspring, like adoptees, have a fear of inbreeding and even unwitting incest. The American Fertility Society suggests that a donor be limited to fifteen offspring and the Warnock Commission in England recommended ten. Sperm banks are in a position to distribute the semen in different areas. Because physicians using fresh semen have limited resources, they often use one or two donors for their entire practice. Articles in the DI literature, for example, have stated that five donors were responsible for ninety pregnancies, one donor "siring" as many as thirty-five. Christiane Northrup, an obstetrician in Maine, told me how she always felt alarmed about the potential inbreeding from her male colleagues at a small-town medical school. Some of these students had donated sperm regularly for up to eight years.

Although many donors exaggerate their estimated number of successes, there is a common fear of "innocent incest" if two offspring from the same donor happened to have a sexual relationship. Actually, the statistical probability is slight; it has been calculated by Curie-Cohen (1980) that a donor would have to be responsible for more than 292 pregnancies. On the other hand, incest may be more of a potential problem in areas with a small population, or within a minority group, where one donor is used a great deal. After two half-siblings nearly married in rural Maine, it was discovered that the donor had been responsible for 807 pregnancies! I know of a "Mothers of Twins" club in a small community where the same donor provided the sperm for three sets of twins. There was also a case in Tel Aviv recounted by Hoffer (1975) where two offspring from the same biological father did marry, but the truth was disclosed to them in the nick of time. *Time* magazine also reported a situation in New York where two DI half-siblings were unwittingly planning to marry.

Lori Andrews, in a 1984 *Psychology Today* article, describes a donor she interviewed. Peter Forbes, a Sherman Oaks, California, gynecologist, provided sperm for thirty-three pregnancies when he was a medical resident at Georgetown University in Washington, D.C., thirty years ago. Mindful of a possible paternity suit one day, Forbes has made a will that any child not borne by his wife will be entitled to only $1 from his estate. He also has advised his children not to marry anyone from D.C.

Knowledge of Outcome

Not only the donors, but also the practitioners rarely have any knowledge of the outcome—a woeful situation for any kind of research. Curie-Cohen found that only 51 percent of DI physicians deliver their patients after conception. Thirty percent never learn whether the pregnancies are carried to term, and almost 5 percent never even learned whether a pregnancy ever resulted from the DI.

Although the mixing of semen is less frequently done today, there are ways of combining the donors to maintain their obscurity. Thirty-two percent of physicians changed donors for every insemination done in one cycle, and the 44 percent who used the same donors in each cycle, varied the donor from cycle to cycle. Only 13 percent used the same donor until pregnancy, and only 2 percent used the same donor for subsequent pregnancies of the same woman (yet the possibility of doing this is one of the main reasons DI is chosen)!

Donors are traditionally not told of "takes" (pregnancies) in case they conceptualize a living child. But in some instances they manage to obtain this information or even to surreptitiously examine the patient's charts. Most of them at least want to know if the inseminations were successful, even if not all of them want more information about their biological children. Often this may simply be a desire to know about their own fertility. However, the donors assume that pregnancies are occurring, especially if they are being accepted for months or even years. It is very disturbing that many DI practitioners would not inform the donor of a defective child, for fear that the trauma and knowledge of that fact would outweigh the benefit of being aware that his future children were at increased risk.

Tekavcic (1973), in Yugoslavia, received answers from two thirds of the donors he contacted. One fifth said that they had thought about the child, and nearly the same number would consider meeting the child. Ten percent regretted that they were ever donors, and two stated that the child's existence, which they found out about, had been a psychological stress for them. The majority wanted to know the pregnancy outcome, to "have been able to share happiness," although some wondered if this were not a secret wish to propagate themselves. Others preferred to think of their sperm being given without specification as to whether it was research or DI. As one donor said:

> Sperm donation is giving some part of my physical being, without any further involvement of myself (or of the couple) as a person.

Schoysman (1975) writes:

> If in the future something happens to his own children it is very likely that later in life he will be troubled by the fact that somewhere there is another child of his alive. He contributes by giving a semen sample and there is no reason whatsoever that he should know the result.

In contrast, donors confided to Achilles:

> Sometimes now when I go by a mother and child I think, Could this be one of them? and sometimes it kills me because I could be.... You know, I am technically his or her father but I am not allowed to be part of their life. At first I didn't think it would bother me ... but I think about it more frequently now.

> You more or less just do it and forget about it and then three years later you start to think back about it.

I'd like to be a father. I wish I could be a social father as opposed to a biological one, but you take what you can get.

I think it is natural to want to know what they look like, what they chose to do with their lives.

One resident delivered a baby with an identical birthmark to his own, in the exact same location. He concluded that he must have been the donor. Another physician, doing his obstetric residency, exclaimed, "I wonder if I am the father of any of these DI babies?"

General Profile of Semen Donors

Nijs and colleagues studied twenty-seven donors (twenty-three of whom were unmarried) in Belgium. They found an interval of about six months between the first impulse to become a donor and the first step. In their group, the motivation to become a donor arose from direct encounters with fertility problems among family members or friends, often with the wife's prompting. The donors typically came from large families and planned to have several children. All were from a professional background dealing with health care or education. They felt that giving sperm for concep- tion was a minimal contribution, merely physiological, compared to the experiences of parenthood, such as pregnancy, birth, and child-rearing. Yet, most felt that being a donor was easier than be- ing a recipient, which would take more time and consideration.

Robyn Rowland, a social psychologist, studied sixty-seven do- nors at a hospital in Melbourne, Australia. In her 1983 study, only one donor was a medical student; their occupations ranged from gardener to computer analyst. The donors were often selected by lab technicians. This will be a surprise to recipients who imagine that their doctor is making a personal endeavor to find a replica of their husband. The donors were from nineteen to forty-nine years old; the median age was thirty-one years. They were mostly middle-class, about one third were married, and one third held a university degree. Twenty-one percent of the donors who were fa- thers did not live with their children.

Donors tend to imagine that the couple will be similar to them- selves. (Likewise, couples hope that the donor will be similar to them, or even "upgraded.") Forty-four percent used negative adjectives to describe the infertile couple like "desperate, lonely, and pathetic." Thirty-three percent used positive terms such as "loving, strong, and courageous."

The interviews and the questionnaires raised issues for the donors that they had not considered. More donors requested interviews than Rowland could see, indicating their need for personal discussion.

Huerre interviewed forty-five French donors, whose average age was thirty-two, with an average of two children. Their occupations ranged from a factory worker to engineer, but were generally ranked socially and professionally above average. In contrast to other studies, the initiative was taken mainly by the husband or the couple. When the wife encouraged the donation it was the result of direct requests from women friends whose husbands were infertile.

Donors' Feelings About Secrecy and Anonymity

The donors interviewed by Nijs felt strongly about discretion and anonymity. They believed this was necessary to keep their involvement on a technical, neutral level and preferred to avoid any personal contact with recipients. In contrast, Rowland's research challenges the stereotype of donors as a secret and reluctant group who demand anonymity and destruction of records. The surprising information was that 42 percent would still donate if their names were available to recipient parents. Yet in response to the question about couples automatically receiving their names, only 15 percent said they should. Donors apparently draw a distinct line between keeping their names available for offspring and parents if they require it, and automatically handing their names out to all couples. Some were concerned about mutual consent and legal problems.

Thirty-one percent of donors living with a partner had not told her and did not intend to tell her. Some who had shared the information were initially encouraged to donate by their wives. However, 77 percent had told others of their donation.

Half the donors felt that only nonidentifying information could be kept, and the other half felt that records should not be destroyed. During interviews, it was not unusual for donors to reconsider this issue and be concerned that they might change their minds later and would allow access by the child to their records.

Ambivalence toward DI was revealed when only 67 percent of the donors said they would approve of their own wives using DI. However only 19 percent would choose DI for themselves if faced with that option, and only 14 percent would choose adoption. More than half the donors felt that they would like to know about the donor if they themselves had been conceived through DI. Twenty-two percent would like to choose potential parents from descriptions of infertile couples applying for DI.

Eighty-one percent wanted to know if conceptions resulted from their sperm; some were just curious, others felt it would give a sense of achievement and purpose to their donations. Half the group believed that they might feel some connection with the child.

Sixty percent of donors would not mind if their DI offspring contacted them after the age of eighteen years to ask them information about family history and other details. Of course, there were 40 percent who did not want to, but we have to remember that the program was based on anonymity; that was the agreement on which the donation was undertaken prior to Rowland's investigation. *The point is that it is possible to obtain donors without anonymity.*

The majority of donors did not want to meet the couples in contrast with a greater willingness to meet the offspring. Similarly, parents often do not want to meet the donors, but would not stop a child who wishes to search.

A 1976 California study quoted by Lifton (1981) found that 82 percent of birthparents would like to meet their child today. They felt that it was helpful for the child/adult to satisfy her need for knowledge about her heritage. Furthermore, with the passage of time, they were more able to handle the prospect of such a meeting.

According to Huerre, only fourteen of the forty-five French donors were going to reveal the DI to their family and friends but forty of the donors were prepared to tell their children.

Attitudes of Donors' Wives

Consent by a donor's wife is not required legally since the United States Supreme Court decision has ruled that one spouse cannot veto the reproductive decisions made by the other spouse. On a practical level, this means that it is a man's constitutional prerogative to become a sperm donor just as it is a woman's private business if she chooses to have an abortion. Nevertheless, consent forms for the sperm donor's wife are presumed necessary by the American Medical Association, as well as medical associations in Britain, Australia, and other countries. Because "marital interests" are involved, DI practitioners wish to have her signature to the statement: "I know my husband may become the father of a children of which I am not the mother."

One woman wrote that when she had to be artificially inseminated with her husband's semen in order to conceive, he was found to have an extraordinarily high sperm count. Her husband was then asked to be a sperm donor, to which he agreed without any payment; money was neither mentioned nor considered.

> It was simply an altruistic endeavour to be accomplished, but not before I was extensively interviewed as to the possible consequences. It turned out that I had no objections but felt, as did my husband, that if his contribution could make others happy, could indeed make another *family,* this was just fine. I asked my husband what he would do or say if someone rang the doorbell and announced she was his daughter. (He is still pondering. . . .) However, I would welcome her and let her see everything in his life that related to her, let her see her father's pictures and that of her grandparents and letters and so on.

A physician's wife told me she occasionally wondered about his offspring as he had told her he donated sperm as a medical student. She said she would welcome any such children "with open arms" if they wanted to meet her husband. Perhaps it is because women carry children for nine months in their bodies that they feel the meaning and bonds of identity at a deep, inextinguishable level.

Achilles suggests that the high percentage of donors who conceal their role as a sperm donor from family members—individuals who are linked to them biologically—may be interpreted at least partially as an indicator of the strength of biological ties. Anonymous sperm donors agree to donate under certain conditions that make it impossible to trace lineage. If biological ties are important to family members, knowledge of potential biological offspring may cause unresolvable curiosity or concern.

Personal Profiles of Semen Donors

> The cultural image of the donor sits somewhere between the altruism of a blood donor and the irresponsibility of a sailor with a "woman in every port."
>
> *—Rona Achilles*

I decided to become a donor while scuba diving. I guess you could call it an ego trip—I saw how vulnerable life really is.

Donor #28 from the Repository of Germinal Choice was interviewed by *Los Angeles* in December 1982.

I got a letter from [recruiter Paul Smith], a nosy note. One of those "Congratulations, you have been selected" things followed by a questionnaire. I thought it was rather tacky and obtrusive, and I threw it away. Then one day I was sitting in my office, and this strange-looking person knocked at my door and said he wanted to talk. He chuckled a lot and I thought he was a crackpot. Later, however, I reckoned if I was this great genius, the least I could do was let others participate in it.

How does the idea of who-knows-how-many little look-alikes running around in the decades to come appeal to him?

I guess in about twenty years I might start wondering, and if a kid in my class bore a slight resemblance to me I'd be interested in finding out his family background. I may feel uncomfortable knowing I have kids out there I may never see, and I may kick myself later. But not now. In terms of improving the world's gene pool, this is like trying to drain oceans with an eye dropper. I have no grand goals to change the universe. If I can do a favor for a few women . . .

A British dentist whose family compiled a detailed genealogical tree wanted to be a donor because his wife, a busy professional, did not want to have children.

Martin Curie-Cohen, after publishing his national DI survey, received a letter from a scientist who felt his superior intelligence and clean bill of health made him an ideal sperm donor. As part of the research for this book, I telephoned this man to explore his motivations. I explained that I was undergoing DI and after a very uncommunicative conversation, it occurred to me that he may have feared I was looking for *him* to be my donor!

Neil

Neil said he became a donor for a "good cause." Aged thirty-one, he works in a hospital and knows people with infertility. He thinks infertility is especially stigmatizing for men. He donated before marriage in case it would cause trouble with a wife; he thinks that to become a known donor would require a very careful discussion with the wife. Neil feels that a husband who agrees to DI must love the wife very much.

> I am thrilled by the idea of putting a child into someone else's life. I come from a broken home so I am one for the truth. If there is any chance of the child finding out, it is better off being straight from the beginning.

Eric

Eric, aged twenty-six, saw a notice on the job board at college and was accepted by a local obstetrician after a physical examination and semen analysis. Eric says his friends, of both sexes, knew very little about DI. They thought he was joking when he told them about being a donor and made comments like, "Did the nurse help you?" and "I thought you used a hose!" Generally, his friends assumed that semen donation was very much out of the donor's control. Some of his friends asked him how to get started, if more donors were needed and so on, but he felt they should find out about it on their own initiative.

Eric usually donates two to three times a month, but one month he gave seven donations. When we spoke he had been doing this for three years, totaling over 120 donations. Commenting on the money, he said, "You might as well get paid for it, you're going to do it (masturbation) anyway." He considered the thirty dollars per specimen "perfect for the amount of work." He also stated that he "strongly wanted to help people who had made a conscious decision to obtain a child by DI." Personally, Eric felt that being a sperm donor and being responsible for "that many babies" added mystique to him, especially with regard to his female friends. He was somewhat curious about the pregnancy outcome, and like many donors, grossly overestimated the actual number of pregnancies that had resulted from his semen (the true number I had learned from the gynecologist). Eric had considered the possibility of consanguinity among the sperm recipients and dismissed it. However, I interviewed several couples in the same community who had all received their children courtesy of Eric's sperm!

Eric said he would be happy to be a known donor and meet the recipients, as long as they wanted it too, and there were no obligations involved. "I'm a people person—a humanitarian. I am not threatened by this, I see fathering as a social, loving, and caring act. It is up to the parents to tell the child."

When asked what he would do if he were an infertile husband, Eric said he would want to pick the donor himself and use a close friend. "I would be much more comfortable knowing the identity." He continued, "If I were a DI child I would want to know my heritage and share the life history of the paternal line." Eric was well known and liked at the gynecologist's office, and if couples in a few years asked the secretary or nurses about the donors, they would surely remember him.

Henry

Henry, an English donor, was interviewed by Hanscombe and Forster for their book *Rocking the Cradle.* Aged thirty-six, he worked with antiques and lived in an apartment in a large city. He volunteered to be a donor after hearing about lesbian women who wanted children.

> I felt very sympathetic toward lesbian mothers. I felt that I could help them in this way to have children, which otherwise would

have been impossible for them. I'm not too worried that I don't know the mother. It's the case that I think of more than the outcome. You see, all the unmarried mothers who go there, I take to be lesbian. I just assume they are, so I think it really doesn't matter who the mother is. I'm doing it because otherwise I'd just be masturbating. This way I feel I'm helping people who want to be inseminated. I'd reached a stage in my life where I thought I might never get married. I might never sire children. This seemed a good opportunity.

When asked about his reactions to the possibility of fathering some children, he replied:

> I'm not quite sure whether I have. I haven't heard, at the moment, but if I knew that I had, it would fill me with a certain satisfaction—that life hadn't been a complete waste, that I had used it for a purpose. I'm rather glad that I'm not getting involved. . . . I would feel that it was her child, rather than my child. I'm just providing a service. . . . There's not a lot of money involved. The doctor said, "I'm not buying your semen. The money is to cover your expenses."

The Many Problems of Anonymity

The worst aspect of anonymity is the denial of the child's paternal heritage. As Rayner said:

> It is through the anonymity of the donor that the child is robbed of the right and ability to accept himself as the child of these particular parents, and thus fulfill the obligation of his existence.

Everyone involved in the DI triangle is affected by the anonymity: the donor who never knows his offspring, the doctor who perjures the birth certificate, the geneticist who has no data on DI to research, the psychologist who counsels the genealogical bewilderment, the psychiatrist who treats the mother's fantasies of the unknown donor, the future spouse of the DI child who may commit incest, and ultimately society in general, which helps to shroud this sorry state of affairs.

Achilles also observed how the "anonymity of the donor and the medicalization of the procedure facilitated denial of the donor." A single mother told her, "It is amazing to see people's reactions when I say he has no father."

Barbara Kritchevsky, an attorney, argued in the *Harvard Women's Law Journal* that single women have a constitutional right to DI and similarly denies the reality of the donor:

> The legal questions raised by DI out of marriage with an anonymous donor are different, since *no man is involved in conception* or child rearing. [Italics mine]

Heterosexual single women and lesbians understandably have problems with patriarchal rules and regulations, but often they deny the underlying social norm of blood ties that are unquestionably linked to those laws. This cultural norm of blood ties presents additional problems for lesbian mothers who are already challenging familiar norms in their choice of female partners.

A further hazard of making the donor anonymous and abstract is that women will more easily submit to mixed inseminations, multiple donors per cycle, and different donors each cycle. This abstracting process gives the practitioners convenient flexibility with the sperm they use. If it is "just" sperm—then all sperm is the same! One DI father commented, "If it can't be my sperm, then anyone else's will do." The more the donor is depersonalized, the more similar it is to just a medical treatment, although one of the ways the DI father typically depersonalizes the donor is to think of him as someone just like himself! If a woman or couple really permitted themselves to be concerned about the donor, then such practices would be completely intolerable. From the outset, I was repulsed by the idea, and now having conceived a child with a known donor, such attitudes seem to me even more incomprehensible. I was amazed when I interviewed a couple with two DI children, and they had not bothered to find out if the same donor was used for both pregnancies!

The Rights of Donors

Should semen be controlled by middle men, such as physicians or sperm banks? Should the medical profession step aside and allow consumers to select from a catalog? Should sperm be advertised? What are the rules of access, if any? How can no discrimination on the basis of age, marital status, ethnic group, or sexual preference be monitored? Can the state regulate mail-order semen from commercial sperm banks?

How does a man feel about his sperm being frozen? Does he have the right to know if it is banked? It is more convenient, and its preservation may be an advantage or a disadvantage. Fresh sperm are not subject to the biochemical treatment and trauma of freezing, but more important to conception are the attitude and feeling of the donor at the time of ejaculation. Perhaps this explains why studies show some donors' semen never results in conception even though the sperm quality is as good as those donors who are successful. I believe a constellation of factors must come together for conception to occur. If our donor had a headache, or was tired after a busy day, then I didn't pursue the insemination that cycle. I preferred to wait another month until the gift came as a blessing rather than as an obligation.

What rights does a donor have with regard to the transfer of his genes? Does he have the right to prevent the use of his sperm for inseminating single or lesbian women? Seventy percent of Australian donors in Rowland's study did not object to their sperm being received by lesbians. Even larger majorities did not object to single, divorced, or widowed women using their sperm for DI.

Could the donor sue for emotional pain and mental suffering caused by the knowledge of the use of his sperm? Some donors are told that the semen will be used for research, when in fact it is sold for "therapeutic purposes" (DI). Does a donor have the right to insist that records be kept, to be informed of successful conceptions? The third National Conference on Adoption in Australia affirmed the right of the natural father to be informed of his paternity and to participate in providing information to the child. Should donors not be informed of any genetic defects in the child?

What special protections should donors have for their service? If a DI couple later separates and neither wants the child, or the wife dies and the husband no longer wants it, or both partners die, should the donor have the right to visitation or even custody? What should happen to stored semen in the event of death or divorce?

Often a birthmother has improved her circumstances in later life, and discovered to her anguish that her child was worse off— psychologically, socially, and economically—in his or her adoptive home.

By donating sperm anonymously (or with a contract between friends to the same effect), a donor shows his intention to waive his parental rights. What if the mother were single and the donor had signed away his parental rights but later invoked them, or if the mother were married, and the donor were known and had not signed away his rights? Although anonymity is traditionally guaranteed to donors, one third of DI physicians do keep records on donors. There have never been any suits against the donor, but the possibility exists, of course.

> The man who gives his seminal material into the keeping and control of an institution is hardly exercising maximum self-determination. Rather, he is courting authoritarian interference in his affairs. Even if he made use of a completely commercial activity, it would be subject to state monitoring and control. His privacy would only be respected as far as computers can be trusted to respect it.
>
> *—Germaine Greer*

A New Kind of Donor

The medical profession assumes that without anonymity and payment, donors would not be forthcoming. Anonymity works against donors too—they are usually not told if children are conceived or if there are any health problems with their offspring.

However, I believe that if donors gave truly *informed* consent, they would not agree to participate *without* an informed choice and unless records were kept.

We need semen donors who have a highly developed sense of ethics. If they are not willing to supply an accurate medical history and heritage to offspring who come of age, or before, then they are not responsible enough to be donors. However, semen is controlled by physicians and sperm bank directors who have the opposite view (except for the Center for Reproductive Alternatives in California, which started an open donor program in 1987).

Ian Johnston (1980), a senior gynecologist at the Royal Women's Hospital in Melbourne, Australia, writes that "an occasional (donor) will not be considered if he seems unusually interested in the progeny that results from his semen." (Likewise, couples who have "too many questions" about the donor are usually not accepted for DI.) In my opinion, this healthy concern would be an essential indication for selection, certainly not a contra-indication! Johnston believes that if donor and recipient meet there would be a risk that the donor might become psychologically attached, because the child comes from his biological material, and he might try to remove the child. Or the wife might become attracted to the donor, which would create stresses within the marriage. Likely or unlikely as this may be, it is still no excuse to deprive the child of her identity.

Donors should have the option of an extensive interview with an expert, do preparatory reading, and go through the decision-making process at their own pace. Counseling for sperm donors would be a step in the right direction, so that they can understand their motivations for donation and think through the consequences later in their own lives of possibly fathering children as sperm donors.

We could assume that donors who have their consciousness raised about the issues and long-term effects of genealogical bewilderment, will think very carefully about donating sperm. Legal liabilities and fears of maintenance and inheritance claims are slowly being resolved by state legislatures, and will encourage donations from men prepared to disclose their identity. We will explore such donors in the next chapter.

8

Known Donors in Collaborative Reproduction

AS WE HAVE SEEN, donor insemination has traditionally been viewed as a medical treatment. However, if you take responsibility for finding your own donor, you can avoid the waiting lists, costs, scrutiny, and judgment of the medical profession, as well as fulfilling the essential need for your child to know her paternal origins.

In this chapter we will look at various forms of reproductive donors—those who donate eggs, or sperm, or an egg along with the use of their uterus (surrogate mothers), or babies (adoption) within an *open* relationship with the recipient.

The relationship may be simply *identified* or, as with some adoptions, progressively *cooperative*, with mutual ties maintained, which mean emotional risks—and rewards.

> Cooperative relationships acknowledge that everyone has equal credibility and should therefore have equal negotiating and relating abilities.
>
> —*Mary Jo Rillera and Sharon Kaplan,*
> *Cooperative Adoption*

Donor insemination introduces a third party into the conception, and a known donor, unlike an anonymous donor, cannot be depersonalized. There are risks involved in any journey into the unknown, and all parties must be open to the possibility of the emotional ambivalence or complications that can occur in any significant relationship. By its nature, human interaction is complex, and creating children is one of life's most powerful experiences. As adults, it is to be hoped that the parties involved in DI can sort out any problems together. Many psychological problems have also arisen with anonymous donors (see Chapter 5), but at least with a known donor the child is not deprived of half of her identity as well. Donors, like birthparents, must also recognize that they have a responsibility to ensure that their offspring will be able to know their identity.

Surrogate Mothers

While there is a stark contrast between donating sperm and conceiving and carrying a baby, both situations have in common a relinquishing of biological material for the creation of a child. In fact, it is interesting to learn how the surrogates cope with their experience, which is much more profound and potentially problematic than donating sperm.

Parker (1983, 1984), the Detroit psychiatrist, has studied several hundred surrogate mothers. He found that all of the surrogates preferred to have some kind of contact with the parental couple during pregnancy and postpartum. However, it was not clear to Parker which arrangements with the couple will lead to any better psychological outcome. Contrary to some people's belief, there is also no evidence to indicate that total and complete anonymity between the surrogate and the couple will lead to a better psychological outcome for the surrogate. Rather, the surrogates seem to need and benefit from making their own arrangements with the parental couple. I am aware of a few cases where a woman became a surrogate for her sister, which is quite different from breeding a baby for a fee. The money is definitely the prime motivating factor, as was found in Michigan when the courts disallowed a fee as "baby-selling," and applicants virtually disappeared. Corea examines these and other issues of surrogate mothering at length in *The Mother Machine*.

One surrogate mother during the course of the pregnancy changed her mind and refused the ten-thousand-dollar fee because she had established a relationship with the parental couple. As the pregnancy developed, the fee became less important as a motivation for relinquishment after birth.

Pregnant surrogates deal with the anticipated loss of the baby in several ways. Most have a need for some contact with the parents, by meeting, phone, letter, and also a need to idealize the parents. One stated that she and the infertile wife were sharing in the mothering process: she was the biological mother while the infertile wife would be the psychological mother. Sometimes the surrogates would become close to the recipient family, staying at each other's houses, going to prenatal visits together, and one infertile wife accompanied the surrogate to the hospital for labor support. A mother who nursed the baby, the only one in Parker's study, did it for a divorced man with no consistent maternal figure in the background. Some surrogates stated that they felt most of their sadness in connection with the loss of the relationship with the couple rather than the loss of the baby.

Most surrogates wondered how the baby would fare in the future. Many wanted periodic information from the couple or someone else. Some planned on maintaining a relationship and were refused by the couple. As a result, they often felt angry and unhappy about the enforced exile from the parental couple and their new child. Most surrogates acknowledged increased thoughts of the baby on the child's birthday.

According to Parker, surrogate mothering may help some women deal with prior unresolved losses of a fetus or a child. One woman dealt with her own biological mother's relinquishment of her for adoption, as well as her own giving-up of a newborn at age fourteen, by becoming a surrogate. As a result of the phone contact with the adoptive couple, she felt more confident about what might be the personality and sense of caring of the unknown couple who had accepted the newborn she relinquished as a teenager.

Parker (1983) has drawn up some guidelines to optimize the psychological outcomes of the process. In contrast with traditional medical and legal viewpoints, he cautions against anonymity.

> The surrogate mother and parental couple should be allowed to mutually arrange the extent and nature of any contact between them. This would permit the development of empathy of the extent desired and needed. Of course, the participants should also be made

aware of the possible problems arising from the desired contacts so that their decision is an informed one.

The pregnant and postpartum surrogate mother should have the opportunity to participate in a support group experience. An important aspect of this experience is to have at least one facilitator-therapist be female.

Egg Donors

Women having IVF undergo ovarian stimulation so that several eggs can be removed at one time and reimplanted after fertilization for an increased chance of pregnancy. Often these women are asked by the medical staff if they will donate—anonymously—extra eggs to other infertile women. Some do, and occasionally a recipient will conceive with a donor's egg before the donor does. Others refuse to donate but have deep guilt feelings as they also feel very indebted to the program. Perhaps if the secrecy were abolished, more of these women would donate eggs.

Interestingly, it is not uncommon for a woman beginning an IVF program to say that she has a friend willing to donate ova (and no one has assumed latent homosexuality, unlike the Lyon group when sterile men brought in male friends to donate, see Chapter 7)! However, no eggs from a known donor have been accepted, as far as I know, and because hospitalization is required, this process cannot be done surreptitiously like DI.

Prior to 1985, eggs could only be stored if they had been fertilized. After a breakthrough in Australia, eggs alone can now be frozen, although further refinement is needed to prevent chromosomal abnormalities before ova freezing becomes a standard clinical service. Since the ethical objections to embryo freezing are thus removed, and women with certain gynecological problems could have their ova banked for later use, it can be expected that there will be major developments in egg storage and donation in the future.

Open Adoption

The concept of open adoption was pioneered in California by Sorosky, Baran and Pannor, authors of *The Adoption Triangle*. They define it as

> an adoption in which the birth parent meets the adoptive parents, relinquishes all legal, moral, and nurturing rights to the child, but retains the right to continuing contact and knowledge of the child's whereabouts and welfare.

This new kind of arrangement is different from opening sealed records as contact is never broken off between the two families involved. The procedure ensures that the new parents and the child will know as much as possible about his biological heritage and the reasons for the adoption. It prepares adoptive parents to deal with the reality that their child has been borne by someone else. The unending grieving of birthmothers in closed adoptions is avoided and the adoptive parents don't have to live in dread that the child's natural mother may return to claim him. The birthmother chooses her child's new family and stays in touch with them and her child directly, or through a third party. This is the opposite of closed adoptions where the agency selects the parents. The adoptive couple, instead of waiting for the agency to find them a baby, searches for their own baby to adopt privately.

With a "shortage" of white adoptable infants, birthparents are in a bargaining position, and as more and more of them become aware of this, they are dictating the terms of the adoption.

Open adoptions are as legal and final as closed adoptions. However, in open adoptions the consent papers are signed within several months after the child is placed in the adoptive home, unlike adoption through an agency where parental relinquishment to the agency is finalized before placement. In an independent adoption, there is usually a time period (six months in California, for example) during which the mother can revoke her consent. This involves going to court and a custody battle with the adoptive parents; only 2 to 3 percent of birthparents engage in this time-consuming and expensive process.

Agencies are also placing children in adoptive homes prior to securing relinquishments from both birthparents. These programs are termed "Fost-adopt." Prospective adoptive parents take out foster-care licenses and take custody of the child from the hospital. When the relinquishment is secured, the adoptive parents proceed with the adoption.

In Hawaii, infertile couples have traditionally been able to adopt openly from friends or relatives who would relinquish one of their younger children. Belonging to a family clan is much more important to Hawaiians than illegitimacy. *The Adoption Triangle* goes on to cite an explanation that

> children could not be adopted without the full consent of both true parents, less some misfortune befall the child, and when consent had been given the child was handed to the adopting parents by the true parents with the saying, "We give the child to you, excrement, intestines and all." This was as binding as any law made in our modern courts. The child became the child of the adopting or "feeding parents" and only under rare circumstance did the biological parents attempt to take the child back unless the adopting parents died. . . . Unlike the modern way of concealing the true parentage of an adopted child, he was told who his biological parents were and all about them, so there was no shock and weeping at finding out that he was adopted and not an "own" child. If possible, the child was taken to his true parents to become well-acquainted with them and with his brothers and sisters if there were any and he was always welcome there.

Now that adoptions in Hawaii are influenced by the American system of secrecy and sealed records, Hawaiians are feeling conflict. Pukui, Haertig, and Lee, in their book *Look to the Source*, describe how

> Hawaiian grandparents and other relatives feel strongly that even the child of unwed parents should know his family background, and object to legal adoption because it blots out the past. The Hawaiian couple who want to adopt a child feel much the same. They are not at all concerned if the child is illegitimate, what they are worried about is taking a child whose parentage is concealed.

Norman Chance describes open adoption as practiced by the Eskimos in North Alaska:

The child's origin never is concealed and in many instances he is considered as belonging to both families. He may call the two sets of parents by the same names and maintain strong bonds with his real parents and siblings. In undertaking genealogical studies, anthropologists often have become confused about the biological parents of an adopted child since both sets claim him. It is evident that whatever the reasons for adoption, the parents usually treat a foster (adoptive) child with as much warmth and affection as they do their own.

Carole Anderson suggests that closed adoptions promote abortions.

Rather than face such unending torment (of not knowing what happens to the child she relinquishes), many a young woman will instead elect to have an abortion. She is likely to reason abortion would mean *not becoming* a mother, rather than becoming a *childless* mother through closed adoption. The adoption literature has revealed that over 90 percent of birthmothers did not want, or expect, privacy and confidentiality.

Carol Sorich and Roberta Siebert, writing in *Child Welfare,* note that many an adoption agency unconsciously communicates its difficulties in coming to terms with open adoption. But as the agency became more comfortable with the alternatives, more adoptive couples expressed a willingness to participate in them. Independent adoption is legal in all but five states (Connecticut, Delaware, Massachusetts, Michigan, Minnesota) and the District of Columbia. More than half of the adoptions in California are done independently, and the rate is much higher in the case of infants. Ninety percent of the two hundred and fifty birth mothers relinquishing babies in San Diego County each year have taken part in the selection of the adoptive couple, and about 10 percent meet with them.

Jean Etter, an open adoption counselor at Open Adoption Resources in Eugene, Oregon, recalls that the biggest task of her own experience was balancing "desires and rights while battling feelings of jealousy and possessiveness." During the birthmother's first visit, Etter resented her acting as the mother of her child Angela (which indeed she was).

Finally I was able to see there was room in this role for two people. I realized there's enough of Angela to go around.

Etter concludes after several years of experience with counseling participants in open adoption that

the kids who have contact with their birthfamilies are healthier. Children who know they're loved by their first family as well as by their second family are happier. It does not confuse them. It just makes them feel more secure.

It seems only natural that we would welcome our adopted child's birth parents into our home and family. He exists because they gave him life and nurtured him until his birth. We think of them as relatives.

What more could anyone share with us? Adoption is probably the greatest form of sharing there is. We think that the baby will have a better understanding of our feelings about adoption if he knows eventually that we were open about "sharing" him ... the most important thing after all is his happiness.

Elizabeth Hormann is an adoptive mother in Belmont, Massachusetts, who traced and maintains contact with her adopted son's birth family. In a 1982 article, "Sharing the Joy," she describes the experience.

I wondered who really benefits from the total secrecy and separation that is taken for granted in adoption. Couldn't the child and his family have a secure home and the birthmother a new start without cutting the child off from an important part of his or her heritage? My conviction grew that I would be cheating Charlie by acting as though he had no life and no background before he came to us.

In the years since Hormann first contacted the birth mother, the families, including the grandparents, get together at birthdays and holidays. She concludes

I'm sometimes asked if this arrangement complicates our lives. It does. Having children or brothers and sisters or second cousins complicates lives, too. It goes with having a family, but joy is also part of the package. With access to his blood relatives, Charlie has a chance to know more about himself. He doesn't share the fantasies, the exaggerated flights of fancy, the hidden terrors that many adopted children have about their birth families. He and his brother and sisters have seen first hand that families by birth and families by adoption are much the same. They are filled with real people—both the pretty wonderful sort and those who fall short. Yes, it's a complex arrangement—intertwining our lives together as we have done. Yet in a time when families are fractured and somewhat out of fashion, we feel blessed that because of a small boy, our two families have come together as one.

A birthmother who relinquished her twins in an open adoption, and visits them frequently, commented

> I've felt good with the decision since I made it, and I've never had any second thoughts about it. I just know I couldn't have handled them. I enjoy going there and seeing them, but I also enjoy watching them (the adoptive parents) love the babies. I think I'll always be close to them.

Another birthmother, Lorraine Dusky, relates in a 1983 article, "The Daughter I Gave Away," how she first made contact with the adoptive parents.

> How could I tell this man that I didn't want to steal his daughter? And that I didn't want to be an emotional kidnapper either. . . . I spoke to her mother again. She asked if I would like to come out and meet Jane. I wanted to kiss the hem of her skirt. And then she said something that will always make me feel twice blessed: She referred to Jane as "our daughter." "I don't own my children," she said. "They're their own people."

Open adoption has also been well received by birthfathers, who are typically thought to be less affected by the adoption decision. In fact, women may consider the birthfather to be unimportant when faced with an unwanted pregnancy, and not even inform him of their child's birth.

The benefits of open adoption are also clearly felt by adoptive parents who have also obtained a child through closed adoption. Such parents deeply regret that they did not have an opportunity to know the first birthmother and birthfather, and feel that they will be at a disadvantage in dealing with this child's feelings and questions regarding his adoption compared with what they know about the second child's heritage. On the other hand, adoptive parents must give up their exclusive position as the child's parents and this may be threatening to some. It takes time, trust, and understanding for them to see that it is in their child's best interests, if not their own, to form an open adoption.

Sperm Donors

Many social scientists today see the most valuable donor as one who feels a sense of responsibility about his actions, concern about the outcome of the pregnancy and welfare of the offspring. As Julian Huxley (1963), the eminent British scientist, stated, "Knowing the donor must be not only a choice but a duty." Curie-Cohen's national survey found that 91.8 percent of physicians did not permit a known donor, and those who did, did so only rarely. Rutgers University researchers Leiblum and Barbrack found that 63 percent of medical students and 78 percent of the infertile couples they surveyed said that DI recipients should be allowed to select the donor.

Using a known donor has benefits for both parents and child. The most important consequence for the DI child is at least the preservation of her genetic heritage, and at best, an open and mutually satisfying relationship with the donor, her biological father. The helpless passivity that inactivates couples or single women at DI clinics can be turned into active control over reproductive choice. The infertile male partner can be actively involved in both helping select the donor, drawing up the arrangements, and physically assisting with the insemination.

Many future problems are resolved when a known donor is used. These include fear of future "innocent incest," genetic diseases of unknown origins and symptoms (which means they may go unrecognized earlier than otherwise), and the worst one of all—deprivation of the child's identity and heritage.

On the other hand, there are unconscious mammalian instincts that may be interpreted as supremacy by the donor and inferiority by the infertile male. These are present whether the donor is known or unknown, and may affect a friendship. In Australia, where the AIDS problem shattered the donor system and sperm banks closed down pending the development of an AIDS screening test, the use of known donors is now being encouraged and requested. For some friends, having a baby together by DI can be a very awkward and somewhat unmanageable thing to do, according to Jan Aitken, a Melbourne social worker who counsels DI recipients. Some couples express their fears that accepting sperm from a friend will change the relationship, and in fact the friendship ended in a couple of cases. Aitken's understanding is that the "usually contained sexual attractions are somehow made too conscious when a friendship has a baby to show for it."

Dunstan wrote that practitioners

> in search of specimens have a duty not to encourage men to trivialize their psycho-genital potential . . . the life potential of their seminal fluid by taking it from them impersonally and for a use beyond their human reach, as though it were no more than a bodily secretion.

When a known donor is used, then due appreciation and respect can be shown for the gift. By handling the semen myself, I treated it as a priceless treasure—I was handling the seeds of life itself.

Donors must surely feel privileged to be asked for their genes in the creation of a child. It can be anticipated that their ego would receive a boost, especially if they were chosen above others. It is a chance to really *give*. I certainly would feel a deep sense of satisfaction if I could give another person the depth and breadth of joy our donor has given us through our child, although at times I'm sure the sharing would be painful.

> I would have preferred a known donor, but at the time I didn't know any men and I had no time to create a relationship. I now feel my daughter needs a man around her and will try to get in to some relationships with men.

> My donor has switched from just doing it as a favor, to really wanting to do it.

> A child can love two fathers just like a father can love two children.

Openness for single heterosexual women and lesbians during the procedure often provides a legitimizing function by avoiding any stigma that might be attached to unplanned or "one-night stand" pregnancies. Some recipients felt that rather than seeing DI as something to hide, they were proud of having taken control of their lives. The known biological tie can be very important for a lesbian as her partner may not legally obtain the right to be a co-parent.

The Center for Reproductive Alternatives in the San Francisco Bay area has been arranging open surrogate births for the past few years, and on Father's Day 1987 was scheduled to begin an open donor program. Donors will meet the recipients, who may be single women or couples (heterosexual and lesbian). According to Bruce Rappaport of the center, thorough psychological screening and counseling will be offered to all parties. Donor births will be limited to three. He feels that the supply of donors will be greater initially than the demand of couples. The address of this pioneering facility is listed in Resources.

Relatives

In the early practice of DI, as Finegold points out in his 1964 edition *Artificial Insemination,* the burden of selecting the donor was removed from the physician, as the husband generally brought along his brother, father, or other relatives. A couple of gynecologists I interviewed in Australia had also experienced such cases, especially with the migrant population. When family members visit from Europe, semen samples can be taken and banked. These physicians happily cooperate with the requests; in fact they are spared any difficulty in matching certain ethnic groups. Candace Turner, founder of Donors' Offspring, recommends that donors be from the husband's family where possible.

Schoysman (1975) reports two cases where a brother's sperm was used without the knowledge or consent of the woman:

> In order to limit as much as possible future indiscretions the wives both of the donor and of the receiving couple were not made aware of this decision. Considering that the result from these two particular cases is the creation of happy family relationships, we have no regrets.

This, of course, is a short-term view. Since the wives did not know of the details of the conception, then they would have no reason to tell the doctor of any dissatisfactions. This is a clear violation of marital confidence, as well as a violation of parent-child confidence. One can only guess what it is like living with a double-barreled secret like that and what the emotional reactions would be in the event of disclosure.

> My husband has three brothers. We thought about mixing their sperm together so no one would know which one was responsible. But then we would always be guessing . . . In cases of identical twins, the sperm is often easier to accept.

Most practitioners feel that relatives should not be used because, of course, it is too hard to keep the secret. Barton et al. (1945), writing in the *British Medical Journal* also add that "experience shows it is conducive to emotional disturbances involving both the husband or wife." They worry also about conflict if the couple run the constant risk of meeting the donor. Unfortunately, like so many writers who dismiss the concept of known donors, no details are ever supplied as to the nature of those emotional disturbances.

There was a well-publicized case in France where a woman carried a baby for her twin sister. In Massachusetts, in 1985, Sherry King carried a baby for her sister Carole Jackson, conceived with Mr. Jackson's sperm. I was recently contacted by a woman in New England who used her brother-in-law's semen. Unfortunately she miscarried, but they were trying again. All members of the family knew of the arrangement and felt quite comfortable. On the other hand, Lori Andrews mentions in her book *New Conceptions* about male identical twins where the fertile brother was going to provide sperm for his infertile twin. However, the wife of the potential donor did not want her sister-in-law raising her husband's children. (It is interesting that although the genetic combination couldn't be closer, nevertheless, there is some "essence" of person, apart from genes, that some people do feel is conveyed to the offspring.)

Sources of Sperm Donors

Afton Blake chose Donor #28 from the Repository for Germinal Choice because he was "the sort of man she could have married." Intending spouses don't usually subject each other to genetic screening and extensive fertility and health workups (although some perhaps wish they had!). Typically, one knows one's partner's family, relatives—the same as with a known donor. In fact, one has even more genetic evidence if the donor has children. Not only is his fertility proven, but the children's attributes can be observed.

I feel that ideal donors are older men with children, or even grandchildren. They are more mature and more emotionally stable, especially if they are married. Also such a man is less likely to be possessive about a DI child he helps create. Another advantage for some couples is that a man ten, twenty, or even thirty years older, is in a different peer group from the infertile male. A donor with longer life experience is likely to be more mellow and philosophical about DI. It is also probable that a mature donor takes a broader view of reproduction and has a more spiritual understanding of human life, compared with a "young and silly lad," which is how one Australian Minister of Health described the typical donor. (I realize that most sperm banks do not accept donors over the age of thirty or thirty-five. This is a very arbitrary division. Many men father children in later life, such as Picasso, and today genetic screening is available for recipients who may be concerned about increasing defects with paternal age.)

Doing DI yourself enables you to choose a donor of your same social background—a friend or a friend's husband. The compromise of a go-between that is common in the gay community may appeal to some heterosexual couples as well. Attorneys, as well as friends, act as go-betweens. Although most go-betweens keep records so that the child at age eighteen can know, the gay community often uses two "sperm runners" to ensure the anonymity of the lesbian. The exchange of gifts for the donor is encouraged by go-betweens rather than money.

Couples and women with less social resources may turn to advertising in personal columns in newspapers, esoteric journals, and societies like Mensa (for those of high intelligence). Other potential sources of donors are sex therapy institutes, vasectomy clinics, the gay community (if the donors can be adequately screened), and sperm banks where permanent records are kept on the donors, such as the two banks in California described in Chapter 6.

Let people know you are looking for a donor. This means giving up privacy and, where infertility is involved, feelings of helplessness.

Some recipients may want to screen the donor, and to send the semen to a sperm bank for analysis and/or storage.

Physicians and clinics are an unlikely source for a donor to be known or *even* recorded, as this runs against the primary credo of DI practitioners. However, before Robyn Rowland's research (see Chapter 7), no one apparently had ever asked donors how they felt about anonymity, so perhaps some gynecologists will find a few donors who will reveal their identity, either to the couple or at least later to the child.

Donor Information Questionnaire

You may want to ask a potential donor if there is any family history of

1. Repeated miscarriages or stillbirths.
2. Congenital defects such as cleft palate, club foot.
3. Mental illness, such as schizophrenia.
4. Hypertension.
5. Diabetes.
6. Rheumatoid arthritis or other auto-immune diseases.
7. Asthma or other allergies.
8. Cardiovascular disease, such as strokes, heart attacks.
9. Chromosome abnormalities, such as Down's syndrome.
10. Genetic diseases, such as cystic fibrosis, hemophilia, Tay-Sachs (in Jewish people).
11. Exposure to hepatitis, sexually transmitted diseases.
12. Cancer.
13. Infectious diseases.

The donor should also be asked about his sexual practices and any drug usage (prescribed or illicit).

Risk Factors for AIDS

1. Multiple sexual contacts, especially anonymous ones.
2. Contact with someone known to have AIDS.
3. Blood transfusions.
4. Warning signs such as a suspicious skin lesion, fever, weight loss, diarrhea, persistent cough, unusual bleeding, enlarged lymph glands.

For more comprehensive screening forms, see Appendix 3.

Sometimes a donor goes looking for the couple as happened in the following case. Noel Keane, a Michigan attorney, represented a single male who wanted to donate his sperm to "an infertile white couple" who would then have his child and raise it themselves. He would set up a trust fund for the child (twenty thousand dollars) and "be like an uncle to it." Ads were placed in newspapers, but after the donor met and came to trust the selected couple, they decided to go ahead without an elaborate written agreement.

The Commitment to Donate

Cooperative Adoption, by Rillera and Kaplan, has excellent guidelines for contacting, meeting, and setting parameters that are applicable in cooperative DI. The authors also cover drawing up agreements, conflicts, mediators, the extended family, and withdrawing. Their aim is to set up a win/win, not a win/lose, situation. Remember, you can negotiate for the child only what you are guessing the child will feel, think, and want. The best negotiation is one that is open for renegotiation as the child becomes able to participate.

The ideal donor will make a commitment, based on a thorough understanding of all the dimensions of DI. Nothing is more shattering than to call the donor around the time of peak fertility and learn that he has changed his mind! If he has a wife, she should be informed about the arrangements and agreeable to them for everything to proceed smoothly, although legally a man has autonomy over his sperm, of course. It would be very hard to explain phone calls and visits to the house at odd hours, to say nothing of the deception, if the donor's wife were not involved. Every aspect of the process should be aboveboard, and affirming, not threatening, the self-esteem of those involved.

Our donor's wife has been an important part of the process. Not only in accepting her husband's actions, but her support and hospitality to us while the inseminations were taking place. She has a keen sense of social justice and an astute perception of the needs of children.

A typical question I often receive (always from men, including our attorney!) is: why didn't you just do it naturally? First, there are the feelings of the uninvolved spouses. Most wives feel very sensitive about their partner's infertility, as well as any threat to the security of the donor's wife. Second, the logistics of arranging a suitable location to consummate the union physically are far more complex. Julia would never have been conceived the night that she was, under natural circumstances. It was hard enough just to arrange sequential visits into the bathroom! Third, direct transfer would blur the legal distinctions between the involved parties as it would be a case of acquiescing to adultery. This was also made clear by our attorney when he drew up the contract.

However, NID—natural insemination by donor—may be perfectly acceptable to all parties in some cases. Gynecologists have informed me of women who just could not conceive artificially, but did so as soon as the donor had intercourse with them. Considering how many acts of intercourse an individual may have in a lifetime, people not confined by "middle class morality" understandably aren't worried about some extra sexual episodes for so noble, and ironically, so appropriate a cause! In retrospect, I must say the means (so transient) seem of much less significance than the results (so permanent)—the creation of a human being. It should be also pointed out that donating semen is a sexual experience for the donor, as he has to masturbate to orgasm. (Amazingly, many men imagine there is some artificial way that sperm can be retrieved from them!) Clearly our daughter has organic memories of her own conception, otherwise how could she have explained it to us the way she did (see Chapter 12)? She was also confused as to why the donor's sperm went into my vagina, but not his penis, and we had to reassure her that penises were OK. One must concede to her logic!

According to Australian psychiatrist Graham Farrant, the great- est start in life—the cornerstone of holistic health—is for a child to be "planned and conceived in ecstasy and passion." With this in mind, the artificial conception that occurs with DI may be re- grettable, albeit necessary for other reasons.

Difficulties with a Known Donor

There may be problems making a sound decision in choosing the donor, or in having an adequate choice. The donor will always be in your life and your child's. It is important to avoid men who are nervous about birth defects, potential suits, and the like. A donor who is intent on legal advice is probably going to change his mind (especially with the present hazy state of the law in most jurisdic- tions). The duty of attorneys is to advise of the worst that can hap- pen and I suspect that very few law students or lawyers become donors!

As well as avoiding fearful donors, take care to choose one that does not have grand plans for your child. This is more of a prob- lem with childless donors. A woman in California complained to me:

> One of the potential donors wanted to have the child for school holidays and had ideas about the child's schooling, so I didn't choose him.

While donors need their heads to be clear about what they are doing, the offer has to come from the heart. If it isn't a good "gut feeling" for the donor—let him go. Using a known donor flies in the face of all conventional wisdom and established medical prac- tice. It has to feel right. Also avoid donors who give out of pity rather than admiration for your creative solution.

One known donor commented in Rowland's survey:

> The recipient, donor, and their families *should all meet*. The donor
> should be a friend of the recipient. However, the donor must have
> no hand in raising the child nor any responsibility . . . it should be
> done between trustworthy friends without interference from doc-
> tors and clinics.

There is also the fear of embarrassment if the donor refuses,
thus it may be more comfortable to ask indirectly. When we first
told our donor, as a friend, about Geoff's sterility, we had planned
to use semen from another friend who had offered. There was no
attempt to "sound him out"; he simply offered spontaneously.
Just like there is always someone who will stop and help a
stranded motorist (most won't), there are just some people in the
world who can really give of themselves, but again, most won't.
You just have to find that one special person.

Since the success of DI depends upon the accurate timing of
ovulation, some of the requests are bound to be inconvenient for
the donor. The stress of imposition is repeated month after month
by those women who do not readily conceive. As well as the disappointment over not conceiving, there is the anxiety of wondering how long the donor will keep donating—six months, a year,
two years . . . another child?

Donor Involvement as the DI Child Grows

The presence of the DI child is proof of the man's fertility and evidence of his genetic endowment, as well as satisfying any unful-
filled generative urge he may have. The unfolding of a human being, especially when it is partly your creation, is one of life's
miracles to share. The donor, like the birthmother in adoption,
has the most to lose in the triangle, although the infertile husband
may feel the most threatened. I think it is important to respect that
"loss," although it can be turned into a gain if the donor has contact with this child, who otherwise would not have been born. It
is not only the donor who may participate in the extra relationships, but his wife and other children who are the DI child's half-
siblings. In these stressful times of transient bonds and a sense of

powerlessness with regard to the future of our species, many of us welcome new and deep meaning in relationships.

The level of involvement may not always be mutual, of course. Donors of organs also have feelings about the recipients. A kidney donor complained that it was unfair that the recipient went back to work, "too soon, with my kidney." The father of a heart donor said to the father of the recipient, "I've always wanted a little girl so now we're going to have her and share her with you."

If emotional conflicts arise, it is important to keep the lines of communication open. It is essential for everyone to keep in touch with their feelings, and to know that allowing themselves to recognize deep emotions is not the same as acting on them.

Relationships can always be renegotiated, and this option must be safeguarded.

> It is interesting to see kids who are as much mine as my own but for whom I have no responsibility. The oldest two will not be told about me until they are ten years old. I don't know if that is good or not. Now I can only wait. I see them about once a week. I am in no way their parent.

The role of the donor may range from secrecy to friendship, and with or without the child's knowledge. The most cautious couples will want no relationship at all beyond permanent records, which acknowledge the biological connection, for the child to have access to at the age of majority (when the connection can be reactivated). Others may inform the child about her DI status, but not the donor's identity until a later age. Some donors are willing to act as a noncustodial father or an "uncle" to the child where the mother is single or lesbian. Others will allow the donor and child to choose their own level of involvement.

Each case of DI is unique, so recipients and donors will have to work out the most suitable arrangements, bearing in mind the vulnerability of the infertile husband. The choice of donor is thus paramount, realizing that all relationships bring potential psychological risks.

Of course, some DI offspring may well choose not to know anything about their paternal genes, just as not all adoptees choose to search. But if the opportunity is there, and the information is available, perhaps the DI adult may want to make contact at a later date, such as after a birth, death, or divorce. At the very least, DI offspring must be guaranteed that opportunity.

Lori Andrews (1984) interviewed a donor at the Northern California sperm bank, who is allowing the release of his name and intends to design a portfolio about himself that the mother can give to the child. He will include a profile of himself, photos of where he grew up and information about his family tree. This donor is also willing to participate with raising the child. "I imagine it would develop along the lines of the role a divorced father takes," he said.

In our case, the donor and his family have become a very special kind of "kin." For me, it is a unique relationship; this man is the co-creator of my child—more than a friend and less than a lover. Certainly very deep emotional bonds are generated and a deep sense of pride and sharing. It is important to point out that love is not finite—like cutting up a pie—so that the husband, for example, receives less love because the donor is known. Love is expansive and self-generating, and I believe with Etter of Open Adoption Resources that there is enough to go around for everyone involved. Julia says, "X gave the sperm and Geoff gave the love."

Our donor describes his emotional response to Julia as a combination of three different levels. First, there is the rational knowledge that she is part of his flesh and blood. Second, there is a subtle bond of heredity which he calls "a kind of resonance, a fine spiritual feeling." Third, there is the social bond that has been generated through visits since her birth. With regard to his other children, the social bond is the most powerful of the three, but because he does not see Julia on a daily basis, she does not engender the kind of belonging that he feels with them or even with his pets. Rather like a grandparent, he can enjoy watching "the little flower unfold," without any responsibility for raising her.

Interestingly, it is precisely this social bond that the practitioners of DI stress as the most significant for the DI father. As it turns out, in our case, to be the least significant link between our donor and the child, then it makes only more sense to be relaxed about the mutual exchange of both social and genetic knowing. That is, if the paternal origin is acknowledged from the beginning, it will be a nonissue, just a part of the information in a biographical package to which the DI child is entitled, rather than a lifetime crusade as we will see in Chapter 11 with some adoptees and DI offspring.

Another, subtle bond relates to cellular consciousness beginning at conception, which I briefly describe at the conclusion to the book. Here we are talking about a biological energy field that can only be sensed by highly intuitive individuals. This was painfully evident when Julia lost a finger in an accident. While our donor didn't suffer sleepless nights of remorse as I did, he nevertheless felt a loss, in a way, of part of himself. I also want to add that at this generative level, he was the only other person who really understood how *I* felt. This accident superseded the DI issue—we were more concerned about reactions at school and in the community to Julia's amputated finger than to her mode of conception. Fortunately, both the disclosure of the DI and the accident happened before the age of four, so she was able to do the necessary integration and adjustment before kindergarten. I am sure that for other DI families, bigger events (good as well as bad) will happen to overshadow the DI experience, which seems so monumental in the beginning. For us, the accident also interrupted our plans to conceive a second child with our donor. I tried for about six months, but my grief was not resolved.

We see our donor and his family several times a year. Since learning of Julia's connection to them, his children have viewed her with more interest. At this point, we guard his actual identity very carefully. Apart from ourselves, only my mother and sister (who live in Australia) know exactly who he is. I must confess there is an element of exclusivity too. If the word got around that he was a "sperm donor," I am sure he would be besieged for his services! He is such a special person, of such courage and generosity, that he probably would not refuse and I might have to wait in line for a second child!

I think that donor loyalty is very natural. I observed that when an anonymous donor was used, couples wanted the same donor for a subsequent child. This is not so much for the children to look alike and be full siblings genetically, but I think parents grow to know and like the features of their children. Or perhaps it is a case of the devil you "know." As a family friend said once, when he saw Julia for the first time, "Wow, next time you'll certainly want to get some more of where she came from."

Single women and lesbians have often used known donors, and many heterosexual married couples have used the husband's twin or brother. However, I know of only one other case than my own in which a married couple used an unrelated known donor. I was able to interview both the DI parents and their first donor.

Sam and Susan

Sam and Susan had been living together before they married and Susan was aware of Sam's infertility. In fact, this was a big stumbling block in the way of their planned marriage. However, they had six months of counseling that helped them communicate better and stop "talking around issues" rather than explore alternative ways of reproduction. Susan had a Resolve pen pal with two DI sons, and she provided tremendous support for them.

Sam and Susan did not set out to find a known donor. After having searched for a physician who offered DI, they underwent seven months of home inseminations with frozen semen. Because they wanted to do the insemination themselves, this gynecologist supplied them with a cervical cap and arranged for the semen to be shipped to the couple's home. Susan remembers fearing that the Federal Express man would ask what were the contents of the strange packages that he delivered so regularly, and one day he did! After that, Sam's mother received the shipments.

So half a year and over $1500 in semen costs later, they returned to the doctor. It so happened that I had met their obstetrician in the interim and persuaded him of the merits of open DI and known donors. Susan remembers she was quite surprised when this doctor said to her, "Don't you have a friend who can help you out?" At first she was shocked and felt like replying "I am not that kind of a woman!" However, both she and Sam immediately thought of the same person, and Sam called him on the phone. A former coworker of Sam's, this older, now-divorced man was honored by the request and said "yes" right away. He gave a detailed health history and all parties signed a contract.

The first (and only) insemination was done in the donor's house. Susan and Sam were alone; he had left the specimen in a Red Cross mug with "We're grateful for our donors" written on it! The donor had also left a photo of his great-grandfather, whose prominent ears made him look like a monkey, and a joking comment — "hope the kid doesn't look like this."

Susan conceived that cycle and was both happy and scared to be pregnant. "I was afraid somehow everyone would know, now that it had happened." They personally called the donor after the birth and see him a couple of times a year (he lives in another part of the country). When the donor first saw the child he experienced the same reaction he had toward his own children, "an automatic concern and affection." He loves children and, yes, he is sorry that she is not "his." He would love more contact but doesn't know what that might mean, what is a "safe" amount, "like once a month would be nice, maybe more would be too much." He made the excellent point that a child is never more than 50 percent of a parent anyway, so he would never think of the child as "his." Without a doubt, he sees Susan and Sam as the parents of the child. Furthermore, his love for Sam and Susan is equal to his love for the child. Before the DI he said he always felt close to them, and now he feels closer. Seeing them so happy was a source of great satisfaction and he stressed to me that he will forever respect the arrangements that they made. Of paramount importance, he emphasizes, is the child, whom he hopes will be okay when she knows the truth. He certainly has no regrets about being a donor, but acknowledges that it takes a special relationship between the parties involved. "Issues like this need to be rethought, but it is hard to suggest rethinking without threatening people that somehow you are getting into a new morality, free love or whatever."

> I hope I did . . . I feel sure . . . I did the right thing and that it will continue to work out well. We all have a rare relationship and I hope other donors have it as easy.

Sam admits to experiencing feelings of jealousy and disempowerment resulting from his infertility. He saw the donor's children growing up and observes the physical resemblance to his daughter. Although saddened by the end of his genetic line, he enjoys his wonderful family life. In the presence of the donor, he sometimes feels strange and awkward and wonders if his daughter and the donor "share a mystical connection."

A man of considerable maturity and sensitivity, Sam expressed his concern for the "pain and emotions" experienced by the donor (who, incidentally, denied that there was any pain!) as follows:

> The infertile husband has painful emotions whatever happens. That is his lot—whether he adopts, does DI, or never has kids. The donor, on the other hand, only develops those feelings when he is asked to donate . . . and even if he refuses, he will still have feelings about that.

A year or so later, Sam and Susan wanted another child. However, this time the donor refused. The donor explained to me that it was a "heavy trip, a big responsibility emotionally. . . . The legal contract and the logistics were the easy part." Most difficult was his feeling of concern, wondering how things will go in the future. He felt that two DI offspring were more than he wanted to cope with. I asked if he would consent to be a donor for another couple. He replied, "I would only do something like this for a *very special* friend, and I don't have any more friends like Sam."

I asked the donor if he would have used DI had he been infertile. "I don't know . . . I don't know how that feels," he mused. When asked how he would react on learning that he was the product of an anonymous sperm donor he replied, "Awful, I wouldn't feel complete." Susan was fortunate to conceive the first time, but the donor said he would have donated for as long as it took—"I made a commitment." He feels no sense of awkwardness when meeting Susan and Sam nor did he feel badly for declining to be a donor a second time.

Susan and Sam were disappointed, but understood his misgivings because donorship had been a bit difficult for him. They had actually anticipated his refusal and thus had a back-up plan of another potential donor.

The second donor also had worked with Sam in the past. He was a little younger than the first donor, had never married, but was in a de facto relationship. His girlfriend, who had a child from a previous relationship, was not willing for him to do the DI. However, the donor later called back and said he would do it anyway and not tell her. Two pregnancies were achieved with the second donor, but the first ended in a miscarriage. As with the first insemination, Susan conceived each of the times with a single attempt. This donor also lived some distance from them, so they met at a midpoint and used a motel room. As with the first donor, they did not physically meet at the time of the insemination. The second donor, "respecting their privacy and perhaps feeling some shyness," left the shade up of the motel room, and the door ajar, so they could enter after he left. This time they did not bother with a health history or signed contracts.

The second donor has never seen the little girl who was born, but has talked to Susan and Sam on the phone. Prior to the donor's move out of state, they would all meet once or twice a year. Because the second donor concealed the DI from his de facto, he needed to talk it out with his brother, who was supportive. However, the second donor has some apprehensions that his parents and other family members might hear about it.

Friends and family do comment on the dissimilar appearances of Sam and Susan's children, who are both dark, while Sam and Susan are both fair. But Sam also experiences many comments about how much they look like him!

Susan and Sam intend to tell their children. He forecasts that he and his children will "lose the connection that we don't have, but it won't diminish the connection we do have." Sam says:

> The child must be told, so she will have the necessary information and the power and will not be defenseless when others question or comment.

Despite the small tensions that have developed with the donors, the friendships are still strong, and "it would be much worse not knowing the donors." Most of their friends knew of their infertility and struggles to conceive in the past, although not all of them are aware that the donors are known. Susan regrets that she revealed the identity of the donor to one friend, who had actually met him, and now Susan worries that she violated his privacy.

Despite the open arrangements in this story, however, each member still carries a burden of secrecy. Susan has never told her parents, and cannot explain what it is she fears in their reaction. The first donor has not told his children that they have a half-sibling (he doesn't feel he has Sam and Susan's permission to disclose this information), and the second donor did not reveal the DI to anyone but his brother. Nevertheless, all parties hope for more contact in the future, so these issues will surely be discussed and resolved.

The DI Child's Feelings about the Known Donor

As I have not interviewed other DI children who know their donor, I can only speculate from the literature on open adoption and adoption reunions (see Chapter 12). Julia certainly is aware of which physical characteristics she received from her paternal genes. At age five she said, "I guess I have two fathers: Geoff is my real father and X is a kind of pretend father because he gave you the sperm." Sometimes she will call the donor her "father" and Geoff her "Dad." At least the option is available for the relationship with the donor to become closer as she grows older, and if and when she has children of her own.

Documentation of Rights and Responsibilities

I believe that every donor should have control over his semen. It is only semen when it leaves his body, but it may create a human being when it reaches its destination. Donors should have the right to evaluate the kind of parents, family, and medical background, life-style, religion—whatever—that this child would have, just as birthmothers in open adoption can interview different adoptive parents before giving up the child. In my opinion, if sperm donors were counseled they would not be donors on any other terms than with a known recipient, or at the very least, with permanent records kept on all parties.

As we have seen, documentation is a controversial issue. Generally the last thing that couples, and particularly single women, want is a record of paternity. For some, the idea of a contract implies a lack of trust, but others feel that a contract helps each party keep their side of the bargain. From the known donor's point of view, contracts and wills may help protect him from future suits for child support if anything serious happened to the mother's husband or the mother if she is single.

A contract between sperm donor and recipient, in the absence of any relevant state laws, has only evidence value in a future court case. However, in the absence of any laws pertaining to DI in Massachusetts, we felt it was the best to define our mutual agreement and to put in writing the intent and purpose of our actions.

A very simple contract was drawn up by our attorney for my husband and donor to sign:

Husband's Agreement to Artificial Insemination

Having been found sterile by my physicians, and having considered and rejected the alternatives, including continued use of available medical therapy, adoption, and continuing my marriage without children I have decided, with my wife, that artificial insemination, using sperm from a donor known by and selected by me and my wife, is my most acceptable course of action.

Accordingly, I hereby agree and consent to my wife's participation in artificial insemination using the sperm of a donor known to each of us. I further agree to and acknowledge my obligation to care for, support, and otherwise treat any child born as a result of this artificial insemination procedure in all respects as if the child were my natural born child.

_____   _____
Date   Husband's Signature

Sperm Sale Agreement

I agree to sell to _____ one or more specimens of my sperm for which I will be paid $1.00 and other valuable consideration per specimen. In consideration of this payment I agree to permit _____ to use my sperm to artificially inseminate his wife, and I hereby waive any and all rights I may have in any child that might result from this use of my sperm.

Date	Seller
	Purchaser

Although only one dollar changed hands (and our donor took over a year to cash the princely check!), our attorney felt that it was important to legally define the donor as a vendor for the purposes of the contract. Both parties retained copies of the agreement.

For those who feel that life cannot be priced, payment (except for the one dollar to make the contract legal) is clearly out of the question. Doing DI yourself with a known donor avoids not just the expense, but the unsavory commercialism. Infertile couples generally feel that by paying the donor for the semen, they have discharged all feelings of obligation, which really amazes me. We have tried to show our appreciation in small ways—dinners, gifts, and so on. Our gestures seem very minor considerations compared with the gift of our beautiful child. At least the donor and his family can share the gift through knowing Julia.

The contract with our donor safeguards him from any obligations or responsibility for the child. We set up a trust so that friends will act *in loco parentis* in the event of both our deaths. However, we would be more than happy to name our donor and his wife as legal guardians if they wanted to assume that role. If the situation were reversed and our donor suddenly found himself without his wife and children, we would certainly share Julia more with him.

The most important aspect of DI reform is being able to know the donor or have permanent records of the donor. Yet single women and lesbians, working with a known donor or a go-between, generally feel that "nothing written, nothing said" is the way to protect their interests. A contract, on the other hand, would acknowledge paternity and put them in a vulnerable position. Furthermore, in some Equal Rights states it might be rejected by a court unless 50 percent of the rights and obligations were shared by the donor. The contract is more relevant for married couples because it certifies the husband's willingness to accept and raise a DI child. However, Karen Kruskal, an attorney in Cambridge, Massachusetts, counsels lesbians as to whether contracts are appropriate, as in the case of a known donor. Some known donors and the lesbian recipients want no contact, and others arrange to coparent the child. (Lesbian couples also sign coparenting contracts between themselves.) Such contracts, which are not legally binding, and which may or may not be signed, are primarily designed as statements of intent, which purport to clarify the expectations of all parties.

Lesbian contracts with known donors deal with such issues as visitation and custody rights, support obligations, donor identity and disclosure, and number of pregnancies by that donor. Usually written into such a contract is the knowledge and acceptance of the lesbian life-style.

Donors for Lesbians

Many gynecologists and clinics refuse to inseminate single women and lesbians so they are obliged to turn to friends, go-betweens, and the gay community.

While some lesbians fear paternity suits, fatherhood is important to others. They feel the need for relationships with men, as the child-raising will be done by women. However, both donors and lesbians may have cold feet about meeting each other when neither is protected by a contract or state law. Gay men may be threatened by being known, as a gay and as a donor, and/or by having their name on the birth certificate.

A lesbian I interviewed said her donor was unhappy about it now, and did not want the child to search for him. "He was afraid that the child would hate him." Another donor felt a "strange loyalty" but received no support from his friends who were very much against his action.

A member of a lesbian couple who used a brother for a donor commented to Achilles:

> I am very happy I used a known donor and particularly that there will be a biological tie between my partner and the child. I had been very afraid of the legal and emotional ramifications, but as time went on I realized that there are major problems with an anonymous donor and that a situation like ours is ideal. I know I can trust the donor and we went to great lengths to comply with the law. The fact that his children understand it all made it a lot more "safe." In addition, my lover's family definitely see this child as theirs. . . . This is exactly how I wanted to have kids, with another woman, and now we are tied together forever. I am the mother of her child and that's forever. I now realize how important honesty is.

The comother commented:

> It was a good decision to use artificial insemination and a good decision to use my brother. I knew it was the only way that the child would be accepted as a grandchild by my mother which is very important to me. *I also wanted there to be a known biological tie and this was the only condition under which I would agree to have a child. An unknown donor was unthinkable to me—a horrible idea.* [Italics mine]

Personal Profiles

The following are personal profiles of donors used by single women and lesbians, for the simple reason that apart from ourselves, I know of only one married couple who has used a known nonrelated donor.

Larry

It is not uncommon for a brother of a lesbian to donate sperm for her partner. Sometimes the donor visits regularly, or babysits, to provide a male role model. One such donor, described in the December 11, 1984, Boston *Phoenix,* wasn't quite sure in his own mind what his role was. "I don't feel like I am the father and Emma is the daughter," he said, "I feel more like I am giving support to friends." As he has no financial responsibilities, he compares his relationship with Emma to that of an uncle. However, he carries her picture in his wallet and says since she was born he feels a lot different. "I marched into my boss's office and demanded a two-thousand-dollar raise. For the first time, I thought I was worth it."

The *Phoenix* reported that Larry doesn't minimize the unknown territory he is charting or the difficulties it might bring him later. He admits the possibility of rivalry with his sister's partner, but says that so far that hasn't happened. "We really connect. There is a strong bond between us," he says. If at some point in the future he doesn't like the way Emma is being raised, he concedes he may have to "grin and bear it." But he stresses his trust in their judgment. About his future relationship with his daughter he predicts, "At times I will be closer to Emma, at other times, less so."

Edward

In *Rocking the Cradle,* by Hanscombe and Forster, Edward, an English donor, describes his experience when asked by a woman friend if he would be a donor for a lesbian couple.

> I was asked about my medical history in great detail. My first thoughts were "What am I doing? What is my responsibility?" Before I agreed to donate I wanted to be assured that the people who wanted the kid really wanted it. So the reply came back that they had one kid of two years and had been trying to get another one and they couldn't. I care about people in relationships. If a child helps a relationship in a situation where, by nature, they can't create a child, then I'm prepared to help that. I am not a breeder. My brother and sister have families, but in no way do I want to have one myself.
>
> I'd read a manuscript that said it's preferable to have forty-eight hours' abstinence before giving your sperm, so I was very good for two days. My friend arrived with a brown paper parcel. This was the first setback. I thought I'd get something like a specimen bottle you get in hospital. This was more a test tube. I thought, "Aiming into that, I'm going to lose it all over the carpet or on the sheets,"

so the tension built up. I lay on the bed with my picture books. I couldn't get an erection. I was sweating. I knew I wasn't going to make it. So I go back to the sitting room. We had a cup of coffee and chatted a bit. She was smashing. Then I went back into the bedroom and looked at this test-tube bloody thing. (Why can't they give you something a bit bigger? I'm quite serious about this, because I think it might put men off.) Anyway, I made it using the picture books. There was no problem making it the second and third times.

Jenny

Jenny, a lesbian living in California, used two consecutive donors before conceiving her daughter. She did conceive with the first donor, but miscarried. Then, after three more attempts he backed down, feeling that "It wasn't okay to produce a child without a father." But after a couple of months he wanted to be involved with the DI again. By that time Jenny had become pregnant by a donor who "nearly collapsed" when she asked him, as he is gay. However, he is apparently very glad to have a child in his life whom he visits once a week, and his parents are also involved. Jenny put the donor's name on the birth certificate and had a lawyer draw up a contract, listing her sister as guardian if anything happened to Jenny. The donor is happy for the sister to have those rights as long as his fatherhood is officially documented and he can enjoy an ongoing relationship with the child.

Jenny is aware of her adopted sister's anguish over the lack of her medical and genealogical history. Thus, in spite of the potential legal hassles, Jenny preferred to have a known donor. She has a high profile in the lesbian community and feels that lesbians who would be dismayed to conceive a boy are "irresponsible—if they want a girl so badly, they should adopt."

Susan

Susan used two married donors and one who was unmarried and gay. She knew their identities and one of them she knew personally. An adoptee friend had stressed to her the need for every child to know his origins.

She had been trying one to three inseminations a month for almost a year, without success, when we spoke. She used a different donor each cycle, because he had to be on "twenty-four-hour call" around the middle of the month. The donors filled out a questionnaire she drew up, "with silly questions like, What is your favorite color?" Susan felt she had received "crummy treatment" at the DI clinic where she had gone originally. "There is enough stigma about lesbianism and artificial insemination, as well as the stigma of being unnatural." She had her first donor, whom she paid one hundred dollars, checked out by a physician, but there were no payments to the subsequent donors.

Susan found that the donors were more willing to trust her and donate directly than work with a liaison. They were curious to see what sort of a woman she was and whether she would be a good mother.

As far as she is concerned, her child-to-be "never had a father and will never have a father." She thinks that it will be easier for the child to have DI origins than it has been for her being a lesbian. Even though she has "come out" it is always an issue whether she is asked, or not asked, about her lesbianism. "Even though I don't feel that I have to explain anything to anyone, I am dealing with it every day." Her parents know about her DI plans and have been supportive.

Susan has tried a syringe, cervical cap, and diaphragm. As well as charting her temperature, she examines her cervical mucus under a friend's microscope. She says she is getting "less angry and jealous" about her failure to conceive and will soon be ready to try again.

Mary

Mary, divorced eleven years ago, chose DI so she could experience pregnancy. Initially, she began at a clinic, but "the worst thing about it was feeling out of control with the physician calling the shots," as well as the time, and the financial burden. "I actually liked the doctor," she said, "I just have a problem with medical procedures."

Mary lives with her lesbian lover in Sacramento where a newspaper article was published about their blended family, called, "And Baby Makes Four." Not only does Adam have two mothers, but they used a known donor because:

> We knew what we were getting. We needed an active father and extra parents . . . and I have seen many adopted children wanting to know their biological parents, and I know there is so much wondering with DI.

Mary knew the donor, but hadn't seen him for two years, so she used a friend as a go-between. The donor called right back after the initial request and thought it was "marvelous, wanted to talk more about it." However, several months passed before he called again and said "Let's talk baby talk." It took two years for the lesbian pair to decide which one would become the mother (their ages were thirty-seven and forty-one) and finally Mary pushed the issue.

She was lucky to conceive the very first time (as a female psychic had predicted). Both the donor and lesbian partner accompanied Mary to childbirth classes and the birth. The donor's brother, an attorney, made sure that the donor's name was on the birth certificate as there was only a verbal agreement made with Mary and her partner. Adam has Mary's last name, but his middle name is the donor's first name.

The donor lives close by and comes over every day, as well as spending some weekends with them. Mary's mother thinks she is crazy and calls the child a "bastard." However, the donor's family have been very accepting and active grandparents. They are such a close-knit group that Mary commented, "If the donor wanted to marry, we would want to check out Adam's stepmother." Like Mary, the donor works as a counselor and said he "wouldn't be a donor without being a father." If the women moved away for any reason he would want to arrange meetings and continue co-parenting in some way.

Samantha and Penny

Samantha, currently pregnant, lives in northern New England with her lesbian lover Penny and Penny's DI son. They both used known, but different, donors. Neither knew the donor prior to the search through the network. "We just called everyone we could think of and asked them if they knew of anyone who would donate sperm." They interviewed many donors over the phone and personally. It was important to Penny and Samantha that the donor had considered the major issues rather than brushing them aside. Some donors were too keen, and didn't hesitate to agree to several donations a month for "such an important end result." Others were prepared to be uninvolved, but then didn't want to inconvenience themselves for two or three specimens per cycle. One donor thought he had to masturbate in front of them; another wanted to come and stay the night and bring erotic magazines.

Penny conceived the first time she tried, with a gay donor from out-of-town, whom they got to know well because they had "imported him for a vacation week." He was delighted to donate, very curious about the pregnancy, and celebrated the birth with a dinner party. After that, however, he stayed away for a year. Penny senses that while he doesn't want any responsibility, which was what they agreed, he nevertheless feels very attracted to the child, who greatly resembles him. "But he's so adorable," said the donor when he first saw him. Penny admits that there is an intense bond, a special intimacy, even though she is a lesbian and has seen the donor only a few times.

Samantha took about seven cycles to conceive with an unmarried donor. They drew up a contract of written guidelines, which no parties signed. Their intent was to begin with minimal donor contact (visitation once a year) but to allow more involvement depending on how the relationships developed. It was very important to the pair that it was clear in writing that the donor, who was not gay, accepted their lesbian life-style.

Penny and Samantha did not expect their child to ask about his origins as early as two and a half, but when he announced that his father was "shot by guns," they told him that he did have a father, who didn't live with them. A couple of weeks later they explained that the donor lived in Boston, but the child did not remember meeting him. However, he appeared to sense that a toy, given to him when he was eighteen months old by the donor, was special and asked his mother, "Who gave me this?" They said, "Your father," and this is the toy he often takes to bed now. Both parents believe it is important not to evade charged words. Likewise they talk about sperm, rather than "seeds," and have informed the donor about the disclosure.

The use of known donors, like the practice of DI, is probably underestimated. However, as more of us who have taken this step share our stories, we may encourage others to protect the child's right to know the identity of the donor.

9

Ethical Questions and Moral Dilemmas

GEORGE ORWELL'S supposedly ill-fated year 1984 has passed and there is certainly a brave new world of reproductive technology, as Aldous Huxley predicted. It was only in 1941 that human fertilization was first observed by scientists through the microscope, and within four decades the world has seen the birth of babies from in vitro fertilization (IVF) using donor eggs and donor sperm, and from previously frozen embryos. The media generally hails the latest development as a modern miracle, "an elegant way to make people happy." Any questions or reluctance that people may have about this reproductive revolution is downplayed because, as one commentator put it, "Each achievement is emotionally and scientifically compelling, given the undoubted human tragedy of infertility." Studies of infertility, which is on the increase, continue to show the depth of longing for children that people suffer when the experience is denied them.

Marriages are presumed fertile until the evidence shows otherwise, and reproduction is considered by many people to be the single most important dimension of their life. It is central to their identity and their concept of a meaningful existence. Such individuals want to contribute to the human race and thus satisfy their own desire for continuity, even immortality, in the enjoyment of a biological connection with future generations. They may also want to maintain that continuity with the gift of a grandchild for their own parents. For women, much of this pressure derives also from the institutionalization of motherhood, which causes women to describe themselves as "incomplete," "disabled," or "unfeminine" if they cannot experience pregnancy and birth. However, male partners may also feel that these are essential experiences for cementing family relationships.

> The proliferation of arrangements that deliberately create children with the intention of separating them from one or more of its parents is alarming.
>
> —*Carole Anderson, Concerned United Birthparents*

Therefore much of the new technology, especially in vitro fertilization and embryo transfer, is designed to allow couples to have their *own* offspring. The profound ethical dilemma here is that these new technologies are based on the same need to continue the paternal lineage that is denied to the DI child. The anonymous donation of sperm is a pretense to a biological tie, a cover-up of the male's infertility. However, he at least knows his biological father, whereas the DI child conceived on his behalf will not. D. J. Roy (1973) of Montreal writes:

> Techniques which modify traditional patterns of reproductive behavior inevitably introduce changes into the relationship and institutions designed to regulate and sustain that behavior. Such behavior touches our fundamental human values. . . . DI is a simple technique but by no means simply a technique.

The Right to Reproduce

Technology is outpacing the law and other social institutions that can no longer cope effectively with the new developments. In this century, we have seen that legislation has granted freedom to avoid conception and birth, and now the question is being raised with regard to the right to become a parent. Both the United Nations Declaration of Human Rights and the World Health Organization have affirmed the "right" of every individual to have a family. However, the right not to reproduce is not, by extension, also the right to reproduce, even with assistance. As John Robertson (1983), of the University of Texas Law School in Austin, points out:

Freedom to have sex without reproduction does not guarantee freedom to have reproduction without sex. Full reproductive freedom would include both the freedom *not* to reproduce and the freedom *to* reproduce when, with whom, and by what means one chooses. However, the developing technology will arouse strong moral and political reactions, and demands for regulations.

Contraception divorced sex from procreation and paved the way for DI, which is conception separated from sex. Along with the liberalization of abortion, attitudes have grown less restrictive with regard to nonprocreative sexual activity such as masturbation and homosexuality. Separation of parental from procreative functions commonly occurs already in adoptive families and those blended through remarriage. Now, the conception, gestation, and rearing of a child can be separated and recombined in many different ways. Some men and women, for example, may not be able to find a desirable spouse or may not wish to marry. Lesbian and single mothers may want to avoid heterosexual intercourse, yet still want to conceive or bear and rear a child. Others, such as volunteer donors, who are often gay men, may want to transmit their genetic heritage without taking on the responsibilities of pregnancy and birth, or rearing, or both. Some women may wish to conceive and parent, but may not want to physically carry the child and give birth. Noncoital "collaborative" reproduction makes it possible for all these persons to achieve these goals. The number of people who may be involved in a collaboration has reached six: donors of the gametes or the biological mother and father; the surrogate or gestational mother; the infertile couple or rearing mother and father.

According to Robertson, included in the positive freedom of an individual to procreate is the right to take on the rearing role through complete or partial reproduction with one's partner, or with the partial or complete collaboration of others beyond oneself or one's partner. It is also the right of parties to agree how they should allocate their obligations and entitlements with respect to the future child, although this will mean overriding legal presumptions of maternity and paternity to redefine the "family" in many novel ways.

The right to avoid or abandon the rearing role is another aspect of this procreative freedom. For example, one can avoid conception with contraceptives, abort a fetus before viability if pregnancy ensues, or divest oneself of responsibility by agreement, as does the semen donor in DI, or place the child for adoption, as single and married women have done.

Feminist author Germaine Greer examines DI satirically within the larger social context.

> It is an axiom of sociobiology that all living creatures, man included, are driven by a need to pass on their genes. Some species, man included, are reproductive opportunists, seeking to maximize their chances of successful transmission by fornication, adultery, and rape. In the bad old days, the children of priests sat by working men's fires and the working men's wives congratulated themselves on having combined their genes with those of a more successful line. The squire who lingered by the stile with the milkmaid was pleased to produce a hybrid of his etiolated strain and a more robust one. Monarchs named their by-blows Dukes of This and Marquesses of That. Nowadays the method they adopted would be called NID, natural insemination by donor. You might have thought, now that adultery has become a parlor game for bored couples, that this cheap and effective method of overcoming a husband's sterility would at least be as popular as ever, and perhaps it is. An experiment involving a sample of families from Birmingham in 1974 had to be abandoned after a preliminary scan of blood groupings in the families selected showed that nearly a third of the children could not have been sired by their mother's husbands. Surrogate fathering has been around for a long time; unfortunately improved techniques of genetic analysis now make it possible for all children and not just the wise ones to know their own fathers. Women shall soon lose their one opportunity to practice genetic sabotage.

Pressing Questions

Mary Kay Blakely, in *Ms.* magazine, pointed out the sexism and racism in the struggle for the "right" child. Ads in city and campus newspapers indicate what kind of donor or surrogate is sought: invariably "white," "northern European," "Caucasian." Likewise, adoption is much more difficult for a baby without those attributes, although there are always plenty of "hard to place" or "special needs" babies and children needing homes. Blakely questions the motivation of a man who married a mother of three children, but still wanted to have his own child through the use of reproductive technology. Similar comments were made when the first IVF baby was born in India, a country where countless children are orphaned or live in hopeless poverty.

Who should receive priority when scarce, usually costly, resources for assisting reproduction are allocated? Are waiting lists the fairest system? Should older women have priority since they have fewer fertile years ahead of them? Should only childless couples be accepted for assisted conceptions? In an English study, couples with up to six children were accepted for DI at a private clinic. What about research physicians who want to patent their techniques? How much reimbursement for reproductive technology should be paid by health insurance? Does a man have a right to coverage for a vasectomy reversal? And if it is unsuccessful, to DI? If abortions may be subsidized by taxpayers, then should infertility treatment be covered too?

Are fees paid for services or for babies? Surrogate mothers may prefer to receive their remuneration throughout the pregnancy rather than as a lump sum afterward, to avoid the label of a baby sale. Does payment mean that the best sperm or embryo will go to the highest bidder? Who is liable if the "product" doesn't match up to expectations? Can defective children be "returned"?

Carole Anderson, writing in CUB's position paper, "Surrogates and Other Non-traditional Reproduction," realizes that people cannot be stopped from entering into such relationships. But she states, "No person should be permitted to sell or rent or to give any payment of any kind for the use of his or her sperm, uterus, or ovum to create a human life."

On the other side of the Atlantic the Warnock Commission also warned that when "people treat others as a means to their own ends, however desirable the consequences, they must always be liable to moral objections. . . . Such treatment of one person by another becomes positively exploitative when financial interests are involved."

Are professionals offering collaborative/noncoital reproduction obliged to screen the recipients? Who should be responsible for selection, if it were possible to agree on the selection criteria? Is it fair to subject infertile couples to rigorous psychological and physical examinations when fertile couples in the general population are not obliged to undergo such scrutiny—and perhaps rejection? Assessment implies selection and, to some minds, social engineering. There is more pressure against positive eugenics (breeding "desirable" characteristics, or excluding a couple who seem inappropriate) compared with negative eugenics (avoiding undesirable traits, or excluding couples for whom DI might cause or increase emotional problems). Should eugenic considerations be made explicit? We can guess how selection criteria would affect single, lesbian, disabled women. Do infertile people have the freedom to pick eggs and sperm as they select mates? (Some selection is already done with marriage licenses in regard to mental retardation, blood testing, and epilepsy.) In Australia, the Melbourne *Age* in November 1983 reported that ten women went before the Equal Opportunity Board to argue that the Victorian State Government's moratorium on the use of donated ova in the IVF program (pending a Law Reform Commission report) was sexually discriminating, since women with infertile male partners were able to receive sperm for DI.

As Germaine Greer notes:

> Resort to artificial insemination by donor, called AID (and actually another way of transmitting AIDS) is only necessary when a couple is revolted by the element of "criminal conversation" involved in NID (adultery). The method has a number of drawbacks unless it is offered by a public health authority, it is likely to be costly, but in any case, it exposes the couple to the scrutiny of authoritarian institutions. . . . On the spurious grounds of public accountability, the medical establishment agrees to "evaluate" candidates for infertility treatments of this kind.

Donor insemination is utilized not just for male infertility, but to prevent the transmission of genetic diseases and to enable single women to experience motherhood. Is DI a medical procedure or a simple "asexual sexual" activity, which needs no more licensing or supervision than copulation itself? What about a couple's right to privacy? Many couples prefer DI over adoption precisely because they wish to avoid the deep personal investigation and probation involved. Yet when conception is brought from the private realm into the practice of medicine, issues of social responsibility and regulation arise. One physician wrote that because DI was a medical procedure, a medical practitioner must act first and foremost as a physician and not probe into personal affairs of the couple such as income. After all, many future problems may befall a couple who are stable, affluent, and committed at the time of the DI.

Do applicants have a right to counseling and knowledge about the personal and social aspects of infertility?

Who owns the sperm once it has been donated? In the event of a donor changing his mind, for example, can he request the remaining sperm to be destroyed? With frozen semen, women can give birth after the death of a husband or donor. What happens to the estates of donors with stored semen in a sperm bank? In 1977 a woman gave birth to a child twenty-one months after her husband's death, by being inseminated with his frozen sperm. Legally the child was not his (because it was born more than ten months after death, the present legal limit), but biologically it was! How long does an executor of a will wait until he is satisfied that there will be no more posthumous conceptions? What if a series of children are born to different women over a period of years by a donor who has died before their conception? Some have even suggested that using the semen of a deceased donor is the safest way to protect the donor against a paternity suit. In France, a widow had to sue to obtain sperm that her deceased husband had banked prior to undergoing chemotherapy treatment; that was 1984!

Who owns the embryo when it is donated by one woman and transferred to the uterus of another? How will ownership of the in vitro embryo be decided and how will that affect the in vivo embryo? Will a man be able to prevent an abortion because he is the joint owner of the embryo even if the woman doesn't want to continue the pregnancy? Each side plays its own semantic game with regard to the "right to life" and "right to choose."

It is not surprising that these situations give headaches to lawyers and clinicians, as well as the infertile couples. Blizzard, a DI father, warned:

> People receiving DI are inevitably taking great risks and entering a difficult, largely uncharted, or incorrectly charted area of human experience. But, we should not assume that our proper, conventional relationships are so optimal and rewarding that we cannot afford to explore the alternatives. DI rectifies childlessness. A single, large problem is replaced by a multitude, but these are all amenable to learning, time, and thought . . . one of the most fascinating attributes a man can discover [is] namely the ability to adapt and the necessity to choose.

Unexpected Outcomes

Reproductive technology leads to all kinds of surprises and fiascos. The lack of legal precedent and social experience enlarges the mysterious dimension of the newsworthy outcomes of some assisted conceptions.

Another widely publicized case in 1984 resulted after the death of a couple who were in the process of IVF. Their embryo, awaiting implantation in the biological mother (now deceased), lay in the deep freeze in Melbourne, Australia. The world watched with suspense to see what the legal outcome would be. As Bernard Dickens of the Toronto Law School remarked at the 1984 American Society of Law and Medicine Congress in Boston, "Is it a case of the gametes inheriting the estate or the estate inheriting the gametes?" (The Rios couple were millionaires.) Finally, the Victorian parliament decided that the embryo should be discarded, as the law has not yet decided the status of gametes.

Another newsworthy case involved a surrogate mother whose baby was microcephalic, born with a small head and brain indicating mental retardation. This infant was put in a foster home because both the contracting father and the surrogate mother disclaimed him. However, blood tests proved that the surrogate mother's husband was the real biological father of the child, and on the *Phil Donahue Show* the Stiver couple promised to bring up this child as it was their own. Mr. Malahoff, the semen donor, who contracted with Mrs. Stiver to carry his child, had hoped that a child would reunite him and his wife following their marital separation.

Several of the six hundred surrogate mothers (according to an estimate quoted in the June 1987 *Life*) have decided to keep the baby and not to turn it over to the infertile couple as contracted. The mothers have succeeded in retaining their offspring until the notorious Baby M case in 1987 ended in a court judgment upholding the contract and forcing the surrogate mother to relinquish her child to the sperm donor and his wife. Many feel, and I share their opinion, that the mother should have the right to change her mind after the birth, as do mothers relinquishing their babies for adoption. Another possibility is a compromise, such as a joint custody, because the child is the product of two biological parents and the husband of the contracting couple in this case is the child's genetic father. Perhaps if Whitehead had been called a *birthmother* (and she *is* the mother; Mrs. Stern is the surrogate), the biological tie would have been emphasized and the contract may not have been upheld. Indeed, proposed legislation in Michigan would allow the mother a period of twenty days to seek a court order to negate the agreement and return custody to her. The publicity around this case has served to bring the humanistic aspects of reproductive technology squarely before the public's attention.

Outcomes may be even more bizarre in the future unless both the public and the professionals can work together on developing guidelines. Unfortunately, the solutions in sight seem few, and too simplistic. It is difficult for legislatures to take action when the basic ethical and moral issues are in such a quandary.

Attitudes to DI

Artificial insemination by donor was the first type of collaborative reproduction to be developed. It is the oldest and the simplest to perform of the reproductive technologies. But its implications are enormous. As Mark Frankel has said, "DI is a technology in search of a policy" and is practiced in inequity.

The procedure of DI has been almost exclusively the domain of the medical profession, which has concentrated more on how to control the biological variables than on worrying about the social and psychological dimensions, short and long term, for parents, donor, and child. The emphasis has been much more on the creation than the result. Artificial insemination by donor is considered acceptable medical practice, particularly when government health care services or private insurance pays for it. However, the practice may be objectionable to some physicians, as it is to segments of the public, on moral or religious grounds. Also, both physicians and infertile couples may avoid DI because of the legal uncertainties.

Some people will always condemn DI outright. Others may approve of DI in principle, but it may not be morally acceptable to them under all conditions (such as single women), or some may even fear that such a procedure paves the way to artificial wombs and genetic engineering. Those who think DI is wrong obviously will not use the procedure, but their attitude may affect people who see it as their last hope. Even couples who have no religious views on the matter can feel personally oppressed by the strong adversarial position of those who oppose the practice of DI.

However, moral views of one group in the community are not sufficient to restrict the reproductive rights of others or to justify state interference. That is, just because something may now be seen by certain people to be immoral, does not necessarily make it illegal. Within this century great social change has already occurred with regard to contraception, as Julian Huxley noted after a 1961 international gathering to pay tribute to Margaret Sanger. A pioneer of birth control, she actually received a jail sentence in 1917 for just providing *information* about contraception.

As attorney Walter Wadlington, in his 1970 article "Artificial Insemination: The Dangers of a Poorly Kept Secret," commented:

> It is in part because of the staggering conceptual problems which artificial insemination poses that some have chosen to sweep it under the rug as long as this could be done, particularly during a time when it was considered that the practice was minimal. Of course the issues involved had far-reaching consequences for the institutions and values which the law has traditionally protected.

Public Opinion About DI

Until recently, public awareness of reproductive technology was limited more or less to the use of artificial insemination for livestock. If the average person had read anything about DI, it was probably about the actual procedure, such as the shortage of donors, or nowadays, some genealogical catastrophe.

Donor insemination has remained cloaked in secrecy and therefore does not arouse the same public energy as divorce or abortion. Also, more people are affected by divorce and abortion, although individuals who are not personally involved in such experiences have opinions and interests to express in public. No such advocacy has been forthcoming from pressure groups concerning the rights of the DI child. They themselves have not formed a pressure group, as the truth of their status is, in almost all cases, withheld from them.

A 1950 survey of student attitudes to DI at the University of Colorado found only 52 percent approved of DI, and a 1970 national poll found a 55-percent approval of DI, an increase of only 3 percent over twenty years. In contrast, a 1969 Harris poll found that only 35 percent approved of DI for infertile couples.

In 1974 *Science* reported an unpublished survey of eighty-eight randomly selected unmarried women aged eighteen to thirty-three. Only 14 percent supported DI or IVF using *anonymous* sperm donors.

A 1976 survey in France found that only 32 percent of those polled both knew about DI *and* approved of it. When asked if any medical or social means possible were acceptable to overcome infertility, 44 percent approved of DI, but of those who did not generally approve of assisted conceptions, only 11 percent approved of DI. Respondents who accepted DI did so because it allowed the wife to be "really" the mother. However, concern was expressed that the child would be only the mother's, and not her husband's, and also that undesirable traits might be passed down from the donor.

Matteson and Terranova (1977) investigated the acceptability of various reproductive technologies to forty-five female undergraduates in the United States. Techniques that maintained the genetic relatedness of both partners were the overwhelming choice, and the subjects indicated that they would seldom choose donor eggs or sperm.

A 1983 study of medical students by Leiblum and Barbrack at Rutgers University showed that they had generally positive attitudes toward DI; 62 percent approved of DI for single women, with 50 percent supporting DI for lesbians. Eighty-two percent of infertile couples interviewed in the Rutgers study felt that single women should have access to DI, and 50 percent of them thought lesbians should have access to DI as well. This survey also showed that there are many areas of disagreement among prospective physicians about the merits and indications for DI. On the other hand, infertile couples are often very well-informed and positive about DI, much more so than student physicians. Females in the survey were more positive than males (no doubt, because DI allows a woman to experience pregnancy and birth).

In a 1984 poll in Australia, 51 percent of Australians approved of DI to create "test-tube babies" (IVF) compared with 42 percent in 1980. Age was a significant factor; only 38 percent of the forty-and-over group approved the use of donor sperm compared with 63 percent of the sixteen-to-thirty-nine age group. However 72 percent felt that the use of donor sperm should be curtailed until all the legal problems are resolved.

Joseph Blizzard wrote that while the procedure is just a means to an end, the "implications are daunting enough for the most accomplished intellect and the most phlegmatic disposition." He observes that

> professional training, whether legal or psychiatric, and religious study, limit the dimensions over which an issue like DI can be explored. It is evident that where DI is considered within these contexts, the learned conclusions are most likely to be prohibitions . . . inappropriate sources of comment and sanction . . . and cannot be taken too seriously or exclusively.

> Distaste and overt or implicit objections are expressed by some of our most powerful social institutions and to stand confident in the face of their condemnation requires qualities that are hard to earn and information that is hard to find.

Religious Objections

The position of the various churches ranges from reticence to reprimand with regard to DI. Religious organizations tend to shy away from recommending regulation because that would imply an undesirable degree of official control. Instead, the decision to become involved in DI is left up to the conscience of the individual member. Realizing that prohibition is unenforceable, the churches try to balance the importance of responsible parenthood and the exclusivity of the marital relationship. Their rationalization is that DI just supplies the genetic material. Usually Protestant churches accept "donor assistance" to a functioning marriage as a last resort.

Depersonalization of human sexuality and a violation of the marriage are the major religious conflicts with DI. Another objection to DI is that the donor abandons all responsibility in an area of human activity that normally demands a maximum commitment.

It is the general view of orthodox Jewry and most Christian churches that the relationship between marriage and procreation is so strong and exclusive that any invasion of it is always wrong. The point is also often made that a couple marries "for better or for worse" and "in sickness and in health." Yet the marriage commitment doesn't prevent a couple from seeking to remedy a disease or to better some adverse condition. Thus, by logical extension there should be no problem in seeking "medical treatment" for infertility.

Judaism

Orthodox Judaism opposes DI as an evil without reservation, considering it an "act of hideousness and an abomination of Egypt." The reasons are primarily moral. There is concern that allowing DI might lead to its abuse, no matter how great the benefit might be in individual cases. Fears include an increase in incestuous marriages, an increase in promiscuity, and the possibility of women "satisfying their craving for children without husband or home." Jewish law bans the conjugal relationship with a husband if a wife is carrying another man's child. Donor insemination is also opposed because it would free the child's progenitor of the levirate bond (to marry the widow of a brother or next of kin especially if there are no sons). However, Conservative and Reform Judaism accept the procedure for overcoming infertility, and Israel has several DI programs and sperm banks.

Catholicism

Catholics may not be donors nor receive donor sperm. The Roman Catholic church's position has been a powerful barrier to the passage of legislation in many countries. Pronouncements beginning in 1897, and carried on by Pope Pius XII in 1949 and Pope Paul VI in 1968, reject DI absolutely. In 1987 the Vatican reaffirmed its condemnation of DI and other practices relating to contraception and reproductive technology. The majority of Catholic theological opinion opposes not only DI but also artificial insemination with the husband's sperm. The church's position is based on an unwillingness to tamper with God's universe, but this view, of course, does not take into account man's creativity in solving his earthly problems, including many life-saving medical procedures. The church views DI as immoral because it combines both the evils of masturbation and adultery (despite the mutual agreement of all the parties involved). All of the medically practical means of obtaining semen are considered "pollution." Any separation of the germ cells from the generative organs is "intrinsically sinful" and therefore wrong, no matter what it seeks to accomplish. (One writer suggested that donor semen could be taken from another woman's vagina to overcome this obstacle!)

The church's arguments have been pronounced specious because they rest on an "independent evil of separation." G. R. Dunstan, a professor of theology in London at the Anglican University, King's College, commented on the Catholic position. He points out that it is for circumstantial reasons that the procreative objective of coitus (one action) has to be attained by the means of two separate actions, masturbation and insemination. The separate moral considerations of those circumstances are the central problem for the Catholic church. However, in DI this separation still leads to the birth of children that the separation was considered sinful for preventing! Furthermore, the Church emphasizes that only persons united in an indissoluble monogamous marriage have the right to beget children.

Others have pointed out that although DI disassociates procreation from conjugal love, the relationship continues for the couple, and the arrangement for the genetic component of their child is done of their consensual free choice, and can be seen as part of the love that the couple expresses for each other. Although the semen used is disassociated from conjugal love, the donor is not simply engaging in masturbation for its own sake, but giving semen for a worthy cause.

The situation with a known donor is much less mechanical. First there is a personal relationship, usually with a married couple agreeing that the man's sperm is to be given to another couple in order for them to have a child. This is very different from an anonymous student selling his sperm for twenty-five dollars and fading into oblivion.

Statistics show that many Catholics, however, do avail themselves of DI. Many Catholic countries such as France, Spain, and Italy have DI programs. Catholics come to terms with DI in much the same way that they resolve the issue of birth control.

However, since the 1987 condemnation by the Vatican of non-coital reproduction, sperm banks have noted a drop in their Catholic donors. The infertile Catholic couples continue with DI, nevertheless, but with a "heavy heart" at disobeying their church's command.

Church of England

In contrast with the Roman Catholic church, the Anglican Church of Australia is realistic in recognizing that DI, rather than diminishing, is on the increase. Arguing from a more constructive position, it has pressed for protection of the interests of the child.

The 1983 Social Responsibilities Commission of the Anglican church in Australia reaffirmed that DI is inconsistent with the Christian moral tradition, where marriage is understood as the exclusive relationship between husband and wife. However, it stated:

> While we recognize that there is no adulterous intent involved in the process of DI it nevertheless involves the intrusion of a third party into the intimate sphere of the marital state as represented by his sperm, i.e., his reproductive capacity.

It recognizes the reality, however, that DI is occurring and calls upon the government to legislate regulation of the practice.

The commission recommended that DI children should be told of their true origins because "deception is damaging to both the parents and the child." Archbishop Rayner of Adelaide emphasized that the call for DI children to be told of their true origins was a very important part of the statement.

> I understand that an integral part of present practice is for the anonymity of donors to be entirely preserved and records destroyed. While I understand the reasons for this, it removes from a child a natural right to know his origins. I do not agree with the principle of DI at all. If, however, programs are to exist in our hospitals, it should only be with the preservation of the right of the child to be given information about his origins when he comes to an appropriate age. . . . Donors should sign a contract to make their identity available to children who might seek them out. Hospitals should be prohibited from destroying donor records. We must also consider the questions of origins and rights of the child produced by DI. Any person is entitled to know something of their personal inheritance, their history, which includes their full genetic background. At present the focus is more or less entirely on the needs of the married couple who make use of the process and there is insufficient consideration given to the child so conceived who might, in later life, wish to know in full his or her origins. This right is presently acknowledged in the case of adopted children. Why then should we deliberately contrive to cause human beings to be born who are denied any chance of knowing their full biography?

The Anglican Archbishop of Canterbury, as long ago as 1948, commented:

If it is of such fundamental importance that certain facts shall be concealed, it is prudent (to say no more) to subject those facts to special and searching scrutiny. It is axiomatic for the champions of DI that secrecy shall be absolute and continuous; this, in a manner which touches the very springs of physical life, the family's pride in its stock, and the community's concern for its future genetic constitution is contrary to the established and unwavering tradition of every known society.

The Three "D"s:
Deception, Dishonesty, Denial

It is because DI is the most private of the reproductive technologies that this privacy has moved into the realm of secrecy. A couple can pretend that the pregnancy is wholly theirs, and can get away with it. This has led to deception in many dimensions. The child is denied the truth and knowledge of her paternal genes; medical records are dishonest and/or destroyed, birth registers are falsified, family and social relationships are based on deception, and the existence of the donor is denied. In addition, the secrecy prevents any real exploration of the outcome for the individuals involved, especially adverse effects. In DI and surrogate mothering, one half of the child's biological origins is a blank. But in IVF, with both donor eggs and donor sperm being used, both halves of a child's origins could be a blank. The resulting child would have neither a legal trail nor a genetic map of her biological heritage. The third National Conference on Adoption in Adelaide, Australia, strongly condemned the practice of secrecy and recommended community education, support groups, and counseling of infertile couples to combat the practice.

The degree of secrecy goes beyond the confidentiality that is normal within a physician-patient relationship. The secrecy extends to the donor, who, even more, remains anonymous. In at least two thirds of the patients confidentiality in the physician's office may be so extreme that there is no documentation of the DI, or whatever records do exist might later be destroyed. This secrecy affects the relationship between the practitioner and other medical colleagues too. Further collusion occurs, albeit often unknowingly, between these parties with falsification of the birth certificate. Kleegman (1954), a DI practitioner in New York, wrote:

> The couple is also counseled against sharing this confidence with anyone—friends or relatives. If the confidence of such contemplated action has already been shared before coming to me, they are advised to inform their confidant that they are starting with a new physician who is referring the husband for further tests and treatment. In order to give the couple a reality background for such a statement, the husband is referred to a urologist for an additional checkup. Then, should a pregnancy result, family and friends accept the child as the lawful issue of the husband and wife.

Anonymity of the donor is always presumed essential to guarantee a supply of semen. This anonymity completes the secret circle by denying the child and the donor any knowledge of their mutual genetic connection. The medical community has a vested interest in maintaining anonymity because the donors, in the United States, come primarily from medical schools. The physicians today who run the clinics and insist on anonymity may have been donors themselves in the past. They take care that the donor's name will never be on a recipient's chart, because medical students become obstetric interns. In a 1975 article Strickler stressed that

> the primary advantage of artificial insemination over adoption in our point of view is that the child need not be informed of the circumstance surrounding his or her conception. We believe quite strongly that the family unit is not a mere biologic relation, but rather primarily involves a deep emotional involvement between parents and child regardless of the circumstances of conception.

Finegold adopts a double standard in his book with regard to physicians and couples.

> Should there be any religious, moral, or professional qualms in his makeup, the physician should never execute artificial insemination procedures. On the other hand, a gynecologist-sterologist, who believes that his DI performances are ethical, righteous, and beneficial, should carry out his practice *overtly. By operating clandestinely, the inseminator, fearing the resentment and wrath of his colleagues, will find the stress psychologically disturbing.* [italics mine]

No wonder couples undergoing DI find it a stressful procedure! No wonder they fear the "resentment and wrath" of the child if she should ever find out she was conceived under such questionable ethics.

Finegold continues:

> An applicant for DI should be honest and should stand in *good repute morally.* Another important trait for which we must search is the ability of the pair to keep confidences. One of the great values of DI is its secrecy. Couples who expose to friends and relatives the fact that their child is not the biological issue of the husband must not be invited to partake of the procedure. [italics mine]

It is difficult to believe that trained professionals could think this way, let alone publish such thoughts as guidelines!

Professor Dunstan (1976) observes that

> it is a matter for serious concern that a medical practice, grounded on scientific research and so upon a high value put upon truth, should in fact result in, and to some extent require, deceit and uncertainty. The secrecy involved in DI obliges the practitioner, the husband and wife, and the donor to conspire together to deceive the child and society as to the child's true parentage, his genetic identity. Truth is violated, credibility is undermined; and this is a serious ethical matter. . . . existing legal categories have had to be bent, and even actively misused, in order to accommodate its consequences.

> Undoubtedly DI adults will increasingly assert a right to know their own identity, particularly as the spread of DI undermines the security of an unquestioned assumed parentage; and I see no grounds on which that right can be denied them. It may be that those who give semen, and those who receive, must soon do so on the understanding that some day their action will be known.

The moral question of the child's right to know her full genetic heritage is just as important to her as her legal rights. Daniel Wikler, professor of philosophy and medical ethics at the University of Wisconsin, told the Boston *Phoenix* (December 11, 1984):

> The ability to trace ancestry is a foundation underlying many parts of society. The threat is that if you shake the foundation, a lot else is going to be jounced about.

Although DI couples may prefer to conceal the infertility, without the donor they would not have had their child. As one donor said, "It is with *my* sperm that *their* child is conceived." That self-evident fact is always overlooked in those who practice secrecy. The excuse is often given that there is no point in telling the child about the DI conception because there are no more details available (such as the identity of the donor). One couple stressed that to tell the child "would serve absolutely no useful purpose whatsoever." Because the infertile couple was forced to compromise in order to have a baby, they then compromise their child's right to the truth for their own self-protection. It is like the situation where adoptive parents destroy the original birth certificate and thereby feel that they have eradicated the circumstances of their child's birth and erased his heritage.

As a physical therapist who has worked with disabled persons, I feel it is hard to go through life with a visible handicap, and endure the stares as well as the inconvenient access to most activities of daily living. These indignities are suffered because disabled and retarded people have been concealed from the public, which views them as outcasts; stigma is the price they pay. Only recently have the disabled united to make their claims heard as they demand their integration into the community. Infertility is an invisible handicap protected by the assumption of paternity according to patriarchal social norms. The traditional cloud of secrecy prevents the public from being informed about the scope of practice of DI. If there is strong community feeling that DI is wrong, then there will be continued pressure for secrecy by the participants in the procedure. Yet that secrecy contributes to the stigma. This is a vicious cycle that must be broken by honest communication. Considering the rapid changes in the past decade in social and sexual mores, DI is due—overdue—to come out of the closet.

Parents guard the secret of DI so closely (in contrast to parents by adoption) that very few of the hundreds of thousands of DI adults in the United States know their status, and only a few have expressed their feelings publicly. Relatives are rarely told of the child's origins. Occasionally the truth has even been withheld from the husband, and in a couple of reported cases, from the woman herself! Much of this deception is rationalized on the grounds that the social father is the one who really raises the child. That is undoubtedly true. However, those who emphasize the social aspects of parenting, and casually refer to DI as "adopting sperm" or a mere "fertilizing agent," are never individuals whose own genealogy is in question.

> Infertility, like blindness or any other physical incapacity, is sad. But just as the blind have no legal or moral rights to be cured with another's eyes, the infertile have no right to cure their infertility with another's child. No child should be created as a product to be sold.
>
> —*Carole Anderson*

Interestingly, some physicians writing on DI refer to the past practice of allowing couples to select their own donors, often family members. It was never explained why the practice was discontinued, and while some physicians will accommodate this, especially for ethnic minorities, most stand aghast at the thought.

When it becomes accepted that the DI child should have the same rights as does an adopted child to know his or her biological origins, the whole framework of deception will no longer be necessary. Adoptive parents are not discouraged because they are expected to inform the child of his status; on the contrary, there are waiting lists for babies available for adoption.

Maintaining Records

With the increase in assisted conceptions, social identity and family history are becoming less reliable evidence of genetic constitution and continuity. Achilles (1986) points out that the "onus of keeping records is not necessarily a legal one since donors are arguably not patients. The Ontario Law Reform Commission (1985) has recommended that "donors are patients for the purpose of record keeping."

In the doctors' fantasy, sperm and ova shall be anonymous; no messy adulterous relationships and multiple parentings will occur. Only the professionals will know who anybody really is, and they, like priests in the confessional, will never tell. Old-fashioned lawyers, like Lord Denning, will muse that a child has a right to know its "real" parents, even though it was English law until recently that adopted children could not be told who their biological parents were and many children know less than their mothers about their "real" father.

—Germaine Greer

Curie-Cohen found that while 92 percent of physicians kept permanent records on the recipients of DI, only 27 percent did on the children born, and only 30 percent did so on the donors. Eighty-three percent opposed any legislation that would mandate records for fear it would make protection of the donor more difficult. But with computers being used to store patients' records that privacy of information is already being threatened. Also, donors at public clinics—especially regular ones—become known to the staffs of private physicians. When I enquired of one nurse if she could trace donors despite the lack of records, she said that by looking back in the cash-receipt books she would be able to correlate a donor with a woman who came for DI that day.

The legal protection of confidentiality between physician and patient does not extend to nurses, social workers, psychologists, and other such professionals. These persons, if required by a court, could not refuse to name a donor, if they knew him. Not all states even guarantee physician-patient privileges. In those states that do, if confidentiality is waived by the patient or the donor, the physician has to answer in a court of law. Thus he would be forced to breach the confidentiality he had promised to the couple and to the donor, if he knows who the donor is.

The late Dr. Alan Guttmacher (1962), one of the famous early pioneers in DI, advised his colleagues to:

Forget signed papers . . . Signed papers serve no purpose and act as a memorial that the child was not conceived through natural means. If the patients are carefully selected, contracts and agreements are unnecessary, and simply act as a permanent reminder of something which should be forgotten as quickly and completely as possible. In the ideal case, by the time the patient reaches term (of pregnancy), the woman, the husband, and the doctor have to think twice to remember that the pregnancy is physically not the husband's for psychically it has become his.

Bayles (1984) also argues against record keeping:

Like many other people, DI children may desire to know their biological parents. Such a desire is emphasized in adoption situations. But is this desire a rational one? Finding out who one's genetic father is means learning his personal identity. *Why would that be important?* The mere knowledge does not entitle one to inheritance, other financial support, or love. What one's genetic father is or was—criminal, actor, politician, industrial worker—does not, except for certain genetic traits, determine or indicate what type of person one is or is going to become. Thus, although this desire is not necessarily irrational, if one fully understands what is involved in such information and its implications for one's own life, it would probably not be a strong desire. Much of the current interest is probably culturally conditioned (and exaggerated by the media). In addition, DI children may be significantly concerned about the possibility of inheriting a genetic disease. Such a concern is certainly rational, but fulfilling it does not require learning the donor's identity. . . . Overall it appears that retaining records of the personal identity of donors after all children have been born from their donations is *not worth the effort.* [italics mine]

If DI fathers are hardly ever interviewed, how does Guttmacher know? In contrast, my husband feels it is important to his integrity that he not misrepresent himself as a biological father to close friends. That does not mean he is any the less of a social/rearing father.

Niels Lauerson writes in his book that he is "far too busy" to record the five to six inseminations a month he does in his office! Haman (1954), in the *Journal of Urology,* advises that consent forms be placed in a safe deposit box to be destroyed in the event of his death—without opening the box.

Not only physicians are so short-sighted. The *Indiana Law*

Journal made the statement that the only real advantage to keeping records is that in their absence the husband might be able to prove that the child is not his. The *Journal* continues naïvely:

> Couples who receive DI are so carefully chosen, however, that there is little chance that this will happen, and doctors may feel that the small risk is outweighed by the advantage of complete secrecy.

The *Journal* speculates that the need for records would be further reduced if even more care were taken in selecting donors (such as the same blood group and Rh factor). The conclusion is that

> in view of the small chance that official records would ever be needed and of the damage they could do, there does not seem to be sufficient reason to prevent doctors from keeping whatever records they consider best.

In Dunstan's view, the practitioner of DI "cannot but regard as paramount the interest of the child which his agency would bring into being." The most crucial aspect of records is that without them the child will never, under any circumstances, be able to determine her genetic father. In the opinion of George Annas (1980), professor of health law at the Boston University School of Medicine:

> The most that can be said for such a policy is that it is in the best interests of the donor. But this is simply not good enough. The donor has a choice in the matter, the child has none. The donor and physician can take steps to guard their own best interests, the child cannot.

I believe that permanent records should be kept on all donors that are used, even while the debate over their existence continues. As well as the identity of the donor, details should include the physical and mental characteristics of donors, any genetic tests, the number of inseminations with their sperm, and the number of successful pregnancies. This way, at least the records will be there when the offspring and researchers decide they need them. Legislation requiring court filing may be necessary, in view of the reluctance of the medical profession to maintain records on DI.

Sealed records protect the confidentiality of all parties concerned, and in most states are "subject to inspection only upon an order of the court for good cause shown." Ironically, as was the case in adoption, the birth child is usually the last person to be allowed access to the information, as many judges never find "good cause." It has been suggested that the record should be available only to the child, or only upon the death of the donor, or only when he has waived his right to privacy in the matter.

Housing records in a central registry creates problems. In all adoptions completed after May 7, 1982, the Department of Health and Social Services is required to maintain a central file of the medical and genetic information contained in court reports submitted by agencies at the time of termination of parental rights. The central registry, however, has made the process of searching for genealogical information slow, cumbersome, and expensive, and adoption activists are not happy with this system. Donor records are best kept in the town or state where the insemination took place.

Records are essential not only for genealogical but for genetic information. Children conceived by DI have a right to know what genetic diseases they may carry or inherit. It is important enough for *every* donor to be asked about his family medical history, but the DI child will never be able to answer those questions. Adoptees have experienced great anguish and frustration at missing half their medical history when their offspring have been born with hereditary conditions. Annas concludes that "congenital disability is much more likely to affect the life of a real child than the highly speculative lawsuit is to affect a donor."

> Documentation . . . is done so that no one can take advantage of any other party.
>
> —*Mary J. Rillera and Sharon Kaplan,*
> *Cooperative Adoption*

Any social, psychological, or genetic research on donors and recipients requires records. In the event of a genetic condition in a DI child, the donor, and any other offspring of that donor, natural or through DI, should be notified. If DI is being done because of a genetic disease in the mother's husband rather than for his infertility, then the child is often told. One case involved a DI boy who witnessed his father's demise through Huntington's disease with tremendous fear and anxiety, until it was finally explained to him he did not inherit his father's genes.

Melvin Taymor, clinical professor of obstetrics and gynecology at Harvard Medical School, disagrees. Quoted in *Science News*, September 1, 1979, he said

> I would like to see more evidence that there is genetic or other harm to offspring before such secrecy is removed. I think that opening the records of sperm donors would cause tremendous harm.

Evidence of genetic harm has already occurred. In England, according to Foss in Bristol, a woman who had a normal child through DI because her husband had fibrocystic kidney disease, later had a second child with another donor, and that child developed fibrocystic kidney disease. Two couples who had DI for eugenic reasons conceived a child with Tay-Sachs disease. I was told of a DI child in Australia who was born with a rare genetic defect. It so happened that the pediatric resident taking care of the infant in the hospital was, unknowingly, the donor. Rather than alert the donor to his relationship with the patient, the DI service at that hospital continued to accept his regular semen donations but flushed them down the sink. Nobody in the triangle was informed of the truth in that genetic mishap.

Falsification of the Birth Certificate

When a DI child is born to a married couple, the birth certificate is entered with the husband's name. This covers up the fact that DI took place, makes the child legitimate, and protects the donor. (Of course, often the obstetrician is not aware of the DI, and the donor's name is invariably unknown.) Interestingly, it is not the actual *fact* of illegitimacy that bothers infertile couples as much as the possibility of anyone *knowing* this fact. This shows the tremendous social pressure most DI recipients feel to appear a "normal" family, conforming in every way possible.

The false birth certificate deceives the child and her relatives as to her identity. Subsequent generations may also be deceived when the false identity affects inheritance, custody, and support. Understandably, a married couple does not want to put "unknown" in the space for "father," although this is invariably the case. With a known donor, parents are equally as reluctant to put his name, especially when the parties have contracted that the donor shall be free of all liability. For that reason, my husband's name was routinely entered on the birth certificate. As our donor is known, and we have told our child, the certificate merely conformed with the laws in Ontario, where any child born during a marriage is considered a child of the marriage.

Although most physicians consider a false birth certificate to be just a white lie or a "mild falsehood," it can be a problem for those who do not like to put their signature knowingly to an untruth. It is no argument that this happens anyway with extramarital conceptions, and that the number of false entries made on behalf of DI children is probably much less than for illegitimate children naturally conceived. As Dunstan reiterates:

> Here we are dealing with a professional practice, with what a physician, whose science is grounded in truth, is asked to do professionally, in circumstances of which the outcome is untruth, injustice, or both.

Furthermore, the false certificate does not really guarantee legitimacy. A court will investigate the real nature of the situation, if necessary. The document will be invalidated if the truth is disclosed. Legitimacy will be revoked, in many jurisdictions, if the paternity of the child is challenged or if the father disowns the child. Even where state legislation has taken care of these problems, and blood descent is not the qualifying criterion for legitimacy, it still does not guarantee the child knowledge of his or her biological origins—the critical issue. Likewise, single women and lesbians prefer to put "unknown" in order to avoid a potential paternity suit; again it is the child who suffers.

Gynecologists have tried to deal with this deception in three ways. One is to mix the semen with that of the husband, or to advise the couple to have intercourse right after the DI, in order that all the parties may fantasize that the husband is responsible for the conception. Another option is to refer the pregnant couple to a different physician for obstetric care, and as Dr. Shields (1950) explained:

> There is no problem because it has not yet become routine for an obstetrician to ask the patient "Is this your husband's child?" He assumes that it is, and proceeds on that assumption.

The challenge is to ensure that the correct information is recorded for the child and posterity. One solution is to redesign the birth certificates so that a distinction can be made between *pater* (the social or accepting father) and *genitor* (the biological father). These options would be convenient not just for DI children, but in cases where a woman marries or remarries while she is pregnant with a naturally conceived offspring. Another suggestion is to record the child's social parents on one register while a separate register would record the child's genetic descent. Like the adoption register, inspection would be restricted to those who could show a "just and compelling interest."

The CUB position paper states that any person created by nontraditional reproduction should have full knowledge of how (s)he came to be and of the identities of his or her parents. A national task force was formed by the Child Welfare League in 1987 to investigate these issues.

Professor Dunstan (1973) suggests:

> Such a provision . . . would better serve the public interest in social identity; it would lessen the incitement to falsification and deceit which impugns the worth of the present registration; it would give reliable general data for genetic research and counselling and—assuming that the practice of DI will continue, and possibly be extended—it would provide material for an objective assessment of the practice.

As is known from blood-group research, the birth register is more social than genetic. Studies in the United States and England have found that from 14 to 30 percent of the children in the samples under investigation could not have been the offspring of their putative fathers.

Rights of Heterosexual and Lesbian Single Women, Lesbian Couples, Disabled and Poor Women

Paradoxically, the law has recognized a single person's right not to procreate, but not his or her right to procreate. Studies show a middle-class bias in selecting adoptive parents (and also recipients of organ transplants). Single women may avoid involuntary sterilization, and have access to contraception and abortion. They also have the right to carry a child to term, to rear a child, and even to adopt in some jurisdictions. Prior to two 1972 U.S. Supreme Court decisions, a single mother could by herself give consent to adoption—the child was considered fatherless. But the courts "have not squarely decided whether these persons have a right to conceive through sexual intercourse," or DI. Robertson writes that strong arguments can be made for extending to single persons the right to conceive.

Many physicians have moral objections and believe that every baby has a right to a "father." In the sixties it was generally felt that DI for an unmarried woman conflicted with the social order and was "inadmissible on medical ethical grounds." In 1972 a British physician, Sandler, wrote that he would not provide DI for a "spinster, a couple of mixed colour, or even of mixed religious denomination." However, the times are slowly changing. In 1970, 90 percent of single mothers surrendered their babies for adoption because they were made to believe, with the same arguments used today, that they could not adequately raise their children. Yet by 1980, less than 10 percent of single mothers gave up their babies.

One professor of obstetrics and gynecology says that the way a patient approaches the doctor would make a difference.

> If a patient comes marching in and demands her right to be a mother outside of marriage, maybe you would stop and think and not do it. But the case of a "thirty-nine-year-old professional woman, who owns a company and is a phenomenal success and has a tremendous need for being a mother," might be viewed quite differently.

While the economic burdens of single motherhood are very real, this is a typical example of the inequal access to DI and other reproductive technologies. Stanley Friedman of the Tyler Medical Clinic in Westwood, Los Angeles admitted, "I guess we do make a moral judgment [with a single woman] that we don't with a couple. . . . With the working couple, as long as they can pay our regular fees, that's about it."

Although it is most unlikely that any court would hold a physician who performed DI liable for child support, for this reason too, some physicians are afraid to provide DI for single women. Dr. William Karow of West Los Angeles told the *Daily News* in 1982 that he fears that if he performs DI on single women, the child could one day sue him as the "instrument of conception." He points out that when a married woman is inseminated in California, the husband must consent to become the legal father, but when a single woman is inseminated in California, there is no legal father. Gena Corea observed in *The Mother Machine* how the role of the sperm donor may "expand" (as in court cases where a donor has sued for visitation rights), but when a married couple is involved, the donor's status "shrinks to one akin to a blood donor."

If consent of spouse becomes a legal requirement for DI offered to married women, this may operate to prohibit single women from having access to the procedure, unless their rights are spelled out. Some women then may be forced to fraudulently present a "husband," as has happened in Quebec.

While many could consider marriage the optimum environment for raising a child, the rising divorce rate indicates that the nuclear family is becoming more and more unstable. Half of American children are likely to spend some years of their life in a one-parent home or with a step-parent, and one third of Australian children will do so as well. Thirty-five million American children now live in stepfamilies. The number of never-married mothers (including teenagers) increased fourfold between 1970 and 1983. The number of homes comprised of two or more unrelated people rose by 73.5 percent between 1970 and 1980. Also, 21 percent of single women interviewed for the 1980 U.S. Census said they planned to have no children. This is a sign that many members of the "me generation" may be abandoning not just the old, but the young as well. Perhaps child-raising should be supported by all those who wish it regardless of their marital status? In 1979, a survey found that 75 percent of Americans agreed that it is morally acceptable to be single and have children.

As women become more assertive and financially independent, more of them will postpone marriage or look for alternatives. Statistics show there are fewer and later first marriages. The New York–based Single Mothers by Choice is an organization of women who are mainly thirty-five and older. Ninety-nine percent are heterosexual, and feel that time is running out for them to fulfill this aspect of their biological potential. In most cases, such single women have carefully contemplated the issues of parenting and made careful financial plans. About half use DI to conceive. A great number of single women have been referred from the Feminist Women's Health Center in Hollywood to the Southern California Cryobank in Century City and have expressed interest in the Alternative Parenting Network in Venice. Indeed, ten percent of the DI practitioners who responded to Curie-Cohen's survey inseminated single women.

Germaine Greer (1985) observed:

> It is the English law that a father cannot legitimize his own child except by legally adopting it, but many thousands of children have been legitimate simply because no one knew any better. Since time immemorial, sisters have borne children for their sisters and servant girls for their mistresses, but *homo occidentalis* now thinks such rich confusion unhealthy, clinging to a notion of the "normal" "nuclear" "heterosexual" family which will be realized by fewer and fewer people.

A 1984 *Parade* magazine report gave figures that one in five babies in the United States and Sweden were born "out of wedlock." In Great Britain the number is one in six. Many married women are now single parents, created mainly by a very high divorce rate. Does it make any ethical or legal differences that single parenthood is planned instead of occurring because of the breakdown of a marriage? It is more threatening to a patriarchal society when a woman becomes a single mother by choice, rather than ending up that way through divorce, desertion, or death?

There was a case in Sweden where a single woman claimed she

had undergone DI to shelter the father of her child from support obligations. She was unsuccessful as there were no records at the hospital where she claimed the DI had been performed.

John Robertson observes:

> Procreation may be as central to a single person's identity and life-plan as it is for a married person. Single parent families are increasingly common, and there is no evidence showing that a marriage environment, though perhaps desirable, is essential for healthful child-rearing. Moreover, the right of single persons to bear and rear children that they have conceived is firmly established.

The next big question concerns the recognition of the right of single persons to procreate, which according to Robertson and Annas, does not necessarily follow given the current legal system.

The state, conventionally, has an interest in the institution of marriage and promoting the stability of the family unit. Is the concern actually about single parenthood or single marital status, or both? How are common-law spouses to be treated? At the time of this writing, a health maintenance organization in the Boston area is under fire because it will provide DI to de facto couples, even when the male is not a member of the health plan, but denies the service to single women and lesbian members. In contrast, the sperm bank associated with the Feminist Health Center in Oakland, California, has inseminated over two hundred single heterosexual and lesbian women. Most gay people know at least someone who has a DI child. Gay health-care centers generally receive a couple of enquiries each week about obtaining DI. San Francisco attorney Donna Hitchens has counseled over two hundred women about DI. A Seattle lesbian estimated that there were over one hundred DI children born to lesbians in that area by the early 1980s.

A thirty-six-year-old divorced woman sued Wayne State University for denial of the DI service, and won an out of court settlement on the basis of due process and equal protection. Even if the law did prohibit DI for single or lesbian women, how could it enforce DI that is self-administered or done with the help of a lesbian friend? In 1978 the Ethics Committee of the British Medical Association decided that it was not unethical for lesbians to have children by DI and that it should be left to the discretion of the doctor and patient. In contrast, Ellen Goodman, a *Boston Globe* columnist, condemned "reproduction without responsibility, and children without fatherhood . . . reducing fatherhood to a set of genes so that lesbians and single women can conceive a fatherless child."

Lesbians fear that they could be financially and medically penalized, for example, if human services benefits were not paid to lesbians with children whose fathers are unknown (that is, donors). Also of concern to lesbians is the fear that the relationship of a nonbiological coparent could be interrupted by a court ruling. Clearly, there is discrimination when a mother's lover is female.

Disabled women have also experienced much discrimination with regard to sexuality and reproduction. Should public assistance enable them to conceive and to support the child?

Germaine Greer speaks of women on the fringe:

> After being exposed, ripped off, and humiliated, feminists in the United States arrived at their own version of DI in which fresh sperm is inserted in the vagina with a turkey baster. The lovers, can, if they wish, make of this procedure an erotic ritual and no earthly authority can interfere with them. Infertile people do not have this option; if they develop a passionate desire to pass on their genes, or set their hearts on "having a baby," they must have recourse to haphazard evaluation procedures. Then, if they are deemed suitable cases, they agree to put themselves through painful, time-consuming, and expensive medical and surgical treatments, which are still attended by high failure rates. The doctors who choose to specialize in infertility tell us that they do so because they are so deeply moved by the unspeakable misery of childless couples (as long as they are not homosexual couples).

Lesbians generally prefer that the donor must be anonymous. It is understandable that both lesbians and donors are more vulnerable for a paternity suit, especially with a homophobic legal system, than when a married couple use DI. Lesbians fear that a known donor, or a biological relative, may have more right to the child than a lesbian partner. Courts have traditionally protected and preserved the right of a minor child to support by her father. Nevertheless, as one attorney pointed out, contracts are not as foreign to judges as DI, and while a document may acknowledge paternity, it is proved (excluded to a very high degree of probability, actually) by blood typing. The ethical dilemma here concerns a minority group who are fighting hard for their rights, yet at the same time are denying the rights of their DI children.

Margaret Somerville (1982), professor of law and professor of medicine at McGill University in Montreal, wonders whether undesirable effects may result from self-help if women cannot obtain access to DI which is regulated? (This is similar to the situation with abortion before it was legal.) Some lesbians are very concerned about what they call "street sperm," as herpes and other infections have been contracted, to say nothing of the fear of AIDS from semen donated by gay men.

Somerville is one of the first to look closely at the rights of "deviants." If DI is refused on the basis of sexual orientation, she queries, is it because "deviant" sexual orientation of the parents is known always to be shameful to any child who will be born, or is it because the physician or society disapproves of that sexual orientation and wishes to express this disapproval? What about male children being born to lesbians, are they suffering "harm"? If DI is refused on the ground of sexual orientation or marital status is it because:

1. It is better for the child itself not to be born in such circumstances?
2. It is better for the community not to have that child born, as it is likely to be a problem because the community will have to support it, or because it will become "deviant" and the community wants to suppress such "deviance"?
3. We should not support or even allow access to birth technology by persons we label as "deviant" because by doing so we are approving the deviant behavior of the parent, and approving such behavior is a threat to our community's overtly espoused values?

Is the physician under any obligation to discover the sexual orientation or marital status before providing DI? If sexual orientation affects the physician's legal obligation, what would be the situation regarding the married lesbian woman? Or what about a heterosexual woman seeking DI who is married to a homosexual man?

Parenting is considered the next phase in lesbian-gay identity. Motherhood is more supported among lesbians than fatherhood among gays, although there have been a few cases where male homosexuals have been awarded custody of children. There was a recent case where a lesbian partner did sue successfully for visitation rights of a child consensually conceived by DI. Can a child sue for having been born to a lesbian or complain of lack of parentage if the mother is single? Experts consider that a child does not need two parents as much as one really good one. The lack of a role model in lesbian units has been found to be similar to heterosexual families where the average American father spends only twelve minutes a day with his child. Wrongful life suits have been typically restricted to situations of instrinsic defects, such as an avoidable prenatal condition, instead of extrinsic factors, such as the milieu of the parent(s). However, some jurisdictions have recognized prenatal torts, and it is a matter of speculation how far the courts would go in supporting a child's suit against her parent(s) over the DI.

Children reunite their lesbian mothers with heterosexual mothers in the wider community. In her unpublished thesis Barbara Bryant's survey of 185 lesbian mothers revealed that the number of lesbians or bisexuals among their grown children was no more than among the general population. Richard Green, professor of psychiatry at the State University of New York at Stony Brook, compared the children of fifty-one lesbians and thirty-four single mothers. He found no evidence of (prepuberty) homosexuality in the vocational play of the children of lesbians. In the June 1978 issue of the *American Journal of Psychiatry,* he tentatively concluded that "children being raised by a homosexual parent do not differ appreciably from children raised in a more conventional setting on measures of sexual identity." Most of them wanted to get married and have children. This shows that the family has less influence than the powerful sex-role stereotyping impressed on children by the wider society. Many studies, but not all, show a higher ratio of males to females born with DI, which is typically done as close to ovulation as possible. This can be difficult for lesbians who generally have a strong preference for a daughter. In one study of lesbian DI children, twelve of the thirteen children were boys!

Will Reproductive Technology Increase Men's Control over Women?

History continues to prove that women's access to control over their reproduction as well as the therapy for the loss of that control (i.e., infertility) are determined by race, class, marital status, and age. Recipients of the new ways of making babies are usually required to be "deserving," "appropriate," or even to speak English. Not all of them have empty arms; some may have a child through adoption or from the wife's former marriage. Physicians in reproductive medicine are portrayed as both miracle workers and father figures, helping infertile couples who are a minority, yet talking as if they represent all couples. The compassion, "new hope," increased options, and greater reproductive freedom touted by male physicians thus remain a fiction for most women. There are also continuing conflicts between government regulation and intervention, and the right to reproductive privacy.

In addition, there is the exploitation of women that goes by the name of "research," and the new reproductive technologies are definitely experimental. This has been powerfully documented in Gena Corea's *The Mother Machine* in which the parallels with animal husbandry are disturbing.

Corea observes that by obscuring the impact of reproductive engineering on women as a class, male physicians emphasize the "rights" of the individual women to use these technologies. The developments are escalating at a rapid rate and the confusion keeps women "speechless and powerless." Semantics adds to the muddle, when research subjects are called "patients," "clinic material," or "receptacles," the experiments are named "therapy," or "procedures," and the baby is referred to as a "product," or even an "investment." Doubletalk also prevails. For example, Corea points out that embryo transfer is justified because the "real" mother is the woman who carries the baby throughout pregnancy and gives birth. But when surrogate mothering needs to be justified, the mother is simply a "living incubator," and the "real" mother is the one who raises it after birth. Maternity today is in question as paternity had been when experts equivocated as to whether fatherhood resides in sperm or social parenting.

There is no tradition of women being guaranteed the right to produce *their* own issue, as for men. In patriarchal societies, the male line is paramount, even if it means lying about DI, and the practice of DI lends itself to the deception. Legislation, as we will see in the next chapter, fits DI into the patriarchy.

However, if a woman cannot reproduce naturally, the societal pressures that define a woman's role as mother are so powerful (the coercion can be subtle) that she feels she must do so technologically, despite the pain, suffering, and unknown risks. Corea notes the similarity between women selling their vaginas, as in prostitution, and selling their wombs, as in surrogate mothering. The background is a society where bodies are what we own, rather than what we are, and paradoxically, the feminist movement's slogans of ownership have contributed to the problem. Bodies are commodities that can be sold and thus submitted to all kinds of social, sexual, and medical interventions. "Ultimately, then, the issue is not fertility. The issue is the exploitation of women," concludes Corea.

Reproductive technology is big business today—an industry in its own right, and like all businesses, it is always looking to expand its market. Like the marketing of infant formula, the product may not be in the best interests of mothers and babies. Although sperm banks operate for profit, and physicians and donors are paid, DI is one of the less profitable pursuits of gynecology. The fees from infertility investigations can be high and are one of the motivating factors for physicians to bother with the tedious business of DI. Such doctors insist on a detailed infertility workup at the outset. Some compassionate physicians, of course, genuinely want to help their patients "to banish the bitterness of barrenness" even in spite of their personal beliefs. For example, one practitioner wrote, "I must say I am not at all keen on DI . . . but who am I to play God?" Another responded to Guttmacher's 1950 survey with "few individual doctors are competent to discharge the tremendous responsibilities involved and certainly are not licensed to do so." Others clearly exult in the power of creating life and reassure their clients that "as in fine animal breeding, healthy offspring result from excellent sires."

In 1955 the American Society for the Study of Sterility voted that

> if it is in harmony with the beliefs of the couple and the doctor, donor insemination is a completely ethical, moral, and desirable form of medical therapy.

Guttmacher (1943), in recommending that DI be kept out of the "mercenary column," made the following patronizing statement:

> View it as a personal medical service, the contribution of an aesculapiad [the Greco-Roman symbol for the god of medicine] to the happiness of some wretched, worthy, sterile couple . . . When a doctor consents to do an artificial insemination from an unrelated donor, it is really the couple's insignia of good character.

As DI becomes more available, consumers will expect and demand it, just as has happened with abortion. Does a physician have a right to refuse to provide DI, especially in states where there are legislative guidelines?

Walter Wadlington notes the growing public concern over the need for more careful scrutiny and control of the medical profession as it moves into new dimensions of life and death. The potential for genetic engineering and sex selection makes the practice of DI even more significant, because of the social and political implications. Physicians controlling DI usually select their own junior colleagues for donors; they believe as Dr. Weisner did that "physicians and true scientists make ideal donors." They are thus practicing their own brand of eugenics.

The Curie-Cohen survey showed that the majority of physicians are not reliable middlemen because of their deficient knowledge and training in genetics and psychology. Although they may revel in the opportunity to create life itself, they do not have the social warrant for such decisions. Virtually no jurisdiction allows an individual to make a lone decision about the selection and placement of a child for adoption or the suitability of a couple. Those who object to the physician's "playing God" in dealing with transplants or artificial organs will see a similarity in mating a woman with an unseen semen donor chosen on a combined basis of availability and the physician's decision as to which hereditary factors are important.

The legal solutions to the challenges of reproductive technology already are reinforcing men's social control over women. Men have long controlled the technology of reproduction, be it birth control or assisted conceptions. New developments are initially promoted as increasing women's options. Choices, however, have a way of later becoming obligatory. Technology, as it gets more available and more "cost-effective," becomes used routinely. Ultrasound and Caesarean sections are examples of screening and intervention in the reproductive process that are increasing annually by their own momentum. There have been court cases over a woman's refusal to submit to surgical delivery (and in at least two cases, the women delivered vaginally despite a physician's testimony that this would be virtually impossible.) Techniques such as amniocentesis and abortion are being used for sex selection. Informal techniques for sex determination are already in use among couples, and sperm selection technologies are described in Appendix 2. This is especially a problem in countries such as India and China, with a long tradition of femicide. Polls in the United States regularly confirm that most couples prefer their first-born to be a male; males are more rewarded in our society, and even more so in other cultures. A Chinese saying describes females as "maggots in the rice." Physicians develop and promote genetic screening, which they sometimes use for eugenic reasons in DI. This is a double standard because genetic screening will be of no use at all to those DI children as they mature. These offspring may unknowingly harbor harmful genes and won't be able to recognize the symptoms without family history on the paternal side. The more a person's genetic nature is a result of the choices of others, the more she must consider herself a social product—the result of a social and political mechanism which will make increasing claims on her. On the other hand, natural selection provides more of a balance between indeterminacy and free will in a person's concept of self.

The pressure on women to undergo genetic screening to ensure a "perfect" baby may soon reach a level where to refuse it and, for example, not to go along with an embryo transfer or a donor gamete, may be seen not only as ethically irresponsible but legally incompetent.

If the new technologies are being developed for women's benefit —to increase their options—then why don't women have more say in those choices? Doctors, not women, developed DES, the pill, and the IUD, which has led to much of the infertility that the new technologies are trying to overcome. Doctors can determine who gets abortions and they decide who gives and receives semen in DI. In fact, more than half of the statutes addressing DI in the United States require this legally. As Barbara Katz Rothman notes in an article in *Test-Tube Women: What Future for Motherhood?*

> We thought the information would give us *power*. What we perhaps overlooked is that it is *power* that gives us control over both information and choice. . . . Society in its ultimate meaning may be nothing more and nothing less than the structuring of choices.

The topic of DI is discussed in conferences by predominantly male physicians and attorneys; input from consumers and DI couples or adults is conspicuous by its absence. Although clearly the situation with DI needs much improvement, it is unlikely to occur unless the reins of power change hands. Do women want laws made by men that will make DI by anyone but a physician illegal and punishable? This is already a felony in three states. Do women want men to legislate that they will never know the identity of the donor who makes it possible for them to bear a child? Most women and couples have not thought otherwise; the conflict between their right to privacy and the child's right to the truth is the central theme of this book.

Lesbians and single women fear that the donor could seek a court order to impose on them a kind of "family relationship." Some feminists feel that if donors have rights (which is different from knowledge of identity) to their offspring, a kind of polygyny could develop with men gaining control over several women and their children. However, terms like "alternative insemination" (AI) or "alternative fertilization" may appear to make the donor invisible, but the fact remains that without him, there is no child.

Donor anonymity and the secrecy practiced by DI physicians is a cause for great concern. Other practitioners may be more—or less—scrupulous than those who publish guidelines for their colleagues. It seems clear that DI should be removed from the governance of medicine. After all, couples are only seeking a discreet professional, who will act as a broker for the semen; medical competence is not necessary. The parties involved need to receive the special legal protection they all desire, and all individuals must have equal access under the law.

Philip Parker takes the moral position that the participants themselves should make the choices, not the professional. Rather than screening the participants, he helps them screen themselves.

> The role of the professionals (e.g., psychiatrist, attorney, physicians, etc.) should be to assist the . . . applicants . . . in making a competent, voluntary, and informed choice (consent or refusal) with respect to their participation in the process.

Infertile couples and others seeking DI could consider arranging it themselves. This book helps infertile couples realize that they do have other options than "medical therapy." They can take back responsibility and control for their reproduction. Those who cannot or do not want to do this, would be better off working with genetic experts who, at least, could thoroughly screen donors. Where the woman is having her fertility evaluated or augmented with hormone therapy, a physician's input would be necessary. However, it would be a cooperative role. There are no good reasons why physicians should be the sole decision makers with regard to the selection and performance of DI.

Parents today need to teach children that not every person can have a baby when they want to. Children will need to grow up considering very carefully the method of contraception they choose. As sperm quality diminishes each year, adolescent men might consider having a semen analysis when they become sexually active. As Germaine Greer (1985) asks:

> If infertility is so dreadful, why do we make no attempt whatever to teach young people how fragile fertility is? Most of the infertility that specialists see is secondary infertility. The patients were fertile once and are so no longer.

Ironically, instead of traditionally expanding male power over women, biological fathering through semen donation may actually empower women to make their own reproductive choices. One booklet written for the gay community about this subject is titled *Woman-Controlled Conception.*

Lamson et al. (1951), writing in the *Journal of the American Medical Association,* expressed some male paranoia, no doubt resulting from jealousy of women's procreative powers:

> Some patients derive a peculiar satisfaction from the cold scientific nature of the operation [DI]. Successful results create a feeling of superiority and triumph over the male, as well as a sense of fulfillment.

The overall status of women in society remains the biggest obstacle to their control of reproductive technology. Corea observes that there appear to be two medical systems operating, an "old" one (which includes harmful developments such as the IUD) and a "new" one (which offers only benefits). But, she concludes, "in fact there is one system and a low valuation of women in it." John Robertson also agrees:

> Major barriers to exercising reproductive freedom remain because procreative freedom for most women depends on having the social and financial means to walk the tightrope of work and love—or career and family. A social organization of norms, work patterns, and social services that enable women to do both is as important as formal rights to collaborative conception and pregnancy. In the final analysis, then, it is the material situation, as much as the formal right, which determines the scope of procreative freedom.

10

Legal Issues and Resolutions

IN JUST A COUPLE OF DECADES our understanding of procreation and our definition of "the family" have been radically enlarged. As we saw in the last chapter, redefinition is far from complete. Both donor sperm and eggs are now involved in many aspects of collaborative reproduction. Russell Scott, an Australian barrister and the author of *The Body as Property,* poses a hypothetical case: "What would and should the law say in relation to a test-tube baby born from the body of a surrogate mother in whom was implanted the egg of a second woman who is married, her egg having been fertilized in the laboratory by the sperm of a man not her husband but with her husband's consent?"

Donor insemination sounds simple in comparison to the hypothetical legal and ethical issues just posed. Because of its familiarity, it has been the accepted paradigm for other reproductive technologies for reports from the Warnock (in Britain) and the Waller (in Australia) legal reform commissions. But the dilemmas inherent in DI have not yet been tackled. Like the other forms of assisted conception, DI is much more than just a legal issue. George Annas, professor of Health Law at Boston University (1980), points out that DI may be an unworkable paradigm because it "potentially places the private contractual agreement among the participants regarding parental rights and responsibilities above the best interests of the child." He also observes how parenthood by contract may ignore the relevance of legitimacy, lineage, and the individual identity tied up in kinship, and thus bypass fundamental questions about the definition of fatherhood and its role in the family and the life of the child. Yet if neither the medical profession nor the courts can satisfactorily deal with DI, then how can they cope with the newer, more complex forms of reproductive technology and their inevitable unforeseen ramifications? Laws that distinguish children on the ground of their mode of conception have not solved the problem, because in enabling one form of conception to be protected they create worse anomalies for other situations.

It is beyond the scope of this book to discuss forms of reproductive technology other than DI, except where they overlap concerning principles such as anonymity, secrecy, and record keeping. While each form of assisted conception has its differences, they are nevertheless intertwined to some degree. Ironically, it is the advent of the other reproductive technologies, and the publicity they receive, that may give the added impetus to examining ways to bring about better public policies on DI. At present, as Blizzard comments:

> DI stands in a legal no-man's-land, in a position of ambiguity that reflects and is reflected in society's view of its principles and practice.

The Legal Dilemmas of DI

Law, medicine, and other social structures have the option to permit a practice, actively promote and fund it, simply tolerate it with or without regulation, discourage it, or actually prohibit it. Donor insemination was first introduced in the nineteenth century without regard to its personal, social, or legal implications. Although its use is steadily growing in the West, most countries have failed to enact laws regulating the practice. Family law was generally drawn up with no concept of the new family constellations that are being created by advances in medical science in today's pluralistic society. The courts, always lagging behind technological and scientific advances, have failed to adequately and uniformly address legal questions in DI such as legitimacy, divorce, support, and adultery. The present system is characterized by the absence of legal control, no comprehensive code of practice, no systematic counseling, problems of illegality, concealment, deception, secrecy, as well as tacit official and medical acceptance. Consequently, there is only an "inconsistent patchwork of rules based on the existing structure of tort, contract, and family law" to grapple with the realities of DI today. For this reason I would advise readers to seek legal counsel in their own jurisdiction.

Physicians have even suggested that because many prospective parents are unaware of the legal issues, why not simply allow the present system of secrecy, anonymity, and presumption of legitimacy to continue? On the other hand, is it possible to legally control and medically supervise DI when natural insemination is not controlled—not even with high risk populations such as teenagers and those who have genetic disease? How does the law monitor a procedure that requires only a "man, woman, a jar, and a syringe?"

The work of the law courts is often confused with the work of the legislatures—which is to lay down laws to govern future activities. A court, on the other hand, must decide the particular case before it. Its judgment affects the same and lower courts in that jurisdiction and may also persuade courts in other jurisdictions too. While legislatures may avoid regulating the practice of DI, the courts will nevertheless have to deal with the effects of the ultimate consequences on family law as cases arise.

Anglo-American courts in theory are bound by the principle of stare decisis, meaning that the law is applied on the basis of decisions in similar cases. With most of the new forms of reproductive technology (IVF, ectogenesis, surrogate mothering, embryo transfer) the facts will be unique, and existing law is very limited in framing the issue. Most of the precedents are already quite outmoded and require much bending of the law. The result is a piecemeal resolution of specific problems as they arise. The courts need to decide such cases in the light of modern scientific advances, but they must also maintain some continuity with the past, which provides stability within the legal system. What is really needed is a comprehensive legislative policy that will ensure the benefits of the new reproductive technologies while minimizing their potential harms, as far as we can foretell them. However, as long as state legislatures remain inactive, the courts will be forced to forge some kind of policy.

Ultimately the welfare of a child must be the overriding, if not the only, consideration. If there is conflict between the interests of the child and the wishes of the adults, the interests of the child must prevail. However, because the child has not yet been conceived, he or she is easily dismissed, except for consideration of legal identity. Instead, legislation has concentrated more on the effect of DI on the marital relationship, the recognition of DI as an acceptable medical practice, and its regulation from a public health viewpoint.

We shall now look at the key questions surrounding DI that have appeared in the legal literature with regard to civil and criminal law. DI is not considered a crime in any jurisdiction of the United States when performed by a licensed physician. But in Georgia, if DI is done by someone else other than a doctor, it falls under the criminal offense of practicing medicine without a license. Also, legal uncertainties exist that restrict the practice of DI, such as by U.S. Navy physicians, for example.

The most common legal matters are civil ones concerning adultery and legitimacy, with the contingent problems of child support, custody, and inheritance.

Illegitimacy

Illegitimacy is a historical sanction of patriarchy. The concept created legal, legitimate parent-child relationships where none had existed, so that blood heirs were not lawful progeny unless the parents were married. As a result, the illegitimate child is punished for the acts of her parents. (It is the parents, of course, who are "illegitimate.") The law has always defined parentage in terms of blood relationships, except adoption, which occurs under specific statutory authority. In illegitimacy, the child is considered a bastard, a *fillius nullius*—son of nobody—that is, having no relationship with his natural father because his mother does not enjoy the civil state of marriage. However, the child is always the child of the mother, and custody is likewise always vested in her. (Custody of a legitimate child is vested jointly in both parents.) A written declaration of filiation, or adoption by the husband, would make an illegitimate child legitimate. However, in many jurisdictions a DI child is illegitimate even if the woman's partner consents to the procedure, although courts today would probably decide that the child is legitimate.

At common law, the natural father of an illegitimate child is not entitled to custody, nor is his consent required for adoption, but as the natural father he may apply for access (and has won it).

The stigma and legal consequences of illegitimacy were designed to control female sexuality and perpetuate the institution of marriage. In today's social climate, illegitimacy brings less indignity, embarrassment, and economic loss than in the past. Together with the Uniform Parentage Act, it is seen by many as a socially useless, outmoded concept. Nevertheless this designation may be a source of unease or distress to many couples contemplating DI.

The DI child is technically illegitimate because her natural parents are not married to one another. Illegitimacy in DI can be held when adultery is found and also when adultery is not found. A DI child is illegitimate even if the woman's partner consents to the procedure in England and other countries, although the law would usually prohibit a husband from divorce on such grounds. However, a Supreme Court decision in the United States protects the illegitimate child's legal rights of substance, that is, to claim inheritance regardless of its social position (as long as the father can be identified).

Inheritance

Illegitimate children have rights against their natural parents. The DI child is in a worse position, because she is not the illegitimate child of the mother's husband and has no access to the biological father. However, in the absence of legal protection of the donor, if his identity is known, the child could make a claim on the donor's estate.

Where the status of illegitimacy has not been abolished, the rights, obligations, and mutual interests of the mother's husband in relationship to the DI child are lost. On the other hand, if it was not established during a man's lifetime that he was not the father of the DI child, then it would be more difficult to do so on his death. Even if a DI child inherits by intestacy from his mother's husband, it does not automatically follow that she is eligible under the wills of collateral relatives who may not know the child's DI status, leaving property to the "child," or "heir" of the husband. The question in these situations is the intention of the testators, and the burden of proof will be to show that the husband had *not* accepted the child as heir. The solution in such cases is to actually name the DI child or children in wills.

It is also possible that the DI status of the child could be used to disprove paternity against the husband or de facto partner for the purpose of disinheriting the child from the husband's or de facto partner's estate. However, proof that DI was performed will not prove that the child was thus conceived, so long as the husband was not completely sterile and had access to his wife. The husband can prove his own sterility in court with medical testimony, but in states that have enacted a physician-patient privilege (preventing disclosure of confidential medical information without the patient's consent) the wife may have to establish his sterility on accounts of his own admission or with other nonexpert testimony, unless the husband puts it at issue.

Presumption of Legitimacy

The child will be considered, in many jurisdictions, to be the product of the marriage if conceived (naturally or through DI) during the marriage or within ten months of its dissolution through death or divorce. This presumption serves to legitimize the DI child in the absence of any testimony to the contrary, such as proof of the husband's sterility, impotence, or nonaccess. Blood tests now can exclude the social father as the biological father with 99.95 percent accuracy. However, this "legitimacy," while adapting DI to the patriarchal system, also serves to deny the DI child truth of her origins, and in the absence of records may make it impossible for her to search for her paternal origins.

Legitimizing the DI Child

Legitimizing the DI child avoids confusion of the legal relationship with the donor and removes the child from being in a position to be able to inherit from two fathers. However, some legal experts complain that legitimizing the DI child would mean an unprecedented change in the concept of legitimacy. In the twenty-nine states where the DI child is legitimate by specific statute, the paternity of the mother's husband can still be challenged by any kin and for an unlimited period of time. Also, if it were possible for the donor to discover the identity of his biological offspring, then the donor would have a case for a paternity suit.

However, in jurisdictions with statutes, because the husband consented to the DI, the law deems a DI child to be legitimate. In U.S. jurisdictions without statutes, the presumption of legitimacy operates. In contrast, the child conceived by DI in Australia is in the same position as a child conceived when a married woman has intercourse with a man not her husband. As Stephen Mason (1982), of the Australian Law Reform Commission points out, the husband's prior consent to that intercourse is irrelevant and

> to treat such a consent as determinative of the legitimacy (and thus the parentage) of DI children, but completely irrelevant as so far as concerns children conceived naturally but in similar circumstances, simply creates further anomalies.

One such anomaly concerns surrogate mothering. In those states where the woman's husband is the legal father, and the sperm donor has no rights, then neither does the male of the infertile couple who provides sperm for the surrogate to bear his child. In such cases, the law should protect the biological rather than the legal father, but preceding DI legislation established the exact opposite protection. Also, the Uniform Parentage Act would be inapplicable if a surrogate chose DI by herself, but if she is not married, then there are no legal difficulties!

The proposal to legitimize DI children has been further criticized on the grounds that it amounts to an adoption outside the adoption legislation. Formal severance of the legal links between donor and child actually conflicts with the status of child legislation which guarantees such links, except in the case of adoption, which unlike DI, has been made subject to regulation and supervision. Adoption legislation provides the only method of severing the parental rights, liabilities, and duties. Adoption of children has been recognized as a serious matter, safeguarded by legislation and conducted under government supervision.

When approval is given to a particular adoption, the welfare of the child is the overriding concern. Thus the laws, while seeming to confer an improved status on the DI child, actually circumvent the kind of procedures required by adoption to protect the child's interests.

Samuels (1982), a British barrister, writes:

> "Deeming" the child to be legitimate, as is done in many states of the USA, may be done from laudable motives, but it is the negation of the proper approach in a free society. If DI is to be a good thing, it should be done openly and lawfully, not surreptitiously. Biological fathering is not essential to parenthood. But concealment and deception are inimical to the human dignity of the child and to the parenthood of the "parents."

Concealment, however, is a separate concept from legitimacy, as in many jurisdictions children conceived with an anonymous donor are legitimate.

Annas points out that the question of legitimacy, which is the only single consistent feature of current DI legislation, is an issue that will only arise if the child discovers the truth of her status, or if the parents raise the issue of legitimacy in a situation of marital conflict. In fact, in all the cases regarding the legitimacy of a DI child, the principal parties have been the wife and the husband.

The main problem for the DI child, in my opinion, is that legislation dealing with legitimacy, maintenance, and inheritance in intestacy, does not protect her against concealment of her genetic heritage. No statutes have mandated permanent records of the donor, and there is no legal process by which a DI child could gain access to the records and search for the donor even if records were kept. The simplest solution would be to abolish the concept of illegitimacy altogether. In that case, the relationships between a child and his or her mother and father would be the same whether the parents were married or not. Laws could be enacted with regard to medical records and birth certificates that would permit open disclosure of genetic parentage to children, while protecting the donor from any liabilities.

Adultery

Donor insemination may be found to be similar to adultery because it introduces into the family a different strain of blood—a child conceived with the help of another man. Adultery was condemned at common law because of the "possibility of introducing spurious heirs into the family and adulterating the issue of an innocent husband by turning the inheritance away from the blood line to a stranger." Adultery by a husband, of course, has no such consequences. Three courts have decided that DI was adultery, one in Canada and two in the United States. (See Case Law, *Orford v. Orford*, page 260.) Yet, in contrast with DI, adultery is not usually engaged in with the intent of producing a pregnancy, but for physical pleasure. Thus, DI may be held *not* to be adultery because no sexual intercourse or physical pleasure was involved. However, child support may still be ordered by the court. (There was a case in New Jersey in 1968 of a "splash pregnancy" where the father was liable for support even though no actual penetration occurred.)

The common law courts have been more concerned about the burden on a husband of a child not his own, than the social consequences of having a wife who committed adultery. However, in DI, the husband has agreed to take the child into his home and assume the duties of parenthood, so an analogy could be made with adoption.

Legislation is beginning to be adopted in many places to ensure that the husband, or male partner, by consenting to DI procedure, is willing to be named as the father in writing and accepts the child in every legal sense. This protects the child, donor, and doctor as well as the social father.

Prior to the recent Supreme Court decision on reproductive

choice, some felt that criminal and civil sanctions of adultery would deter physicians from doing DI on a woman without her partner's consent. Of course, the doctor is not usually using his own semen (although this has happened), and the donor has no knowledge of the use made of his semen or may even be dead. If the inseminating physician is a woman, that also would hardly be termed adultery! Infertile couples are generally disgusted by the idea of DI involving any marital misconduct. As with illegitimacy, their feeling about the charge of adultery from outsiders is more significant to them than the actual fact of it.

Where irretrievable breakdown of marriage is the only ground for divorce, adultery is merely an academic concept, and this is mostly the case in no-fault divorce. However, problems of maintenance, custody, access, inheritance rights, and other issues relating to the DI child—as with any child—arise when the marriage breaks up. They are just more complicated when the paternity of the child is in question.

Informed Consent

Informed consent may be required by several parties involved with DI. It would be assault and battery if the physician did not obtain the consent of the woman undergoing DI.

Forms of consent for the infertile couple are standard practice in the United States, Australia, U.K., and many other countries. These forms have served as the closest thing to lawmaking, a kind of "private legislation" that the individuals involved can achieve. Practitioners of DI have expressed the fear that if the physician has not obtained the husband's consent, it could be argued that he took the place of the parent in creating the conception. One article warned physicians that they should be wary of forgery or an imposter when obtaining the husband's written consent. It was recommended that the husband appear in person and provide photo identification! Where statutes require the husband's written consent, this must be documented by the physician. Understandably, there are uncertainties about the rights and obligations of the parties involved where no legal sanctions operate.

In Quebec, for example, consent to DI is necessary to prevent disavowal of paternity. Somerville raises the question whether it could be argued later that if a physician failed to get the woman's consent to approach her husband for consent, this could constitute damage to the child. This is because the child lost an opportunity of being placed in a situation where her paternity could not be disavowed. The American Fertility Society recommends that the consent of a woman's partner be obtained, as is required by many statutes.

Under California Civil Code (Section 7005), if sperm of a known donor is provided to a licensed physician, the donor is deemed not to have parental rights. With self-insemination this is not the situation as was established in a court case, *Loftin v. Flournoy.* (See page 266.)

While written consent may have value in establishing the reproductive intent of the parties at the time of execution, without a statutory basis they may provide mere "evidence" in the event of a suit. Nevertheless, judges usually have more experience with contracts than with DI, and consent forms would undoubtedly impress a jury. Such forms may also serve as a deterrent to legal action. Although many clauses in such forms purport to absolve the physician from liability arising from injury to the mother or child, or from hereditary defects suffered by the child, these clauses could be declared unenforceable if physician negligence can be proved. As one couple said to me:

> We never signed any legal consent or release forms. Some of the donor clinics don't bother with it. If there is something wrong with the baby, they know the couple will sue—release or no release— and they are probably right.

The defect in the child would have to be significant to force a couple committed to secrecy about the DI to take legal action.

Consent forms usually have served to protect the doctor and the donor more than the recipients and child. However, the donor is not a patient and not really consenting to anything (unless he may specify the destination of his genes, for example, "only married women"). The form may require the donor to state that he is in good physical health and has no family history of hereditary disease. The typical AMA form does not provide for the physician's signature to guarantee the anonymity that is implied. Ideally, a contract of indemnity is drawn up between the donor, and the husband and wife or the single woman. However, for those who adhere to secrecy, documentation is usually rejected, so the consent has to be between the doctor and the donor. Austin Asche, senior judge in the Family Court of Australia, conceives of a possibility that a court might rule such a contract "illegal as against public policy" on the basis that a third person cannot relieve a biological father from his responsibilities for his children (if the court could determine the "public policy").

Can a mother consent in advance to a waiver of any paternity action that her unborn child may ultimately want to bring? Even though the parents might sign such a waiver, they are not able to sign away a child's rights.

Some DI practitioners require the consent of the donor's wife. She may be required to acknowledge that her husband may become the father of a child or children of which she is not the mother, and to agree not to try to learn the identity of such offspring. Couples using a known donor may feel the same way, and in such cases I believe it is psychologically a sound policy. However, George Annas calls this a "paradigm of legalism based on fear and ignorance." He explains that such consent is not a legal requirement and does not seem to serve any useful social purpose.

Below is a typical form to be signed by a couple embarking on DI, which was reprinted in the literature by one of the active, early practitioners.

Sonia Kleegman, M.D.

I, the undersigned, cosigner with my wife Mrs. _____, hereby request Dr. Kleegman to inseminate my wife with the sperm of a foreign donor for the purpose of making her pregnant. The choice of the donor is to be left entirely to the discretion of Dr. Kleegman. We shall not hold Dr. Kleegman or her associated physicians responsible for any untoward results as a possible outcome of this procedure. I also declare that should my wife bear any child or children as the result of such insemination(s), such child or children shall be as my own before all men, and shall be my legal heir(s).

Signed _____ (Husband)

Signed _____ (Wife)

Date: _____

Witness _____ (Secretary)

Witness _____ (Physician)

Here is another consent form, which was created by Sarita Gilbert and printed in the February 1976 issue of the *American Journal of Nursing*.

WHEREAS: _____ and _____ of _____, husband and wife, desire to engage the service of _____ (hospital) to perform one, or more if necessary, artificial insemination(s) with sperm from a stranger-donor, and it is desired that an agreement be made in order to fully protect the interests of Dr. _____, any assistants he may desire to assist him, the husband, the wife, the _____ (hospital), and any child or children produced as a result of this program. NOW THEREFORE: It is agreed by and between the above-named husband and wife that the said Doctor is hereby engaged to perform the procedure of artificial insemination upon the wife, said Doctor to obtain the necessary sperm from a donor who shall not be advised of the identity of the husband and wife. The husband and wife shall rely upon the judgment and discretion of the Doctor to choose a donor whose physical and mental characteristics are compatible with those of the husband and wife. We understand that even though insemination may be repeated as often as recommended by Dr. _____, there is no guarantee on his part or assurance that pregnancy or full-term pregnancy will result. It is also agreed that on occasion donor sperm will be used that has been frozen for purposes of storage over periods of weeks to months. The husband fully understands, if pregnancy shall result, there is the possibility of complications of childbirth or delivery or the birth of an abnormal infant or infants, or undesirable hereditary tendencies of such issue, or other adverse consequences; and do hereby absolve and release the Doctor and _____ (hospital) from any and all liability or responsibility for the physical or mental nature of any child or children so produced. It is further agreed that from the moment of conception the husband hereby accepts the child as his own, and agrees:

1. That such child or children so produced are his own legitimate child or children and are the heirs of his body, and
2. That he completely waives forever any right which he might have to disclaim such child or children as his own, and
3. That such child or children so produced are, and shall be considered to be, in all respects including descent or property, child or children of his own body.

It is further agreed that the nature of this agreement is such that it must remain confidential; therefore, the husband and wife agree that the sole copy of the same may be given to the Doctor for his confidential files.

WHEREFORE: The said Doctor, the husband and the wife have hereto set their hands and seals this _____ day of 19

Husband _____
Wife _____
Doctor _____

Kleegman advised the use of the above consent form for "legal protection." She recommended that no duplicate be made and that it be kept under lock and key. The couple are told not to keep any memo among their records or personal papers, and they are counseled to the strictest secrecy. Kleegman would even go to the lengths of referring the husband to a new urologist (to help fabricate white lies) if the couple has inadvertently mentioned DI to any family members.

Couples reading consent forms, such as the two samples here, may mistakenly assume that they are signing a legal document that will make the child legitimate. Legitimacy, however, is a matter for state legislation, and they should suspect something is awry in that no copy of the document they sign is given to them. Many couples are sure to be put off by the emphasis on the possible untoward effects, and the use of the terms "foreign" and "stranger" for the donor.

I have selected additional clauses from other consent forms that give rise to much discomfort, such as:

Nor as husband and wife shall we ever be advised of the identity of the donor. Furthermore, as husband and wife we relinquish, waive, and disclaim any privilege or right we may have to determine the donor's identity.

We fully agree and understand that Dr. _____ or any other professional who may be associated with him or her or the _____ Center shall neither be responsible, nor shall have given any guarantees or warranties of fitness for the sperm.

We do hereby absolve, release, indemnify, protect, and hold harmless the above-named center and doctor from any and all liability for the mental or physical nature or character of any child or children so conceived or born, and for their affirmative acts or acts of omission that may arise during the performing of this agreement. It is further agreed that unavoidable defects or infections, sometimes contagious, may result from the insemination process.

We agree that following the insemination, Dr. _____ may destroy all records and information concerning the identity of the donor or donors.

Husband and wife further stipulate that Dr. _____ has advised them in the presence of each other as to the potential psychological implications that the birth of a child or children through the artificial insemination donor (DI) procedure may have on both their marital relationship and the child or children.

Husband and wife specifically release Dr. _____ and the donor or donors whose semen is finally selected for the artificial insemination of _____ (wife) from any and all liability and responsibility whatsoever for any psychological consequences that the procedure may have on the marital relationship of _____ (husband) and _____ (wife).

Potential Litigation

Paternity Suits

The medical mismanagement of DI is supported by some legal views which imply that paternity suits can be avoided by not keeping any records of DI, by matching the blood groups of the donor and husband, and by mixing their semen. Sophisticated blood analysis now has taken care of that illusion, although not all courts admit the evidence or weigh it sufficiently to overrule the presumption of paternity. In fact, paternity is more often denied, especially if the courts believe the family peace may be disturbed.

On the other hand, others have suggested compulsory adoption, which would safeguard the child's property and inheritance rights, even the idea of adoption in utero. Many DI couples would balk at the idea of adoption, even in a closed hearing, because the act of DI would be revealed.

The donor does not choose to conceive the child. Without the request of an infertile couple or single woman, he would not be a donor. The mother and her partner decide to create and raise the child. By consenting to DI, the husband has voluntarily agreed to bring a child into existence, and should have the same duties of a biological parent, as is the case in twenty-nine states.

Nevertheless, in states where there is no legislation to relieve the donor, especially the known donor, of his rights and responsibilities, legal channels are potentially open for his claiming them, especially where single women are concerned. Despite verbal agreements or written contracts, the donor may later decide to claim paternity. Visitation rights may be awarded to him and even his parents by the court. The donor may request certain types of education, health care, and upbringing. Custody may be decided on the grounds of the mother's divorce, or her single or lesbian lifestyle. In the event of the mother's death, custody may be awarded to the donor, even if the mother has named another family members, or a male or female lover. The donor may gain access to the mother's estate for the benefit of the child until the age of majority. There is a case where a donor had given semen to a single woman friend, and later won visitation rights to the child. (See Case Law, *CM v. CC,* page 265.)

With regard to divorce, husbands have been granted visitation rights to the DI child. More and more husbands today are receiving custody of their biological children, depending on whether the courts are looking at the child's welfare or the rights of the contesting parties for custody. Recently a partner in a dissolved lesbian relationship won visitation rights to the DI child consensually conceived. (See Case Law, *Loftin v. Flournoy,* page 266.)

Negligence

Physicians are required by a legal and ethical duty to exercise reasonable care with any medical procedure, on behalf of individual patients in particular, and society in general. However, when determining "reasonable care," the physician is held to that standard of care observed by other qualified medical specialists. This creates a catch-22 situation because there is no agreed-upon standard of care in the practice of DI.

Although DI presents an opportunity for preventive medicine and eugenics, the selection process is no more thorough than that used with blood donors. Most donor screening is deficient, and done only for some of the communicable diseases rather than genetic defects. In the event of a genetic disease, failure to have done a genetic workup may make the physician liable to the parents for the special costs of raising the handicapped child. A mother might be able to sustain a civil action of damages for negligence, misrepresentation, or breach of contract if the DI child had a congenital defect, hereditary disease, or different racial origin. (In London, a white woman obtained sperm from a private sperm bank and unintentionally gave birth to a black child.) The physician could also be held liable if he did not diagnose a physical problem in the mother like diabetes, which complicates a pregnancy.

Kleegman wrote that "every specimen of semen is always examined under high magnification to make sure there is no pus present." She describes two cases of acute trichomonal vaginitis that resulted from an infected semen specimen divided between two patients. Another two women developed streptococcal pelvic infections, and one was hospitalized with acute salpingitis and pelvic peritonitis (inflammation of the Fallopian tube and lining of the abdominal cavity). Fortunately there were no conceptions from the polluted semen and uneventful pregnancies later resulted. Nevertheless, she concludes that "the rich resources we have of finding donors in the superior levels of our community make the hazards of such infections less than in the general warp and woof of our society."

At least one woman in Australia has contracted AIDS from DI, and as a result all sperm banks in the country were closed in 1984 until the screening test was developed. A Pennsylvania clinic in 1985 recalled all the women on the DI program when it was found that a donor tested positively for AIDS, but the disease was not transmitted.

Physicians assume that acceptance into medical school automatically means having top quality sperm and genes. However, in a 1975 editorial in the *New England Journal of Medicine,* Herbert Horne admitted that in his practice the transmission of disease was more of a problem than other practitioners suggest. Horne especially singled out the organism Mycoplasma and thought it was the cause of the increasing number of spontaneous abortions in his patients who had successful DI conceptions.

Some lawyers suggest tightening the laws of malpractice to better safeguard the "medico-legal" process of DI as the medical profession has shown only "lethargy and benign neglect" with regard to setting its own standards. These advocates want the duties of the physician defined and their infringement to carry civil as well as criminal liability, as well as some legal provisions to protect the physician from being sued for malpractice or breach of contract.

Suits for "Wrongful Life"

There is also the possibility of an action for damages against the doctor by the child. A child who is the product of assisted conception may be subject to physical, psychological, and legal difficulty or disability. There is a chance that the child may sue the physician who performed the DI. Almost without exception, DI practitioners have avoided collecting any follow-up data on DI offspring and their families. They lack both interest in and awareness of the child's development. "Wrongful life" suits have been allowed in only three states because courts are not able to determine whether it is better to have been born under certain circumstances (such as being born illegitimate, or by DI with unknown paternal origins, or with a genetic defect) than not to have been born at all. In any event the parents are obligated to support the child, and unless the child is placed for adoption, then the money from the suit would be used to care for the child anyway. (Adoptive parents may have a case to sue for wrongful life to obtain financial assistance with the care for a disabled child, for example.)

Recent laws in Minnesota, South Dakota, and Utah, for example, prohibit lawsuits charging wrongful life where abortion would have eliminated the damages. Despite legal reluctance to accept these suits, the trend is changing. In Michigan a child collected for dental damage resulting from the antibiotic tetracycline, and in California a suit was brought on behalf of a child with Tay-Sachs disease. This case involved erroneous laboratory results that had indicated the parents were not Tay-Sachs carriers. As Lori Andrews put it in her book, *New Conceptions,* "The suit against the laboratory claimed, in essence, that she had a right to be born healthy or not at all." Other states which now accept such suits include Washington, New Jersey, and Pennsylvania.

Suits for "Wrongful Birth"

On the other hand, "wrongful birth" suits are more common and more successful. Such suits claim negligence of the physician over prenatal issues, such as providing incorrect information or failing to inform about genetic screening. One couple with a Down's syndrome child sued their doctor for not informing them about amniocentesis. Andrews explains that while courts are showing more sympathy for couples who give birth to a seriously ill or defective child due to physician's negligence, some legislatures are protecting physicians.

Nonsupport of a Minor Child

Child support may be a civil or a criminal action, and could involve either the husband or the donor depending on how the issue of legitimacy of the DI child was decided. Statutes vary with regard to inheritance and support. Generally, under law, a man is not liable for support of a child born to his wife unless he was the natural father. However, if the child does not have a natural father, as the term is generally understood, the mother's husband can be seen as the lawful father. At least there is a social if not a biological relationship. In several divorce cases, however, the husband was ordered to support the DI child. No court has imposed liability for support of a DI child if the husband did not consent.

On the other hand, the U.S. Supreme Court denied review of a decision of the California Court of Appeal which held that neither the custodial father's statutory visiting rights nor the biological father's constitutional interest in his children, permits the right of an illegitimate child to compel her adjudicated, noncustodial father to visit her. This means that a child could probably not later enforce contact with the donor.

Donor Litigation

Legal complications could arise from the donor's biological tie with the DI child. A single or separated woman could succeed in a legal claim for child support, if the state were interested in avoiding public expenditure. The DI child/adult could seek part of the donor's estate, or compensation for any disease or defect thought to be linked with the donor. The donor's disclaimer would have to be evaluated by the court.

Some medical students become wealthy or famous physicians and there is a remote possibility that they might be sued for inheritance if their paternity could be proven. If they have given a large number of semen donations they may be fearful of liability for support and inheritance. Lori Andrews quotes a donor's response to this in a 1984 article on reproductive technology in *Psychology Today.*

> Peter Forbes, a Sherman Oaks, California, gynecologist, provided sperm for thirty-three pregnancies when he was a medical resident at Georgetown University in Washington, D.C., three decades ago. Because of the possibility that one of his "children" could prove his paternity, Forbes amended his will. Any child not borne by his wife will be entitled to only $1 from his estate.

However, in the United States, where one third of physicians keep permanent records of the donors, there have been no suits so far.

Falsification of Public Records

When a DI birth is registered with the mother's husband as father, it is obviously a falsehood. A false declaration of paternity is a criminal offense in many states, and it can affect property and tax claims, custody, support, and other familial obligations. The physician may be liable to lose his license, and have to pay a fine or spend time in prison, or both.

There is also a technical possibility that parties who falsify public records could be held as a conspiracy to commit a criminal act. However, this is only likely if intent to defraud can be proven. Likewise, the physician may be in a vulnerable position in the absence of legislation where performing DI could theoretically expose him to the charge of criminal conspiracy to produce an illegitimate child. However, there is nothing unlawful in itself in producing a child, nor in the means, unless the mother is under age or in a prohibited degree of blood relationship.

Legal History of DI

The question addressed in DI litigation has been the legal identity of the child who was conceived extramaritally, and the effect of this identity on the five participants—the child, mother, husband (if there is one), donor, and doctor (if there is one). The law usually has been evasive about drawing up a legal framework because it was never clear if DI was a desirable activity for the law to promote. Two pieces of legislation designed to reform the practice of DI have been introduced recently: the Sperm Bank Licensure and Regulation Act of 1985 in Washington D.C. and the Alternative Reproduction Act in Michigan. The proposed legislation would establish requirements for keeping records and would make medical and genetic information about the donor available to DI offspring at age eighteen. The donor would be informed prior to donation that in the future his identity may be revealed to any offspring conceived. The Washingon bill would set the age limit for donors at sixty and restrict the use of one donor to one DI child. Payment to donors would be prohibited although "reasonable and documented expenses incurred by the donor for transport or other purposes directly related to the donation of semen" would be reimbursed. Unfortunately, this welcome reform has aroused great controversy and the medical profession fears that no donors will be forthcoming under such circumstances. Nevertheless, consequences are forcing legal action that must go on while the social and ethical questions continue to be pondered.

Case Law

1. *Orford v. Orford* was the first case on the issue of artificial insemination in Canada. It was an action in 1921 for alimony in Ontario by the wife who was living in England. The couple had never consummated their marriage because of painful intercourse, and the wife claimed that the child was a product of DI, which she had undergone without her husband's knowledge. He claimed adultery. The court ruled that the wife was not entitled to alimony payments because she had committed adultery. The court's view of adultery was "voluntary surrender to another person of the reproductive powers or faculties of the guilty person; and any submission of those powers to the service or enjoyment of any person other than the husband or the wife comes within the definition of 'adultery.' " The court further continued:

> Sexual intercourse is adulterous because in the case of the woman it involves the possibility of introducing into the family of the husband a false strain of blood. Any act on the part of the wife which does that would, therefore, be adulterous.

This was considered a very strange ruling as adultery presupposes direct physical contact between the partners and insemination is a clinical procedure that involves neither physical contact nor sexual gratification, which is the usual motive for adultery. By similar interpretation of the case, one commentator pointed out, adultery would not be found if a contraceptive were employed during intercourse with a man other than one's spouse.

2. *Hoch v. Hoch* was a 1945 Illinois case in which the husband alleged adultery and the wife said she had undergone DI. The court held that DI without the husband's consent was not adultery as there was no sexual intercourse. The lower court indicated that DI would not have been adultery but the judge refused to believe that no sexual relations had occurred. If the DI could have been proved (i.e., physician documentation), then no adultery would have been found.

3. *L. v. L.* was a 1948 case in England. The wife sought annulment because the marriage was not consummated. Later she had

a child by AIH, which became illegitimate when the court annulled the marriage. English law, unlike that of the United States, did not provide for the legitimacy of the child of a void or voidable marriage.

4. In the 1948 New York case of *Strnad v. Strnad,* the wife sought to revoke her husband's right of visitation with the DI child, which had been granted in the separation decree. The court confirmed the previously awarded privileges because they found that the child had been "potentially adopted" or "semiadopted" and therefore the husband was entitled to the same rights and privileges that he would have had if the child had been officially adopted. The court applied the guidelines that the best interests of the child were the same as a child born out of wedlock and subsequently legitimized by marriage. By defining the child as "not illegitimate," the court stopped short of calling the child legitimate. The court did not rule on the property rights of the child. This decision was criticized because the court, instead of defining the rights of the DI father as the same as those of a natural parent, tried to justify its rationale within the legal doctrine surrounding adoption. Thus there was no clarification of the issues inherent in DI. The court simply applied guidelines as to the best interests of the child.

After this decision the mother moved to Oklahoma where she obtained a divorce and was given exclusive custody. The court, according to newspaper reports, ruled that the husband had no rights of visitation because he was not the biological father.

5. *People ex rel Abajian v. Dennett* was a 1958 New York state case. The court held that the wife could not deny the legitimacy of a DI child who had previously been considered legitimate. The court upheld the husband's right to enforce his customary visitation privileges as provided in the separation agreement and divorce decree. His former wife was "estopped" from asserting that the child was conceived by DI, because the court did not permit the child to be stigmatized as a bastard by alleging its conception to DI. "Estopped" means that a person is precluded from a course of action by one's previous behavior. This doctrine is used to stop a husband denying support or a wife denying a husband access to a DI child. It means that if a husband has consented to the proce-

dure and registration of the child as his own, he could be prevented on the basis of his previous behavior from later bringing evidence to dispute his own paternity. Regardless of paternity, the doctrine could be used to stop a husband denying child support or to stop a wife denying access.

6. *Doornbos v. Doornbos* was a 1954 divorce action in Illinois sought by the wife. The court held that "heterologous artificial insemination . . . with or without the consent of the husband is contrary to public policy and good morals, and constituted adultery on the part of the mother. A child so conceived is not a child born in wedlock and therefore not legitimate. As such it is the child of the mother and the father has no right or interest in said child." This was the strongest condemnation of DI, done with the husband's consent, by a court, to date. (The judge was a Roman Catholic.) The couple were apparently unable to be persuaded to take the case to a higher court.

7. However, in 1958 the Court of Session in Scotland declared in *MacLennan v. MacLennan* that DI did not constitute adultery whether the husband's consent was given or not.

> The idea that a woman is committing adultery when alone in the privacy of her bedroom, she injects into her ovum [*sic*] by means of a syringe the seed of a man she does not know and has never seen is one which I am afraid I cannot accept. . . . Self-adultery is a concept as yet unknown to the law.

Furthermore, the court could not hold that a woman who inseminated herself had engaged in the unlawful practice of medicine.

8. In *Gursky v. Gursky,* a 1963 New York case, the court declared the child illegitimate despite the fact that it was conceived through consensual DI. The wife was granted separation and amendment for annulment on the grounds that the marriage had never been consummated, due to impotence. The DI was performed with her husband's written consent. In addressing the question of legitimacy, the court chose to rely on the common law concept that "a child who is begotten through a father who is not the mother's husband is deemed to be illegitimate." Consent to DI was considered not to meet the statutory requisites for adoption,

which contrasts with the case of Strnad where the child was considered "semiadopted," (showing the legal inconsistencies within the same state).

Despite the court's position that the Gursky child was illegitimate, it compelled support by the husband with the doctrines of implied contract and equitable estoppel. (The husband's prior conduct indicated that he had promised to support the child. Also, the wife's prior recognition of her husband's parentage estopped her from reopening the issue of illegitimacy.) Although the court refused to label the child legitimate, it did find that a husband consenting to his wife's insemination was obligated to support the child. There was no decision on personal or property rights.

The *Cleveland Law Review* stated:

> The Gurskys' court's basic failure lies in its ability to modify common law concepts so as to render them compatible with a situation engendered by modern technology. Moreover, it seems inequitable to place the entire burden upon the husband. If a husband who consents to the DI can be estopped to deny his obligations of support, when then should the wife and mother be permitted to have the marriage annulled? Sound public policy would dictate that in order to preserve the family unit and give the child the benefit of two parents, a mother who has consented to DI should be precluded from later asserting the husband's impotence as grounds for annulment.

9. In *Anonymous v. Anonymous,* a 1964 New York case, the court considered the husband's consent to DI as an implied promise of support. The husband was ordered to pay temporary support to the two DI children.

10. *People v. Sorenson* was the first of three, to date, appellate decisions on DI. This was a 1968 divorce case that legitimized the DI baby. The husband's refusal to support the child born to his wife through DI was not upheld. The couple divorced four years after the DI child was conceived, and the wife did not ask for child support. She subsequently became ill and was unable to work and applied for public assistance. The state sought to serve a support order on Mr. Sorenson. The court determined, under Statute #270 of the California Penal Code, that the meaning of the word "fa-

ther" was not limited to the natural or biological father (who obviously could not be found), but extended to the legal father, a relationship to be determined by the court. The court held that a DI child does not have a "natural father" and "the donor is no more responsible for the use made of his sperm than is the donor of blood or kidney." Thus, the husband was determined to be criminally responsible for not supporting a child conceived by DI with his consent. As no law prohibited DI, the child was considered lawfully begotten, and no purpose was served by stigmatizing the child. The court also noted the intentional planning of the DI in contrast with the lack of foresight that causes most illegitimate births.

> On the question of adultery, the court decided, since the doctor may be a woman, or the husband himself may administer the insemination . . . to consider it an act of adultery with the donor, who at the time . . . may be a thousand miles away or may even be dead, is equally absurd.

However, the court did not explicitly hold that such a child is legitimate. A husband who consented to a child's birth, through artificial insemination, the court continued, cannot create a temporary relation to be assumed and disclaimed at will, but the arrangements must be of such character as to impose an obligation of supporting those for whose existence he is directly responsible. The court did not rule on the child's inheritance rights.

11. *Adoption of Anonymous* was a 1973 New York state case in which a woman's second husband wanted to adopt a consensual DI child of his wife's first marriage. Her first husband was listed as the child's father on the birth certificate. Both the separation agreement and the divorce decree referred to the child as the "daughter" or "child" of the couple. He had been granted visitation rights and had fulfilled his support obligations. The second husband argued that the first husband was not the "parent" of the child so his consent was not required. The court held that the consent of the first husband was required for adoption and he refused to consent. In contrast with the Gursky decision, the court stated that "a child born of consensual DI during valid marriage is a legitimate child entitled to the rights and privileges of a naturally

conceived child of the same marriage." The court noted that illegitimacy is based on history and that the statutory concept of a child born out of wedlock developed long before DI was even contemplated:

> It serves no purpose whatsoever to stigmatize the DI child, or to compel the parents formally to adopt in order to confer upon the DI child the status and rights of a naturally conceived child.

12. *C.M. v. C.C.* was a 1977 case in New Jersey between a single woman and a known donor. The woman, C.C., received semen from C.M., with whom she had a dating relationship for at least two years, and inseminated herself. The court found that the couple had had a long-standing relationship, that he fully intended to assume the responsibilities of parenthood, and that the evidence did not support C.C.'s claim that C.M. had waived his parental rights.

> If an unmarried woman conceives a child through DI from the semen of a known man, that man cannot be considered to be less the father because he is not married to the woman.

There was nobody else in the position to take on the responsibilities of fatherhood. The courts generally feel that it is in a child's best interest to have two parents whenever possible, and in unmarried persons the point is not to distinguish whether the child was conceived naturally or artificially, but to decide the best interests with regard to custody and visitation. In considering C.M. to be the natural father, the court granted him visitation rights.

13. *K.S. v. G.S.* was a 1981 New Jersey case where the wife underwent DI because her husband had had a vasectomy prior to the marriage. A couple of months after the wife conceived, the husband could not accept the pregnancy and they separated. The husband, who had never seen the infant or contributed to its support, denied his obligations on the grounds that during the insemination process he had revoked his initial consent. The physician did not get the consent in writing, which is not required by New Jersey law. However, the court found that there was no clear and convincing evidence that such consent had been withdrawn.

14. *R.S. v. R.S.*, a 1983 case heard by the Court of Appeals in

Kansas, also involved oral consent to DI by the husband, even though the physician should have obtained written consent under the state law. In this divorce action, the husband's argument was that the Kansas law required written consent from a husband if he has a duty to support the DI child. The court concluded that the husband was liable for the support of the child "whether on the basis for an implied contract to support or by reason of application of the doctrine of equitable estoppel."

15. *Loftin v. Flournoy* was a 1984 custody case in California involving a lesbian couple. The court ruled that Loftin, whose brother's sperm had been used to inseminate Flournoy, had the right to petition the court for visitation rights to the six-year-old child. This is the first time that the courts have protected the right of a lesbian nonbiological parent of a DI child. The court upheld the child's need for continuity and consistency with parental figures.

16. *Jhordan C. v. Mary K.* was a 1986 appellate case in California where a DI mother sought legal custody and visitation rights for her lesbian partner. The donor, who had been personally selected by the mother, had previously filed a successful action to establish paternity and visitation rights and was subsequently ordered to reimburse the county of Sonoma for public assistance paid out for child support. The Court of Appeal held that because the semen was not *obtained* through a licensed physician (although a known donor may be used and the DI done at home), the donor retained paternal rights. The mother was awarded sole legal and physical custody, and the donor received substantial visitation rights, but he was denied any input into decisions about the child's schooling, medical care, and day-by-day maintenance. The court held that the female partner was not a de facto parent, but visitation rights were awarded to her.

There have been no cases involving DI that have centered on the right to inheritance. No cases to date have dealt with either donor or physician negligence or malpractice. Some day there will be, when DI offspring can show "good cause" as have adoptees.

Legal Regulation of the Practice of DI

The technical aspects of DI have been left to the medical profession in most jurisdictions. Most doctors and lawyers feel that DI couples are satisfactorily self-selecting by their great desire for the procedure, and that physicians would not perform DI unless the couple appeared "stable" and any child so conceived would have a "good home." Of course, these are value judgments by physicians, who are usually male and may not necessarily take into account the constitutional rights of single, divorced, and widowed women, especially if lesbian.

There is more legislation on DI for domestic animals than for humans. Bills to legitimize DI children were introduced in New York for four consecutive years beginning in 1948. They failed, as did similar bills at that time in Indiana, Minnesota, Virginia, and Wisconsin. Georgia was the first state to regulate DI, in 1964. Many state legislatures have adopted an attitude of indifference. Several states have witnessed the unsuccessful introduction of DI legislation as well as proposals that DI be outlawed. A 1960 bill in Massachusetts, if it had passed, would have made DI a criminal act, similar to abortion at the time. Similar actions were tried in Minnesota in 1949 and Ohio in 1955, but they also failed.

The following chart attempts to make orderly sense of the legislation which has been described as "a crazy quilt of diverse rules denying facile generalization."

No state guarantees the child knowledge of her genealogical heritage because there is no requirement for documentation of the donor, except in Ohio, and those records must be kept for only five years. Only a handful of states has minimum health standards for donors and only two require AIDS screening. Georgia is the only state with a penalty for noncompliance, a one- to five-year term of imprisonment for anyone other than a licensed physician who does DI.

State Laws Concerning

DI to be performed under supervision of:	AL	AK	AZ	AR	CA	CO	CT	DE	DC
1. Licensed M.D.	X	X			X	X	X		
2. Consent of husband and wife	X	X		X	X	X	X		
3. Written consent	X	X			X	X	X		
—acknowledged by M.D.	X					X			
—signed by court									
4. Filed consent	X				X	X	X		
—kept confidential	X				X	X	X		
—opened only under court order						X			
5. DI child legitimate if husband consents	X	X		X	X	X	X		
6. Couple to notify M.D. of birth if not OB									
7. Donor has no legal rights or duties w/r child	X					X	X		
8. Minimum donor health standards									
9. M.D. or hospital may refuse DI									
10. Statute retroactive									
11. Penalty for noncompliance									
12. Donor treated as natural father if he and woman consent in writing									
13. AIDS screening of donor sperm									
14. Records to be kept by M.D.									

Donor Insemination

FL	GA	HI	ID	IL	IN	IA	KS	KY	LA	MA	MD	ME	MI	MN	MS
	X		X	X										X	
X			X	X										X	
	X		X	X										X	
	X		X	X										X	
			X				X							X	
	X		X	X			X							X	
X	X		X	X			X		X		X		X	X	
			X												
			X	X										X	
			X												
											X				
	X														
			X												

State Laws Concerning

DI to be performed under supervision of:	MO	MT	NE	NV	NH	NJ	NM	NY	NC
1. Licensed M.D.		X				X	X	X	X
2. Consent of husband and wife		X				X	X	X	X
3. Written consent		X				X	X	X	X
—acknowledged by M.D.		X				X	X	X	X
—signed by court									X
4. Filed consent						X	X		
—kept confidential						X	X	X	X
—opened only under court order						X	X		
5. DI child legitimate if husband consents		X		X		X	X	X	X
6. Couple to notify M.D. of birth if not OB									
7. Donor has no legal rights or duties w/r child		X				X	X	X	
8. Minimum donor health standards						X		X	
9. M.D. or hospital may refuse DI									
10. Statute retroactive						X		X	
11. Penalty for noncompliance									
12. Donor treated as natural father if he and woman consent in writing							X		
13. AIDS screening of donor sperm									
14. Records to be kept by M.D.									

Donor Insemination (Cont.)

ND	OH	OK	OR	PA	RI	SC	SD	TN	TX	UT	VT	VA	WA	WV	WI	WY
	X	X	X					X	X			X	X		X	X
	X	X	X					X	X			X	X		X	X
	X	X	X					X	X			X	X		X	X
		X	X													X
	X															X
		X	X						X				X			
		X	X						X				X		X	
	X	X											X			X
	X	X	X					X	X			X	X		X	
	X		X						X				X		X	
	X															
	X															
	X															
	X															

Legislation in Other Countries

Australia

Until 1984 there were no laws specifically regulating the legality of the DI. It was all left up to the doctor involved. Paternity of the mother's husband could be challenged under the existing legislation, and the donor had certain rights by which he could bring an action to have his paternity recognized if he knew the identity of his offspring. Similarly, with regard to paternity, the "balance of possibilities" operated instead of "beyond all reasonable doubt."

Roberts v. Roberts was a 1971 case that involved right of access by a mother's husband to the child, who both parties agreed was the product of DI. The husband had been sterilized some years before. The Supreme Court of Victoria proceeded on the basis that the child was legitimate, although it did not make any specific ruling on the question.

The Artificial Conception Act was passed in 1984 in New South Wales. The act deals with the paternity and legal status of DI and IVF children born as a result of donated sperm. Thus children conceived through DI are legitimate, and it is an irrefutable legal presumption that a semen donor is not the father of any child born from his sperm. However, this same act, by attempting to solve legal problems in DI has created further problems—"legally fatherless children"—in situations where a fertile husband donates his sperm to a surrogate for gestation. The Victorian Status of Children Act (1984) is similar, although it designated the bearer of the child as the mother, which calls to task the "mother" who donated the egg where the two are not the same. The Medical Procedures (Infertility) Act of Victoria, 1984, requires records of IVF and the use of embryos to be kept at a central register at the Health Department. Although this regulation specifically relates to IVF, the practice has been extended to DI while the regulations for that procedure are being drawn up.

Key provisions include:

1. A fertilization procedure may only be carried out in accor-

dance with the Act (which would require DI to be done by a licensed physician).

2. It will be unlawful for a person to accept semen from a donor unless the donor and the donor's spouse (if any) have consented and have received counseling from an approved counselor.

3. Payment for semen is prohibited.

4. Hospitals are to keep a register that must contain prescribed particulars of donors and consents, and expenses incurred in giving gametes.

5. Provision for the disclosure to a donor upon his or her written request of nonidentifying information regarding possible recipients of gametes given by such a donor.

6. Records of artificial insemination procedures to be kept where the procedure is carried out in a hospital other than an approved hospital or by a medical practitioner in a place other than a hospital, and where a child is born of a pregnancy occurring as a result of the procedure, for a copy of the record to be sent to the Health Commission.

7. No gametes to be used by an unmarried person under 18 years.

8. No mixing of semen in DI.

At the time when these state laws came into force, a surrogate mother in New South Wales was refusing to hand over the baby she had conceived for an infertile couple. The husband had left his semen specimens with the woman who artificially inseminated herself and agreed to hand over the baby at birth. He is hoping to raise the issue of her husband's consent to contest his right of access to his biological son. The Act specifies that its provisions of paternity of an artificially conceived child depend on the consent of the mother's husband to the procedures of DI. However, in the absence of documentation, the child of a marriage is presumed to be the child of the husband.

After this complicated incident, the Law Reform Commissioners were planning to give the question of surrogacy close scrutiny. They anticipated that the law would recognize surrogate arrangements some time in the future depending on certain conditions.

One of the suggested conditions was to limit surrogacy to a particular class of people, such as members of the family, to carry the child. This, of course, would establish a personal relationship which is in contrast to the traditional arrangement of anonymity in reproductive collaboration.

Canada

The only legislation in Canada pertaining to DI is in the Yukon, which protects the donor, and Quebec, where legislation has been passed to make the child legitimate and ensure the rights of the social father. In 1985 the Ontario Law Reform Commission issued a report entitled "Human Artificial Reproduction and Related Matters."

Great Britain

A Church commission was set up by the Archbishop of Canterbury in 1945, and it reported against DI in 1948, judging DI to be wrong in principle and contrary to Christian standards. In 1958, a committee was set up by the Secretaries of State for the Home Office and for Scotland, chaired by Lord Feversham. This committee reported more favorably in 1960, saying that DI "falls within the category of actions known to students of jurisprudence as liberties, which, while not prohibited by law, will nevertheless receive no support or encouragement from the law." However, this lay committee held the practice of DI to be an undesirable and immoral "liberty" comparable with fornication and adultery, and to be strongly discouraged. (One dissenter, the Dean of St. Paul's, thought there might be some benefit to the procedure.) The report also questioned the "morals" and sense of "responsibility" of the donors, and expressed concern that these characteristics might be passed on genetically!

Only in Britain could the following position be taken with regard to DI and inheritance!

> If the child of DI were declared to be legitimate, the consequent devolution of entailed property, titles, and dignities of honour might provide an additional motive for resort to DI. This would, of course, be against the interests of those persons who would other-

wise have succeeded in default of a legitimate child being born to the husband as a result of normal conception. It would also, we think, be against the interests of society as a whole. Succession through blood descent is an important element of family life and as such is at the basis of our society. On it depends the peerage and other titles of honour, and the Monarchy itself. The Monarchy has not always proceeded by direct descent, but the exceptions only serve to illustrate how much reliance was placed on descent through blood and how much was done to maintain that position that even an apparent usurper should be closely related to the previous Sovereign. The view has been put to us that for a child of DI and his descendants to succeed to a hereditary title through his mother's husband should not only be an injustice to persons who were related in blood to the first holder of the title, it would be an imposition on the Sovereign and a frustration of his original intention in granting such a privileged status not merely to an individual, but to a family or group of persons who for ever after could trace a legitimate descent in blood from the grantee. However small the incidence of DI, we do not feel that these considerations ought to be overlooked.

In 1971, the British Medical Association appointed Sir John Peel, a former president of the Royal College of Obstetricians and Gynaecologists, to chair a panel of six members to investigate DI. The committee recommended that DI should be made available within the National Health Service, and called for the definition of legitimacy to be expanded to include a child born by DI to which the husband of the mother had consented. Lord Kilbrandon was against this for it would change the meaning of legitimacy.

In British law, a "child" includes an illegitimate child in will settlements and if either parent dies intestate. Clearly the DI child is indeed the illegitimate child of the donor and thus could inherit.

If a DI child is accepted into the family, then the husband is responsible for his or her maintenance, irrespective of whether the child is illegitimate in law. A child is legitimate provided the parents are later married, and remains so if the marriage is annulled during the gestation period. The only difference with a DI child is that it is not related by blood to both parents.

Sometimes courts, as in the 1972 English case of *S. v. Mc.*, don't feel that it is in the best interests of the child to order blood tests that might establish its illegitimacy.

Now that DI is offered by the National Health Service in over forty centers in Britain, and regulated by law, the process is thus implicitly legitimized—although the child is still actually illegitimate. A woman must consent to the procedure in writing, she must be over sixteen, and there is no legal requirement for her to be married, or if married, to have the consent of her husband.

In 1981, a Committee of Enquiry into Human Fertilisation and Embryology was set up by the British Government to investigate the questions posed by the new reproductive technologies. The committee, headed by Dame Mary Warnock, gave its report in 1984, which was published as *A Question of Life* (1985). The results were termed "legal overkill" because among the sixty-three recommendations there were twenty-three new laws, and seven new crimes!

Anonymity was recommended for gamete donors, but there was some support for keeping a detailed description of these donors:

> It is argued that they would provide information and reassurance for the parents and, at a later date, for the child. They might also be of benefit to the donor, as an indication that he is valued for his own sake. A detailed description also offers some choice to the woman who is to have the child, and lack of such choice can be said to diminish the importance of the woman's right to choose the father of her child.

> The contrary view, also expressed in the evidence, is that detailed donor profiles would introduce the donor as a person in his own right. It is also argued that the use of profiles devalues the child who may seem to be wanted only if specifications are met, and this may become a source of disappointment to the parents if their expectations are unfulfilled.

> As a matter of principle we do not wish to encourage the possibility of prospective parents seeking donors with specific characteristics by the use of whose semen they hope to give birth to a particular type of child. We do not therefore want detailed descriptions of donors to be used as a basis for choice, but we believe that the couple should be given sufficient relevant information for their reassurance. . . . We recommend that on reaching the age of eighteen, the child should have access to the basic information about the donor's ethnic origin and genetic health and that legislation be enacted to provide the right of access to this.

Though the Committee agreed that absolute anonymity of the donor should be maintained, it recognized that a privately arranged donation, such as between brothers, would not be subject to regulation.

The Committee admitted that its recommendation that the husband be registered as the father on the birth certificate was "legislating for a fiction." They did not deal with this situation when a woman is not married. On the issue of eligibility, they declined to take a position, but instead recommended that the decision be placed on the physician consulted:

> We recognize that this will place a heavy burden of responsibility on the individual consultant who must make social judgments that go beyond the purely medical, in the types of case we have discussed. . . . We recommend that in cases where consultants decline to provide treatment they should always give the patient a full explanation of the reasons.

The Committee had "grave misgivings" about the use of a deceased husband's semen by his widow, fearing that this "may give rise to profound psychological problems for the child and its mother." Yet later the Committee equivocated over the issue of a person's death during the storage time. It was recommended that the "right use or disposal of his or her frozen gametes should pass to the storage authority." They did add that this authority "should bear in mind any previously expressed wishes in relation to disposal."

Europe and Sweden

Generally, in Europe a husband, wife, child, or any interested party can bring an action to repudiate the child's legitimacy. However, the Swiss Civil Code prevents a husband from bringing such an action if he consented to the conception by the act of a third party.

In Italy and Switzerland, the practice of DI is illegal. In France it is deliberately not recognized by the law and left to the persons concerned. The DI child is legitimate unless the husband denies paternity within six months. No laws govern artificial insemination in Germany, but the total responsibility rests on physicians who may be sued, which makes them generally reluctant to offer the service. Legislation protecting children's rights in Germany would conflict with legislated anonymity for donors.

The Council of Europe is attempting to set up uniform regulations for "ensuring the welfare of the child," mainly by stressing secrecy. Apart from prohibiting payment to donors, the regulations are not progressive at all. They specify that DI may only be done by a licensed physician, and that donors should be anonymous, and that a child is legitimate if the husband consents to the DI. The situation regarding single women is left to domestic law, if the woman meets "appropriate conditions."

I telephoned Dr. Kirsten Hagenfeldt at the Karolinska Institute Department of Obstetrics and Gynecology in Stockholm to find out how the practice of DI has changed in the past two years since the legislation was enacted in 1985. Sweden was the first country to legislate the DI offspring's right to know the identity of the donor, and all anonymous semen stored in sperm banks was ordered to be destroyed. Although the supply of donors fell initially, this was also due to other aspects of the law including the prohibition of the use of fresh semen and of DI by private physicians. In addition, some hospital clinics stopped their programs because the physicians did not want to perform DI without anonymity.

The legislation does not permit DI for single women or lesbian couples—"the child must have a father" says Dr. Hagenfeldt. The identity of the donor and his social security number must be kept on file for seventy years. The offspring has the right to that knowledge when grown up—no age was specified in the statute. Married and de facto couples must undergo psychosocial assessment prior to acceptance for DI and they receive counseling throughout the procedure. Semen must be quarantined for six months to allow AIDS screening and karyotyping is done on all donors.

Most donors are married men with children who donate altruistically because they have infertile friends and relatives. Hagenfeldt estimates the number of DI births in Sweden prior to the 1985 legislation as four to five hundred, and in 1987 about two to three hundred. The numbers are steadily increasing again. She agreed that single women wanting DI and couples wanting anonymous donors probably travel abroad to conceive.

In Poland there is no notion of legitimacy. Every father has six months after the birth to deny paternity. In Portugal, DI is insufficient by itself to be a dispute about affiliation.

Suggestions for Legal Reform

The dearth of case law has been considered an argument against the need for legislation. However, some legal experts feel that the infrequency of litigation to date is probably not indicative of the future. The number of possible parties that could be involved in a "collaborative reproduction" has increased to six. (The gestational donor or surrogate, her spouse, two separate genetic donors (egg and sperm) and two separate rearers.) Annas (1980) comments on the efforts of the legal profession to amend the sorry state of affairs:

> Most of the legal literature [on DI] reads like an answer to the following exercise: review all of the case law and statutes relating to DI and discuss all possible lawsuits any participant or product of DI might have against anyone. If time permits, suggest a statutory scheme that might minimize these problems.

Suggested control of DI includes: (1) control by statute; (2) control by the medical profession within a legislative framework; (3) continuing with present status, judicial control when cases arise in addition to "informal control by the medical profession"; (4) a combination of any of all of the above; (5) legislating DI outside the medical profession.

Schatkin (1954), writing in *Fertility and Sterility*, reassured his colleagues that

> knowing that the law cannot be hurried, the wise doctor will continue this happiness-bestowing procedure with the conviction that the law will ultimately give its blessing.

Legislation to date has attempted to deal with the legal identity of the DI child and the rights and obligations of the parties involved, from the time of conception through to divorce or custody matters. The United States Uniform Parentage Act of 1974 deals with DI in Section 5: donor insemination is to be done only under the supervision of a licensed physician, with the consent of both the husband and wife. Records are kept confidential in sealed files and the donor has no legal or financial rights or responsibilities with regard to the child. The actual regulation of the procedure is a much more difficult question.

As George Annas points out:

> The need for "a better public policy" is not synonymous with immediate legislation. The problem with DI is that there are many unresolved problems with it, and few of them are legal. It is time to stop thinking about uniform legislation and start thinking about the development of professional standards. Obsessive concern with self-protection needs to give way to concern for the child.

Supreme Court decisions in recent years have upheld the right to privacy in the area of reproduction. Physicians doing DI, as we have seen, go far beyond privacy when they counsel secrecy, match blood groups, and provide anonymous donors. Among those who call for legal reforms are people who want to safeguard the secrecy and keep DI in the hands of the medical profession and others who would legislate just the opposite. Some will complain that regulation will mean less anonymity, and others will cry "Big Brother." Most statutes permit only licensed medical practitioners to perform DI, although as we have seen they usually do inadequate screening and follow-up. Such legislation makes DI more difficult for single women and lesbians, and drives DI underground, as happened with abortion in the past and home birth today.

My first recommendation is that DI be arranged openly between the individuals involved. However, the current practice of DI will be slow to change and better safeguards must be instituted in the interim for those individuals who cannot make their own private arrangements. Legislation concerning reproduction and parenthood in the United States is primarily a state matter and more than half of the states have some limited statutes. I would argue that legislation dealing with donor screening and record keeping, which is now absent from most statutes, is needed right away. This would protect the child as well as the infertile couple, and would provide the foundation for genetic and psychological research. The President's Commission on Bioethics in 1983 recommended that DI donors be genetically screened and that records be kept of the semen source and sample. Annas recommends that "uniform and complete standards for donor selection and screening (including genetic screening) should be developed and made public."

Records should be kept of all parties so that donors can be matched with offspring and so that in the future the child can have access to these confidential records. Payment for donors should be abolished.

As the preamble of the United Nations Declaration of the Rights of the Child states, the child needs "special safeguards and care, including appropriate legal protection before as well as after birth." I also feel that extensive education and counseling should be mandatory for those undergoing DI, which would also involve professionals other than physicians, as well as families who have experienced DI.

11

The Burden of Secrecy

> If you want to keep a secret, you must also hide it from your-self.
>
> —*George Orwell*, 1984

COUPLES UNDERGOING OR PLANNING DI not only have the psychological burdens of unwanted childlessness and medical in-tervention, but they also have felt obliged to enter a pact of silence as well. Before we look at specific cases of how secrets affect the lives of individuals, we will examine the characteristics of secrecy. Sissela Bok, who has taught medical ethics at MIT, explores the philosophical dimensions of secrecy in her two influential books *Secrets* and *Lying*. Mark Karpel, assistant professor of psychiatry at Tufts University, looks at the family dynamics that result from secrets.

Secrecy—The Philosophical Dimensions

Bok compares the two elements of secrecy and privacy, defining secrecy as "intentional concealment" and privacy as "the condi-tion of being protected from unwanted access by others—either physical access, personal information or attention." She points out that secrecy and privacy overlap when efforts at controlling access to one's personal domain rely on hiding. "Privacy need not hide; and secrecy hides far more than what is private."

The danger of secrecy, however, obviously goes far beyond risks to those who *keep* secrets. If they alone were at risk, we would have fewer reasons to try to learn about, and sometimes interfere with, their secret practices. Our attitude changes radically as soon as we suspect that these practices also hurt others. And because secrecy can debilitate judgment and choice, spread and become obsessive, it often affects others even when it is not intended to. This helps explain why, in the absence of clean criteria for when secrecy is and is not injurious, many people have chosen to regard all secrecy as potentially harmful.

When the freedom of choice that secrecy gives one person limits or destroys that of others, it affects not only his own claims to respect of identity, plans, action, and property, but theirs. The power of such secrecy can be immense. Because it bypasses inspection and eludes interference, secrecy is central to the planning of every form of injury to human beings. It cloaks the execution of these plans and wipes out all traces afterward. It enters into all prying and intrusion that cannot be carried out openly. While not all that is secret is meant to deceive, as jury deliberations, for instance, are not—all deceit does rely on keeping something secret. And while not all secrets are discreditable, all that is discreditable and all wrongdoing seek out secrecy.

Secrecy interferes with rational choice by preventing people from adequately understanding the situation, from seeing relevant alternatives clearly, from assessing the consequences and arriving at resolutions. How can secrecy make an action right which otherwise would not be seen as such? Putting forth a public discussion forces people to determine, before they act, what might be brought out if they were called to account for their actions. Publicity is crucial to moral choice, so that views become explicit and open to criticism, and errors and ignorance can be challenged which helps perspectives to change.

A major problem with secrecy is the emotional cost involved. Bok says we must ask whether it was right to make the pledge in the first place, whether the premise is a binding one, and even if it is, what circumstances might nevertheless justify overriding it. Secrecy creates barriers between people but at the same time it offers the temptation to gossip or confession; there is always the possibility and thus the fear of revelation. Secrets are for telling, as the saying goes.

Bok observes that conflicts over secrecy, especially between the parent and child, are conflicts over power: the power that comes from controlling the flow of information. Secrecy and power are always closely linked, especially with physicians and governments. Lies can often seem the only way not to disappoint or injure families and friends. Deception, Bok notes, is "never more zealously perpetrated than by those who believe that the welfare of those deceived is at issue." (Erikson termed this "loving deceit.")

> Lies don't just affect the child, but other family members participate in the deceit or are themselves deceived as well. It is rare that one lie will be sufficient. One has to keep shoring up lies, adjusting them, and living with the effects of the deception on the liars, anxiety and tension about disclosure, further complications to the story. "Living a Lie" often turns out not to be worth it for the liars as well as the deceived, especially if the price is loss of trust and self integrity.

Adults tend to distort the truth when it suits them to have a child conform to certain expectations they have about behavior, eating habits, and so on. Bok points out that the need to shield and encourage, the low priority on accuracy, and the desire to get meaningful information across in spite of difficulties of understanding or response contribute to the ease with which children are deceived. But she argues that because they have so few suspicions, children should receive the greatest protection.

Children also need to learn the difference between the "truth" and "truthfulness," for example, confusing jokes and fiction with lies. Bok notes that such confusion "fails to recognize the fact that fiction does not *intend* to mislead, that it calls for what Coleridge called a 'willing suspension of disbelief,' which is precisely what is absent in ordinary deception."

Bok suggests the following format for examining lies.

1. Ask whether there are alternative courses of action that will achieve the aims one takes to be good without requiring deception.
2. Set forth the moral reason, thought, or excuse to justify the lie, and the possible counterarguments.

3. Test these two steps by asking how a public of reasonable persons would respond to such arguments.

Bok explores the problem of *consent*, especially the doctrine of "implied consent" in paternalistic lying, meaning that those deceived would acknowledge that it was for their own good. Exactly who is being protected—the patient, the professional, the donor, the child? Confidentiality often stretches beyond the client or patient to include what professionals hide *from* patients, clients, and the public at large. Deception among family members and friends is the form of paternalism in which most of us encounter the hardest choices between truthfulness and lying.

Bok concludes:

> The way to tell rightful paternalistic lies from all the others would then be to ask whether the deceived, if completely able to judge his own interests, would himself want to be duped. If he becomes rational enough to judge at a later time, one would then ask whether he gives his retroactive consent to the deceit—whether he is grateful he was lied to.

> The bond between liar and deceived does not in itself justify paternalistic lies, nor does the liar's belief in his good intentions, in the inability of the deceived to act reasonably if told the truth, and in the implied consent of the deceived. In assuming such consent, all the biases afflicting the liar's perspective are present in force.

> In summary, paternalistic lies, while they are easy to understand and to sympathize with at times, also carry very special risks: risks to the liar himself from having to lie more and more in order to keep up the appearance among people he lies with or sees often, and thus from the greater likelihood of discovery and loss of credibility; risks to the relationship in which the deception takes place; and risks of exploitation of every kind for the deceived.

Manuel (1973), studying the effect of secrecy upon couples in a DI program in France, observes:

> Despite the protective function of secrecy, its preservation may have a high psychological price. If the very deep and legitimate need to communicate and share has to be defended against constantly, the secret itself may become a toxic and burdensome factor which is related, at times, to mood or behavioral disturbances, and even to

more severe symptoms such as paranoid fears, projection and isolation.

The Nature and Context of Secrets

In view of these pressing ethical questions, those who hold secrets need to come to terms with their sabotage. The secret paternity in DI, in spite of, or perhaps because of, the promises of silence, raises fantasies in all involved—the couple, child, donor, and doctor. Legal uncertainties foster the secrecy and are fostered by it, and physicians collaborate in driving the process underground. We must seriously consider the importance of the secret for the unaware child, and view the situation from the child's position. As Ingrid Ursing, writing in the Swedish medical journal *Lakartidningen*, asks, "How can we gain perspectives on this question if we don't speak openly about it? It is time to clean up the secrecy games and the effort to pretend that DI does not exist." David Berger, a Toronto psychiatrist, stresses that the present state of affairs in DI lends itself to being abused in ways that are "indeed socially unacceptable." As one couple expressed to Achilles:

> It has been something that has been very painful to work through. It's not something that has been easy to discuss . . . we haven't been able to discuss it with anybody. . . . If you decide to tell them the question is when . . . because can that child go to school and say that she is a DI baby and not be different from her peers? . . . Somebody had bought us a book that has, you know, a baby's first lock and your baby's first walk and all this and on one page there were family trees and I thought, What am I supposed to fill in on this? I am supposed to fill in my husband's family tree? I suppose I am, but that has a lot to do with genetic inheritance and I couldn't do it because, again, I was feeling we were living a lie . . . or I felt like we were supposed to go home and pretend that this never happened and you can't do that. Every time we bring it up, it's very painful, it really is. We've been through a tremendous amount of pain because of it. The other day my husband said, the agreement was that we would do this and not say anything about it, and now I am wanting to be open about it and I said, "Yes, but Bill, you can't hold that against me because when that was put to us, that

was before we had this human being to consider . . . and, many many things alter when that human being is here in your lives. . . . I have a sense of her being rootless . . . there's a part of her we don't know.

Karpel defines three types of family secrets: (1) individual; (2) internal family secrets (which create a subgroup within the family); and (3) shared family secrets (which separate the family as a whole from the outside world). Secrets, Karpel explains, tend to be about facts, real happenings or incidents, rather than thoughts or feelings. At a factual level, secrets result in lies and distortion, and on an emotional level, they generate anxiety. The target of the secret is the unaware child who is likely to experience confusion and negative feelings with regard to explanations that she concocts as she tries to understand the atmosphere of shame and guilt that exists. However unpalatable the truth may be, the fantasies so created are always much worse.

Secrets set up loyalty dynamics that help create and maintain family secrets that in turn may generate or increase split-loyalty patterns. For example, a woman tells her sister about DI, but not her mother. The sister then feels disloyal to the mother, but cannot share the secret with her or she will feel disloyal to her sister. There is also a dangerous and unstable tension inherent in the power dynamics of secrets that pushes toward destructive disclosures. An example would be the angry husband who screams at his teenage DI son, "You're no child of mine."

> The child swears to the secret and because children take such promises seriously, she never discussed with her adoptive father the one subject, that, had it been aired, might have made them close. So she and her mother are conspirators now.
>
> —*Betty Jean Lifton,* Twice Born

Secrets within the family, such as between the DI parents, strengthen their alliance, but estrangements can develop between the secret-holders and the unaware child because of the deception, mystification, and difficulty in discussing subjects relating to sex and reproduction.

Dynamics of Communication in Secrecy

Communication around secrecy occurs at many levels. Sharing may be done directly or indirectly through hints and acknowledgments. Manuel talks about "leaking."—behavior patterns that are consciously aimed at preserving the secret but indicate the existence of the secret and point toward its content. Secrets may also be shared in the form of confessions, or even acting-out behavior. Some individuals are compulsively honest and share information with just about everyone. Others create a false reality by simulation and partial information. But usually in DI the secrecy is completely preserved through denial and lies, and the result is no communication at all. These parents typically express their attitude with such condescending rebuttals as "Why tell the child—it would serve no purpose at all" and "What he doesn't know doesn't hurt him." But as one adoptee said, "What we don't know *does* hurt us."

Manuel looks at three pressures that secrecy can bring to DI couples:

1. Psychological pressures from defending against various conflicts that are brought up by the DI, infertility, and wish for a child.
2. Pressures from family and society, forcing the couple to adapt and conform in a way that protects them, or the infertile male, from rejection and guilt within relationships.
3. Pressure with regard to long-term consequences that may affect the child and future generations.

His research concludes that "a positive point is reached . . . in the acceptance of DI by the husband when he believes that the child can know his origins."

The American culture considers privacy in reproductive matters to be paramount. In fact, personal freedom with regard to abortion and contraception has been protected by law. Yet the rapid changes in reproductive technologies are affecting society in unforetold ways. The interests of the child and those who produce him are in conflict where privacy extends into anonymity and secrecy. Karpel points out that the distinction between privacy and secrecy hinges on the relevance of the information for the unaware. The more significant the information—such as a child's genealogy—then the greater the compulsion for secrecy.

DI parents popularly use the excuse that they are "protecting the child" when choosing not to tell her the truth of her origins. It is, of course, the parents who are protecting themselves— against the embarrassment of infertility and the fear that their children will abandon them without the "blood knot." It is interesting that the secret is designed to protect the child not from some act that might happen in the future, but simply from the *knowledge* of an act that has already occurred in the past, or feelings he or she might develop about that act. This paternalistic protection (lying) is also a way to avoid taking responsibility for one's own actions. Instead, the DI couple try to conceal their infertility and "forget" that the procedure ever happened.

Everyone lives the lie—those who know the secret and those who do not. The child may not know it whereas the others do, but the fact of the deception exists in all their lives. The family group may even go into therapy "living a lie" either by not disclosing the DI status of the child to the therapist, or including the therapist in the secret but continuing to exclude the child. Karpel concludes:

> Secrets mean that trust is not in fact merited by trustworthiness, and for this reason, whether the secrets are revealed or not, they harm the balance of fairness, the overall structure of trust and trustworthiness, within the system. This violation of trust may constitute the most devastating consequence of secrets.

Secrets—A Violation of Rights

In contrast with most physicians, many psychologists and social workers agree that keeping the DI a secret is a violation of the child's right, a right that others do not have the right to violate. Betty Jean Lifton, an adoptee herself and a pioneer in adoption reform, stresses that no one, not even a parent, should have the right to tamper with a child's history. Lifton explains that parents then raise the child with the "perilous *as-if* factor" (that is, as if she had been conceived by both parents in a natural way). The "right to heritage is in effect the right to reality," she writes. Lee Campbell, a birthmother and founder of Concerned United Birthparents (CUB), stresses that "the creators should know the welfare of their seed and the children their origins." George Annas suggests that "if DI is seen as a loving act for the child's benefit, there seems no reason to taint the procedure with the lie that could prove extremely destructive to the child." Pediatrician Burton Sokoloff writes (1987):

> The secrecy involved in the family using alternative forms of reproduction proves to be a self-perpetuating, all-encompassing problem and a springboard for many others . . . the secrecy surrounding DI is detrimental in resolving the couple's reaction to the husband's infertility and may play a role in the genesis of later family problems.

In contrast, the Ontario Law Reform Commission (1985) stated that the continued secrecy respecting the child's origins and the anonymity of the donor are generally thought to be of substantial importance to the stability of the family and the welfare of the child. For a good many children, to be confronted at some point with the existence of the donor, or with the donor himself, may well be disruptive.

The Warnock report (1984) recommended that "anonymity protects all parties not only from legal complication but also from emotional difficulties." Snowden and Snowden (1984) commented that "if there were any contact between the donor and recipient couple it is very likely that conflicting emotional ties might arise and cause trouble." The American Fertility Society stresses that "if the doctor and the child's parents are the only people who are aware of the nature of the conception, how can the child find out this information and how can he question his identity?" Guttmacher (1962) suggests that

> the procedure should be known to only three people: the doctor, the husband, and the wife, so that to all intents and purposes the child is the biological as well as the legal child of the couple. *Unless we can achieve this attitude, it seems to me that the procedure has little merit.* [Italics mine]

Feldschuh (1978) was aware that "adopted children have identity problems that vary from minimal to serious ones requiring psychotherapy," but he believes "when anonymous donor insemination is used, these identity traumas need never occur. . . . Under these circumstances no one need ever know that this particular child is not the natural child of a particular set of parents."

The medical profession hoped that secrecy would enable all the issues about DI to be swept under the rug. Finegold incorrectly prophesied that

> we find very little reason to suspect that a child who is the product of DI needs to concern himself with any emotional consequences. Unlike the adoptive baby, the insemination offspring never learns of his "test-tube" origin. To him, his mother and father are his true parents, not his foster parents.

(Note that a medical doctor is incorrectly using the term "test-tube" babies and also overlooks that fact that the biological mother is certainly not a foster parent.) On the other hand, the offspring have a different view of the situation. Betty Jean Lifton lamented, "It is a lonely and awesome responsibility being someone else's answer," and Ariel raises our consciousness with her insights:

> When you talk to people who are talking about infertility, it is always, "What do I do to get a baby?" No one talks about the adult the baby will become and the rights that the adult has to know his or her true parentage. But I'm the baby they talk about and I have something to say.

One DI mother complained to Achilles:

> The way they put it to you in the clinics is: "We can find you a donor who looks like you, of your blood type." Basically what they are saying is that there is someone else who is like you out there and you have to pretend that it was you, but it's much deeper than that and I think to live with that all your life . . . and when your child is thirty and you are still living with it . . . I think the secrecy is a terrible thing. I just feel the child has a right to know. You are its parents and you owe it honesty and everything else. . . . To think that child might walk away from you because of that . . . I don't believe that's true. It might walk away from you if you've lied

to it for thirty years. ... I'm feeling now that the deception is worse than not knowing the donor. We want her to be honest; it's a contradiction.

Another DI mother explained to Achilles:

I've noticed a strange thing has happened since we've decided our daughter will know the truth. Before, when we were pretending that Bill was biologically related to her, every time grandma, or aunts and uncles from his side were mentioned, I would cringe inside and think, They are not really her aunts and uncles and grandma. Since we've decided she'll know, I can talk about these relatives and feel now that they are her aunts and uncles and grandma. Does that make sense? As long as doctors continue to counsel secrecy, DI will never be out of the closet. It produces negative feelings of shame and guilt and why not? It must be a terrible thing we did if we're not supposed to ever tell anyone. I truly believe there wouldn't be any conflicts and dilemmas if it was shared from the beginning and the child was raised to know. Doctors are saying "Why tell the child?" and I say, "Why not?"

Achilles concluded that if there were "no point in telling," then there would be no investment in secrecy.

The Psychology of Heredity

In 1952, Wellisch coined the phrase "genealogical bewilderment," which refers to no knowledge, or uncertain knowledge, of at least one biological parent. He found that the resulting state of confusion and uncertainty undermines the child's security and affects his mental health, meaning that he has no stable concept of himself and his status.

Sants (1964) believes that in adolescence, when the normally maturing child is satisfactorily weaning himself from his parents through displacement of feelings and bonds onto wider groups, such as clan or family, the genealogically deprived child is handicapped by not knowing to which clan or family he belongs. Such children appear to be disturbed by this blockage of possible displacement, and the preoccupation can be distressing. A sense of belonging is necessary for emotional security, and thus not knowing appears to be incompatible with a secure self-image. He quotes an eight-year-old foster child who said, "I do not know nearly enough of my Daddy, I want to find out someday where he is. I'd like to know his address and send him a letter."

Let us explore the reactions of adults who were denied access to their full genetic heritage. The vast reservoir of people denied the truth of their origins includes both adoptees and children conceived by DI. Also, there is a certain percentage of children in the population, revealed by blood-group studies, who are unknowingly of unknown paternity. It has been estimated that about five million Americans are adoptees, and that there are over a half million DI offspring, with at least 25,000 being conceived each year. Considering the family members also involved, between 10 and 20 percent of the population is directly touched by the issue of confused heredity.

Betty Jean Lifton (1975) notes that while most families have secrets, the adoptee is in a special position because "his quest for the most fundamental details of his existence is a direct source of guilt. He has no choice but to adapt to a pervasive sense of separatedness and half-life." The same occurs with the DI child, with regard to her paternal heritage if she is aware of it and wishes to search. In both cases, society (parents, physicians, social workers) try to remake reality, replacing fact with fantasy, beginning with the falsification of the birth certificate and continuing around most of the adoptee's life processes.

The adoption experience has proven that it is of enormous significance to the child, especially during adolescence, to explore his heritage. His identity and self-image are built on knowledge of his past, the kind of people he came from, as well as his sense of continuity of the family line with himself. Fantasies about the origins of the father (for instance, that he was famous or suffered an early death) are common in children and create a frame of reference for assimilating clues about the truth in the family relations. However, when the truth is not available the fantasies further alienate the child from reality. Social worker Fernando Colon (1978) writes that

> the desire to know one's biological origins and parentage results from a deeply felt psychological and emotional need, a need for roots, for existential continuity, and for a sense of completeness. To know who one's biological parents are or were, to know where

one's skin color, facial features, body build, temperament, and talents come from is a powerful human desire that drives a person as he seeks to achieve a sense of wholeness about himself.

Lorraine Dusky, a birthmother, examined the plight of individuals who are missing part of their heritage in a *Newsweek* article "Brave New Babies."

> Those of us who take our backgrounds for granted cannot imagine what it feels like to have only questions instead of facts. What does it mean not to know if your father wrote poems or ran the mile or fashioned beautiful objects from wood and played the penny whistle? Or that your mother was a talented cellist and smoked cigars or was a terrible cook but a master at bridge? Or on a more practical level, whether your father developed heart disease later in life and you are at risk? It seems that no one—the would-be parents or parent least of all—is bothering to consider what all this might mean for the child.

Numerous philosophers, from Sophocles to Erik Erikson, have pondered the question of identity. The consensus is that a strong sense of identity is charted both by the past, (heredity) and the present (environment). An individual who lacks either is incomplete. A genetically bewildered person is usually, at some level, a troubled one.

Dusky observed that some very destructive members of society have been adoptees.

> Lacking a full human parentage, that connection with our past that forms such a large part of our present, they fill the hole in their identity with rage. More often the void is filled with alienation and anomie. Even in the best of circumstances it is filled with pain. As an adoptee poignantly expressed it this way. The suspense of not knowing is deeper than frustrating. It's dislocating. Nothing quite fits. You can never establish yourself as a person.

Evasive attitudes by parents about sex and reproduction, for fear that they will lead to a discussion of DI, will be sensed by the child. One adoptee was well aware of such a taboo in her home.

> For almost seventeen years I lived with the concealment of my adoption. At the time I did not comprehend it, but I can still clearly recall the disturbing effect any reference to my birth or heredity had

on my parents—embarrassment and guilt were literally hanging in the air.

The reproduction dilemma becomes more acute when the woman suffering genealogical bewilderment becomes pregnant. All kinds of fears about unknown hereditary illnesses and labor complications and birth defects begin to surface. The experience of motherhood (also death, divorce, or illness) is often the precipitating factor leading adoptees to search for their roots for their own peace of mind and so that they may have something to share with their offspring.

The Cruelty of Deception

Although adopted children have to deal with the fact that their birthmother surrendered them (as we now know, usually under great duress and with deep reluctance), they feel great anger and resentment if the adoptive parents deceived them. The DI child may feel upset that money was involved in creating her existence, but the deception is a worse stress. When there is a lack of biological information about the child, or an unwillingness to convey it, parents create family tension that prevents questions and feelings about the state of not knowing from being raised at all, much less discussed.

Viola Bernard (1963) writes in an article on adoption:

> The child who senses the half truths, evasions, and lies will feel upset, anxious, and confused, and instead of receiving his parent's support and guidance, will be cut off by the conspiracy of silence.

Pauline Ley, an adoptee in Australia, describes her anguish and frustration:

> In my family, my parents attempted to deny their infertility altogether by pretending to me, to the community, and I think to themselves that I was their naturally born child. My parents destroyed the adoption order which contained information concerning my preadoptive identity, as though by actually obliterating evidence of my biological roots, it was possible to deny them altogether. Despite this conspiracy of silence, I grew up sensing that

there was some secret concerning my existence from which I was excluded. My parents, who under no other circumstances would tell a lie to their child, deceived me cruelly. Well-intentioned though that deception may have been, its effect on my dignity as a child, and their integrity as adults, was not without far-reaching consequences.

There should be no more trusting relationship than that which exists between a child and its parents. Children have an implicit and profound sense of trust in the two adults on whom their security, physical survival, and emotional well-being depend. A most fundamental aspect of that trust is the child's belief that he belongs in his family because his mother and his father are his biological kin. In early childhood, the DI child will trustingly accept that because he was born to his mother, he is therefore the biological product of his father, unless he is told otherwise. Our experience suggests that it is folly to exploit the trust of a child. We believe that in DI families where the "big secret" is being maintained, the child will be adversely affected.

If a child feels she does not "fit" in the family, she assumes that there is something wrong with *her*. An adoptee recalls, "I grew up knowing something was missing, like I had an empty spot but could never pinpoint what it was."

Some adoptees recognize that information is withheld or distorted because parents want to protect the child. Most, however, maintain that truth and honesty, however painful the facts, would have been easier than living with lies and would have enhanced their respect and trust in their parents. Triseliotis found that secrecy and evasiveness gave adoptees the feelings that adoption was something shameful, and that this feeling contributed to the development of a poor self-image and a reluctance among adoptees to reveal their adoption even to close friends.

The Adoption Triangle is a poignant book written by a psychiatrist, Arthur Sorosky, and two social workers, Annette Baran and Reuben Pannor. The authors detail the effects of sealed records on adoptees as well as both birth and adoptive parents. An adoptee wrote to them:

I knew my thinking, my independence, my emotions came from somewhere else. I was in no way like the family that adopted me, yet brought me up normally. People that have not been through it simply say, "Forget about it, you could find your mother to be a streetwalker or criminal." The thing that an outsider fails to understand is that you can identify with another human being that made you. Up to that point, you know nothing about yourself and what makes you do the things you do, bad or right as they may be. No matter who raises you, there are certain things that you inherit.

Another adoptee said:

I feel like a test-tube baby. I have asked my adoptive parents what is my background, who am I? All I get is two hurt people that I love very much. So I no longer question them on the subject. Isn't it natural for me to wonder about my past? I feel that it couldn't harm me to know. My adoption seems like a highly guarded secret. Even secrets are told to people with the need to know. I have the need to know.

Genealogical bewilderment is greater when there are differences in appearance and intelligence between the child and his parent(s). One study, quoted by Lifton (1981), found that 60 to 70 percent of sons with the same body type as their fathers had a good relationship, whereas only 20 to 30 percent of those men did whose body type was different. Physical features within families are also important as they orient a child to one side of the family or another.

Dear Ann Landers:
This is for the grandmother with the red-headed grandchild. She was embarrassed because no one on either side of the family had red hair. People kept asking, "How come?" The same thing happened to me. I found myself going into detail about an aunt on my husband's side and my grandmother's sister who came from Ireland. The longer I talked, the more smirks I noticed. Finally I decided to stop being a damned fool. I didn't owe anybody any explanations. From then on I replied, without batting an eye, "It must have been the milkman!" Then they did the squirming.

A DI mother said,

> My daughter looks so like me that people sometimes ask me (jok-
> ingly and unknowingly) if my husband was involved at all. Once I
> startled someone by saying, "No—I cloned her!"

Suzanne Ariel is a DI adult and a birthmother who has become
an activist in both DI and adoption reform. Her saga began when
her mother died in 1979, after which Suzanne began to wonder
about her own daughter, whom she had given up for adoption at
age fifteen. She realized that tomorrow is never guaranteed and
that she needed to communicate the events surrounding the relinquishment to her daughter before time ran out. Within six months
she found her, and two weeks later her father told Suzanne that he
was not her father and that she would have to do another search if
she wanted all the questions answered about her heritage (and her
daughter's). Suzanne recalls that her pregnancy completely shattered the relationship with her father.

> I never understood the degree of his fury about my pregnancy until
> I learned (fifteen years later) that *he was infertile*. I don't believe he
> had ever come to terms with his infertility and therefore could not
> tolerate his fifteen-year-old daughter and her sixteen-year-old boy-
> friend being able to have a child since he could not.

> During the pregnancy, I know my mother suffered. She knew she
> was going to lose her grandchild, but she took charge of the situa-
> tion and handled it in the best way she knew how. My home life
> was very unhappy and I knew that I could never allow my daughter
> to be raised in such an environment. I spent the better part of a
> year mourning the loss of my daughter, although I still graduated
> from high school with a 4.0 grade average and proceeded on to
> UCLA at age sixteen.

Within two years of returning home after the birth, Suzanne left
her parents' home. There was no communication with her parents
for over five years, although she later reunited with them and
worked through most of the issues surrounding them in analysis.

In the office of a therapist that he was seeing, her father told
Suzanne that he had lived with this secret for thirty years and
couldn't live with it any longer. During those years he had spoken
to no one and had lied about family medical history when giving
information to the adoption agency.

It was interesting that the therapist's husband was a physician who had been a donor and she seemed to think that because her husband had been a donor, it was okay, although to me, it was anything but okay. My father terminated our relationship shortly after when I did a newspaper article about the search for my birthfather. He told me he never wanted to see me again, and I was greatly relieved to be able to comply with his request. The relationship had become a burden that I no longer felt compelled to carry. I felt sorry for my father, for his pain, I felt he was a victim of circumstances with which he did not know how to cope. He suffered greatly, and I suspect will continue to do so until the day he dies. At the core of it, the relationship was built on a deception and I was betrayed. Although I understood the circumstances, I could no longer trust him. If my mother were alive, I suppose I would have found the heart to forgive her, but I never would have forgotten the betrayal. I feel certain that she would have supported the search for my birthfather. I know I could have educated her to my point of view, and that she would have understood my position.

The lies and deceptions upon which DI families are built, warp and poison family relationships. No healthy family can be built upon such lies and deception; and in the DI family, deception is at the very core of the relationship. It is a cruel hoax to be played on a trusting child. Do parents have the right to deceive said child of its true heritage for the entirety of that individual's life, knowing that the lies will cripple the parent-child relationship? Is this what parenthood is really all about? I think not. DI sounds wonderful in the textbooks, but what it can do to human lives is something else.

What they are really protecting is the secrecy of infertility, the willingness of a couple to take genetic potluck, and the anonymity of a donor who's just in it for the bucks. The rights of the child are not even considered. I am missing one half of my heritage. I most probably have brothers and sisters, which for an only child is very important. And one half of my medical history is undefined.

I do not believe I will ever reconcile my parents' decision to use DI. The one word which would most accurately describe how I feel about being the product of DI is *anguished*.

Ariel takes to task physicians such as Sherman Silber, who in the April 1982 issue of the *Saturday Evening Post* gratuitously assumes that children born by DI usually "bond closely with the husband and wife and are integrated into the family as closely as any routinely conceived biological child." The same was believed about adoption; in fact, it is still a prevalent social belief that it is "better" for children of young, unmarried mothers to be adopted by usually older, married, supposedly economically and emotionally stable "approved" couples. (The criteria are similar to those set up for couples requesting DI.)

However, adoption does not always provide a better life, as birthparents have found out to their lasting remorse. Thousands of testimonies are surfacing with regard to pressure to excel, molestation, negligence, abandonment, corporal punishment, termination of rights after death of spouse, murder, and suicide. The public is not generally aware that 15 percent of adoptions fail outright and adoptees are more heavily represented in remedial and psychotherapeutic institutions than the population at large. Much of the need for counseling and psychiatric help is due to anxiety over blood ties. So often problems with adoptees are simply brushed aside with the axioms of "bad environment" or "bad seed." But more significantly, as Dusky points out, "It's hard to know where you are going when you don't know where you came from." The Scottish social worker Triseliotis in his book *In Search of Origins* (1973) has found that where families can accept the adoption of the child, those children are not more prone to psychological problems.

The sparse information about DI families indicates just the opposite from what Dr. Silber assumes. The DI children who became aware of their origins and have been interviewed as adults virtually knew there was an "awful secret" to which they were not privy. In almost all cases, the disclosure was made under the most undesirable circumstances. Ariel continues:

> Those of us who were produced by DI and have become aware of our origins are left to face the devastations of our losses, and we are enraged by practitioners like Dr. Silber who present DI as a benign, painless, and perfectly and universally acceptable procedure. IT IS NOT.

Betty Jean Lifton (1981) explains that

> An adoptee's past is like a mummy bound in layers of shroud, wrapped in years of secrets, mysteries, lies, deceptions, confabulations, mythology.

Baran and Pannor report that one of the nineteen DI offspring they interviewed had finally figured out the secret herself and confronted her parents. But it was a long process. First she thought she was adopted. Then she wondered if her mother had had an affair. DI was the last possibility she considered.

A twenty-four-year-old English DI child wrote to the authors of *The Artificial Family* that even before the age of four there were allusions to her father's lack of sexual contact with her mother.

> She said that as he was unable to "put his seed into her, a doctor had put it there with a test tube" or words to that effect. I remember the discussion quite clearly for I wished to know exactly what a test tube looked like.

Later on in puberty, her mother asked a lover to explain the situation more precisely.

> He asked me if I knew about cows being "injected" with test tubes of sperm—I said that of course I did, never being one to admit to ignorance. There was obviously something more to all this but still I did not predict what was to come next. "That's the way your mum fell for you." There must have been more questions from me, answers from him, but essentially I felt like escaping, carrying this great, shattering boulder of information away with me.

> I had a picture of grunting farm animals, test tubes, sperm, and me. God the Father had deserted me, I was the child of the devil, a pubescent melodrama that I acted out in hate and revenge. . . . Never did I worry about being a bastard. No, what upset my whole sense of being was that nobody knew my "real father": as though half of me did not, does not, exist.

> But my mother clearly felt a sense of shame for I was sworn to secrecy. Therefore I told everybody the circumstances of my conception at the earliest opportunity. I sought out my most garrulous cousin and told her "everything" in return for her juicy family secrets. She spread the news throughout my mother's family. To this day maternal aunts, who showed me affection in my early years, dislike and ignore me. Doubtless my personality has contributed greatly to this state of affairs, but I do wonder. . . . My grandmother always finds occasion to speak darkly about "blood" in my company, blood and its mysterious capacity to "carry" talents and traits. She always knew just how my mother had conceived me for she had paid the necessary fee for my conception.

> My father died of Huntington's chorea four years ago. Mother's family commiserated warmly with my (adopted) sister and all but ignored me. They knew logically I was no carrier of the dreadful disease but my "father's" family have never been told. They avoided my eyes, pretended I did not exist. Thank God that an anonymous donor, with good blood, is my father and not a carrier of Huntington's chorea.

The ironic end to this woman's saga is that she later married a man who was sterile, and the question of DI came up as an option for her.

> In discussions with my mother it came out that she had worried about what she was carrying when pregnant, had looked at me and wondered about my origins, my father from whom I had inherited all undesirable traits. ... Subsequently I came to understand my mother's decision to have a baby by DI. She was no thoughtless ogre but a woman who craved her own child. But me, how can I make such a decision? My child would lack two generations of fathers. I could not hide the circumstances of my own conception for it might well find out about my "father's" inherited illness and be full of fear. Friends and relatives all know that my husband is sterile. (He has had a biopsy to confirm that his condition is irreversible.) Children sense the unsaid—it would have to be told and told young. My husband and I have been unable to resolve the dilemma. Instead I went to Teacher Training College and now teach nursery children thus detracting from my desire for a child, not that this helps my husband in any way.

> One thing I do know—the initials [DI] come to haunt me every day of my life.

Another DI child, Lillian Atallah, experienced a much less eventful disclosure. Her mother paid her a visit when she was a freshman in college to announce that she was leaving her husband.

> Almost as an afterthought, she told me a story that began with "Do you remember that nice Dr. Seymour?" and ended with the realization that I'd been what the newspapers called a "test-tube" baby. ... At first I was incredulous that my parents, tradition-bound Arab immigrants, had done anything so radical. On second thought, it made perfect sense. They had chosen DI out of a problem-solving approach to infertility, not out of any desire to join the

space age. In the Arab culture, there was no such thing as "no fault" infertility: barren wives were objects of pity and contempt, while their husbands were regarded with similar condescension, for having chosen "damaged goods." To choose adoption would have been to advertise physical infirmity in a society where "face" was everything. From my mother's point of view, the problem came down to these terms: "I wanted a baby, and I could never bring up someone else's child." Curiously, my father saw parenthood in a different light. Once, when my sister (before she knew about our donor parenthood) joked with him about taking the "wrong" baby home from hospital when she was born, he answered with a smile that the child you raised was your own.

Knowing about my DI birth did nothing to delete my feelings for my family. I felt grateful, especially to my father, for all the trouble they had taken to give me life.

I found a lot of humor in our situation, as did my sister in her turn. It was like having the childhood fantasy of being kidnapped by gypsies or being left on someone's doorstep come true. Though I never had any serious desire to know the identity of my genetic father, the fact that such a person existed sometimes served as a kind of safety valve in my adult relationship with my actual father.

Someone asked me once if I didn't feel a need to know my medical history on the paternal side, and my answer was that it was enough to know that I wasn't subject to the serious hereditary diseases that had showed up in my father's family.

My own feeling is that the manner of conception is only one variable in the life of that child, of the marriage of the family. Like any major life decision, DI can turn out badly or well, depending on the values and attitudes of the individuals, on how they feel about what they've done and the effectiveness of their problem-solving approach in general.

Candace Turner, another DI adult, has founded an organization called Donors' Offspring to make the public aware of the abuse of DI. She was thirteen years old when she found out; her mother had divorced Candace's "father" and remarried. Candace's relationship was not as good with her mother's second husband. As she was packing to visit her "first father" for the summer, the "second father" told her, "He's no more your father than I am."

This also had an effect on her brother, who, when he later considered medical school, wanted to search. However, today he does not share his sister's zeal and pays no attention at all to his biological origins.

Candace has been searching for her biological father for many years and every year she sends a Father's Day card to the doctor's office.

> On the Donahue show I appealed nationwide for my donor father to contact me, or his lawyer to contact me, and give medical information. I was thrilled that the nurse who had worked with the doctor called and she said she'd quit because she was so horrified about what the doctor was doing. She said there was no record keeping.

Candace feels strongly that records concerning the donors, recipients, and offspring should not only be kept but should be regularly updated. She is angry that her mother did know the donor's name (under atypical circumstances) but forgot it.

> She didn't bother copying it or remembering it. She wants to think that I'm all hers. She had the name because she had to write out a separate check to the donor.

> I told my mother I wished she had gone to one of her four brothers-in-law so I'd be genetically related, and had the doctor test all the male relatives on the husband's side of the family and he then pick whoever was best. Then nobody needs to know exactly who because you know that nephews and nieces are genetically linked.

> I go to these adoption conferences and I see these people who just met . . . birthparents and children. They haven't seen each other in thirty years . . . and they had no idea that they would walk the same way, hold a cigarette the same way, have the same taste in their clothes and hairstyles. There was so much that I didn't understand was genetically inherited. I thought these things were environmentally influenced . . . and I just feel real cheated.

Donors' Offspring has a list entitled, What Do Donors' Offspring Wonder About?, from which I have selected the following:

1. Am I adopted?
2. Was I created through a virgin birth?
3. I've studied biology, Dad, and considering mine and your eye coloring, you can't be my biological father.

4. Dad is so sick, will I develop his illness?
5. Dad has so many health problems, who would want to marry me and have children?
6. Why, Mom, did you and Dad really divorce?
7. Why do I have so little in common with Dad? I can't talk to him.
8. Why do you drink so much, Mother? Why do you seem to hate me?
9. Why did you two wait so long to have children? Why am I so different from my sister?
10. Why do I have so many strange nightmares?
11. Mother, why were you depressed for so long when I was young?
12. I'm so glad I was a wanted baby, but why did you wait so long to tell me?
13. I wonder if the donor is musically or otherwise talented?
14. I wonder if the donor is married, if he has natural children, if my grandparents are alive? I wonder what his career and hobbies are?
15. I wonder why the donor did it and why he accepted money?
16. I wonder if the donor has myopia (curly hair, dimples) like me?
17. I wonder if the donor has developed diabetes or other diseases?
18. I wonder how many half-siblings I have? Will I ever meet them? Would I know it?
19. I wonder why I can't meet my donor-father, now that I'm an adult?
20. I wonder if the donor knows I exist, if he'd like to know about or meet me?
21. Since my mother never remarried after the divorce, I wonder what having a father would be like?
22. Why would Dad have a vasectomy? He must not really have wanted me at his age.
23. Why did Dad work at such a dangerous place and become sterile?
24. You two never seem to get along well, why did you marry, or stay married, to someone who was sterile?

25. Why did you intentionally produce me without any paternal roots?
26. I wonder, did you leave the synagogue because they disapprove of DI?
27. Why didn't you adopt? There are so many lonely children, what's so important about a newborn, anyway?
28. If Dad suspected you were committing adultery, why didn't you, instead of paying all that money for an artificial conception?
29. I wonder why you pressured me to become a doctor, why didn't you let me be?
30. I wonder what motivates DI doctors?
31. I wonder if Dad will write me out of his will?
32. I wonder if I should search for my donor-father and what would come of it?
33. I wonder what it feels like to have been naturally created?
34. When I see adoptees reunited with relatives they look and act like, I wonder how much I'm like my unknown relatives.
35. I wonder if my boyfriend is related to me? Since he's adopted, we'll never really know, but he sure looks like me.
36. I wonder who I shall tell about being a donor's offspring, and how?
37. Oh, my child, someone who is like me! I wonder why no one told me what it is like?
38. Now that I have studied and thought about DI, I wonder why the nightmares have stopped? I wonder why it is such a big secret? I don't think DI should be handled in that way.
39. I wonder what was amiss, since my sister was adopted?
40. After I was told the truth, I wonder why suddenly it was as if a huge weight had been lifted off my shoulders?
41. I wonder if I should tell my mother that I've known the truth for years?
42. I wonder why they kept it a secret? To me, he's my father.
43. I wondered why Dad bothered me sexually? Is it because we weren't really related?
44. I wonder if and when I should tell my children, and explain why grandfather is so old and disinterested in them?
45. I wonder why my parents didn't use a male relative of Dad's to be a donor? I would so have liked to have roots.

Alan and Shirley Pratten are DI parents in Vancouver who were counseled by their physician to secrecy but as the years progressed they found it an impossible burden. The Prattens described their experience of DI "traumatic, to say the least." In fact, being interviewed by Rona Achilles was a turning point for them and they kept in touch with her over the years as they came to renounce the secrecy. As Alan said, "You don't start a relationship with a lie, do you?" and Shirley added, "If you can't tell the child then you can't tell anybody."

The Prattens' experiences with the medical profession have made them zealous advocates for reform. Prior to undergoing DI, they had been trying artificial insemination with Alan's sperm, as he had retrograde ejaculation (semen enters the bladder, but it can be collected and washed for insemination). However, the urologist was "too busy," and after a couple of cycles, as Shirley relates, "He said, 'Why don't you go upstairs and see Dr. K — he does DI,' as if there was no difference at all between the two procedures."

Shirley strongly disapproves of the denial that is encouraged at the DI clinics, and the way women get pregnant in isolation and are sent off never to see the doctor again.

> They should accept that DI exists, and deal with the experience and its ramifications, or else stop it. Let's do it properly and use a whole team of people, like with adoption and surrogates.

After the Prattens decided to "come out," Shirley wrote to her DI physician suggesting how his clinic operations could be improved, plus she offered to set up a support group for DI participants.

> He actually referred one woman to me, who was about three months pregnant, feeling suicidal and depressed, as I did at that time, too.

In April 1987, the Prattens held a press conference at the Granville Island Hotel, together with a donor and his wife and attorney Carey Linde (who led the class action suit in Canada against the Dalkon Shield manufacturers). The donor, Wayne Sebastian, is hoping to bring pressure on the physician in order to gain information about the use of his semen and resulting offspring. At the time of the press conference, Dr. K posted a security guard outside his office. Due to the media publicity around their press conference they received phone calls from various DI participants. Attorney Linde placed an "Artificial Insemination Alert" in newspapers across Canada, requesting contact from dissatisfied recipients of DI. A society is being formed that will not only push for reform of DI practices in Canada, but all aspects of alternative reproduction. In addition, they are a support group to inform and counsel participants.

> We want to keep the medical profession honest and take away some of the B.S. For example, at the same time that this doctor is claiming that he allows only eight pregnancies from one donor, a donor called in and said he had been donating for seven years! We contacted the Ministry of Health for information, which decided that since the heat is on, DI questions should be turned over to the Ministry of Social Services! . . . The genie is out of the bottle and we want answers . . . and we will take legal action if necessary.

The Prattens have also corresponded with the College of Physicians and Surgeons and provincial bodies involved in the regulation of DI. They are especially trying to have their own DI records kept longer than the statutory requirement of six years in British Columbia (their daughter is now five). If you wish to contact them, the Prattens' address and Carey Linde's address are listed in the Resources.

Donor Insemination

Donor Insemination Alert

If you are a recipient mother who
—would like to know who the donor of your D.I. child is, and
—whether that man has or will come down with physical or mental illness potentially inheritable by your child.
—had a gynecologist who failed to fully inform of increased likelihood of post partum depression with D.I. child or increased risk of marital problems.
—is concerned your D.I. child doesn't grow up and marry his/her half sister or brother or first cousin.

—thinks your D.I. child has a right to know who his/her biological father is.

—falsely believed that D.I. donors donated only a few times, rather than several times a week for several years.

—believes that only medical students are D.I. donors.

A D.I. donor who

—is concerned that your own children don't grow up and marry their own half sister or brother or first cousin.

—was misled by your doctor-patron on numbers of successful pregnancies and that only married women were your D.I. recipients.

—fears being sued in Family Court for financial support by mother of your D.I. child or having your D.I. children make a claim against your estate when you die.

—wants to know who your D.I. children are in case of parental death, welfare apprehension or divorce and custody fight.

A D.I. Child who

—wants to know who your biological father is and who your half sisters/brothers are.

—wants to know what your legal rights are or should be to inheritance and other possible claims.

The Wife of a Donor or Spousal Equivalent who

—is experiencing problems as a result of D.I.

—wants to know who your childrens' half brothers, half sisters and first cousins are.

A Doctor, Religious Leader or Member of the Public who

—recognizes the valuable role D.I. can play in society, but is concerned at the total lack of laws and regulations governing the practices and ethics of D.I. in Canada.

A D.I. donor and his wife in Vancouver are personally involved in all these issues and intend to take legal action to deal with them.

They need your help by knowing who you are and what your experience has been.

Write in complete confidence to
Law Offices of Carey Linde
208-1650 Duranleau St.
Vancouver, B.C. V6H 3S4

Secrecy in DI:
The "Advantages" Are the Disadvantages

As we have seen, the very advantages stressed by physicians (secrecy and genetic matching) are actually the disadvantages from the child's point of view. The secret of the DI conception is facilitated, and then if the adult wants to search, the truth of her origins is not available. Joan Holland, supervisor of Adoption Services of the North Carolina Department of Social Services, observes:

> These matching attempts have obvious merit, but even if a DI child would have all the genetic characteristics desired by his parents, he would bring them little happiness and would have small chance of it himself, if conflicts with the parents prevent their accepting him as their own.

Another woman put it this way:

> No matter how perfect the physical characteristics of the semen, it will all be wasted if there is not the right attitude.

It is well known that many couples choose DI because it is secret and reject adoption because of the obligation to tell the child of her origins. Let us now tally the burdens that secrecy entails.

1. *Anxiety* about ridicule, stigma, rejection, ethical and legal issues when making the decision to undergo DI.

2. *Feelings of isolation and tension* around being seen in the infertility clinic or gynecologist's office. Many couples also are worried about a breach of secrecy by the hospital, or refuse to have a nurse present during the DI. Often there is a fear of being pushed for an explanation when asking for repeated time off from work. The rare television interviews that have been done with couples undergoing the process have shrouded the individuals in masks or shadows so family and friends will not recognize them. (On the other hand, surrogate mothers have more often been prepared to appear openly in the media.)

3. *The pregnancy may be an anticlimax,* with everyone congratulating the husband, making him feel foolish and dishonest. (If

the truth were known, then congratulations of a different type would be in order.) Some women suffer depression following DI, and may feel that they have been "violated" as in rape. Some men feel almost as if they had paid a stranger to "rape" their wives.

4. The couple can be persuaded by the physicians to get away with the lie, because—unlike adoption—there is a pregnancy, which means that *the mother's partner is assumed to be the father.*

5. Pledging secrecy about the conception allows *the deception of others, most significantly the child,* while the parents share the secret. Løvset in Norway mentions cases where the DI was even kept secret from the husband. One woman regretted this, saying, "I would have preferred my husband to know that he was not the real father." Another woman felt that such deception might be justified to maintain the "self-respect of the husband," but not otherwise. (If readers are becoming upset to think about the husband being so deceived, this will help you identify with the plight of the DI child.) One woman went so far as to say, after she went from doctor to doctor to find one who would inseminate her without her husband's knowledge:

> I look upon my child as my husband's and never give a thought to the way in which I became pregnant. ... My husband doesn't know that I had DI performed and he is sure that the child is his and he is very proud of him.

In contrast, Blizzard wrote:

> Our major error was the conviction that our situation at that early stage was a secret and needed to be kept a secret at all costs. We had plenty of friends and colleagues of considerable wisdom and discretion. If we had chosen to air our troubles and speak with one of these people, then the perspectives might have altered and they might have become less alarming and less oppressive. Having assumed or been persuaded that these were issues to be concealed, we deprived ourselves of a counsel which we badly needed and we committed ourselves to a sequence of deceptions which could have filled up our lifetimes. Once committed, these deceptions could not be erased at will. A whole network of social existence would be built upon the nonsense of our false assumptions. We are ourselves to blame for interpreting this blemish as a leprosy which might exclude us from normal human convention. We were walking igno-

rantly towards a dungeon; obedient to ruthlessly mechanistic jailers.

6. Because families and kin networks are deceived, *pseudo-bonds are created, with rights, obligations, and expectations based on false premises.* The donor and his kin are related to the DI child but they have no knowledge of those relationships. The family is structured around a lie when the decision is made not to tell friends and relatives, in the mistaken belief that you can build a healthy family unit on fraud.

7. The donor is anonymous and in most cases *there will be no recourse for the offspring under any circumstances to gain knowledge of her paternal origins.*

8. There is a *fear of unknown hereditary diseases,* especially if the child develops health problems or deviant behavior. What do parents tell a DI teenager who gets a rare disease (symptoms that may be belatedly recognized because no one else in the family has those genes) when there are no records at the doctor's office or the sperm bank?

9. Community resources, such as social workers, psychologists, and genetic counselors, are rarely utilized. Although group support would be ideal, couples could at least benefit from individual counseling. A Danish study in 1981 found that about half of the couples did not want an open discussion of their own experiences of DI. But all felt the pronounced dilemma of a personal wish for secrecy and *the need to share experiences with other couples.*

10. Secrecy is very likely to increase the temptation not to cooperate with others to reduce shared burdens so that DI parents *raise the child in a degree of isolation.* As Joseph Blizzard writes:

> The couple with a donor child always have a secret to guard from relatives, acquaintances, and neighbours, which may soon impel them to loosen the ties and avoid social intercourse with these people as much as they can. This, again, may have repercussions. Should difficulties arise in bringing up the donor child, the couple will think twice about seeking the advice of their close associates and will have to grapple with the problem by themselves. . . . there were probably a number of people around who knew us and must have caught wind of our problem if only one of them had discreetly and insistently offered advice.

11. *Fear of possible incest.* While some geneticists feel that the problem is remote, it is impossible to know how many donors contribute to different clinics in the same area.

12. Secrecy has meant there is little research on the psychological interaction of parents and the DI child and sparse examination of outcomes. Likewise, there can be *no predictions based on past experience for assessing couples, guiding them with disclosure, and recommending "scripts" as in adoption.*

13. There is a lack of community support groups for DI parents and DI offspring. A national organization, Donors' Offspring, is described in the next chapter, and some Resolve chapters offer DI support groups. In 1987, a divorced DI couple began a support group in Vancouver. See Alan Pratten in Resources.

14. The child has *no or inadequate records to consult* in later life, and her *birth certificate is false.*

15. There is *family embarrassment with regard to subjects like sex, reproduction, blood groups.* Many trivial aspects can also be drawn in to the secrecy as well.

They are playing a game. They are playing at not playing a game. If I show them I see they are, I shall break the rules and they will punish me. I must play their game, of not seeing I see the game.

                                                            –R. D. Laing, Knots

---

Contemplating DI– Coming to Terms with Secrecy

Let us now look at how some DI couples deal with the burden of secrecy, which may be imposed by the woman herself, her partner, or her physician, or all three. Until recently, in Sweden couples were not accepted for DI unless they gave a unanimous pledge of silence. In England and the United States physicians counsel the couple not to inform the child, but some leave it to the parents to decide.

Berger points out that the little psychological investigation that has been done with DI couples focuses on the process itself, rather than on the *secrecy* surrounding that process. The difficulties are not so much because of conflicts, but because conflicts are not worked through. Berger feels that some DI researchers, who have concluded that adoption is preferable, do so because adoption is conducted openly. Berger disagrees with psychiatrist Rubin that controversy and secrecy will always surround DI because of incestuous fears aroused in the women. Berger points out that oedipal fathers in dreams are linked to *strangers,* and that more knowledge of the donor would allay such fears.

One woman corresponded with me, but did not sign her name because her husband, as a condition for consenting to DI, made her promise never to reveal the DI to anyone. Likewise, in magazine articles the real names of the infertile couples are never used, which contributes to the secrecy and shame.

A DI mother wrote:

> The secrecy issue is the hardest for me. When we were going through it all, it was almost the only thing on my mind. I really had a need to talk about this terribly important issue. It seemed sort of dishonest not to talk about it, but I must say I think many family and friends would rather not know.

Another couple said that the husband's parents were not very sophisticated medically and didn't seem to grasp what was being explained, so with them the subject was dropped. All the DI couples I have interviewed expressed a desire to discuss with other couples who told, or didn't tell, and how they handled the disclosure. *This burning issue has been totally neglected by the professionals involved in DI.*

Secrecy drove some couples to pay cash and thus to avoid health insurance claims that would establish the fact they were trying to conceal. (Several were successful the first cycle so that the secrecy was not an economic drain as well.)

Most DI couples seem to be polarized on the issue of secrecy, almost all vowing to keep it, but a few feel it is wrong.

> I think my husband should have the credit for being the father. He's been through so much, he deserves it. We'll just tell people "time did it."

Harry and I have decided to tell the child one day. We don't know how, where, or when but we feel it's important to the child to know. Keeping secrets and this is a big secret, from a child can be dangerous later on. I feel that the child can feel something when a secret is kept. In case anyone finds out for one reason or another, I would hate the child to hear it from anyone else but us.

We had to abandon the idea of DI. The secrecy was for us an unmanageable burden.

I am an honest person by nature. It feels terrible lying to my own son.

A Swedish couple went over to England for inseminations because they could not accept the secrecy rules that existed in Sweden before the 1985 legislation requiring records and disclosure. The man had been told of his adoption at age twelve—"too late"—and was determined not to repeat that experience with any child he might raise. The couple had also discussed their infertility and plans with family and friends.

Toward Opening the Records

We live in a society that is greatly concerned with information—computers, data banks, wire taps. Yet we still cannot grant adopted or DI adults the knowledge of their true identity. The recent Freedom of Information Act demonstrates a new trend toward more candor in society. Citizens now have right of access to medical records, credit reports, and files kept on them by government agencies. One of the special features of human existence is the possession of a historical lineage. Most people take for granted that they can obtain their birth certificate, but currently only four states allow an adult adoptee some access to her birth records without a court order. Nearly all states have statutes requiring courts to seal the child's original birth certificate and all records of the adoption proceedings. Although adoptees may be told something about their parents, such as "your mother was a college student," there is usually no distinction in the records between identifying and nonidentifying information, nor are the records updated at intervals. One adoptee, like thousands of others, who failed to produce "good cause" in New York to open her records, said, "I feel cut off from the rest of humanity. . . . I want to know who I am. . . . I have no ancestry. Nothing." The work of the adoption rights movement has been to unlock the citadel of power and secrecy that severs adoptees from their personal history. The great dilemma is that the courts feel the relinquishing mothers were promised (rather than burdened with) anonymity, and that they need to judge a conflict of interests. Adoptees and birthparents "overwhelmingly support open records, while adoptive parents almost reject them," according to Ganson and Cook. Adoptive Parents for Open Records (see Resources) is an organization for those who have adopted and can put the child's interests before their own.

Sealed records in adoption, legislated between 1917 and 1929, were necessary to deal with unplanned dependent children in a society that discriminated against such overt evidence of a woman's sexuality. With social change and the supply of adoptable babies diminishing, secrecy is not necessary to ensure adoption today. The stigma around DI (mistaken assumptions about a loss of male virility) has similar sexual undertones and is similar to the issue of illegitimacy for adoptees when they were born.

Most legislatures continue to favor sealed records despite the regular introduction of proposals for reform. Some states have made provisions to release nonidentifying information. Others have gone further and established procedures for updating information and for revealing the identity of birth parents through court orders, review boards, intermediaries, or registries. Of course, individuals bewildered about their genealogy would like more nonidentifying information than just medical and genetic data, such as hobbies (not just "enjoys sports and music," for example, but which kinds), years of education, occupation, and information on any biological siblings.

The Child Welfare League of America issued the following statement in 1976.

> Today's sealed record controversy cannot be dismissed as simply the expression of a few vocal dissidents; it must be viewed as a moot issue. In this debate open-mindedness is essential and such open-mindedness has to include consideration of the possibility that

adult adoptees may be right in demanding elimination of secrecy. Regardless of ultimate decisions, social agencies cannot evade the issues. They must confront them. Among the groups involved there will no doubt be struggle and differences, but these can be handled if there are respect and a beginning understanding each for the other. In these beginnings lie the evolution of future solutions.

Betty Jean Lifton (1975) forecasts:

> The records will be open when society comes to understand that it is in the best interests of all three parties to give up the double lifestyle they have been leading for one based on honest reality.

In adoption today, the importance of telling the truth to the child is based on the conviction that the secrecy and lies, and the atmosphere they create, are more difficult and create worse problems. It is extremely difficult for family members to live through the years with an emotionally charged secret without it being revealed in some way or being otherwise affected by the need for deception. The darker the secret, the more the child will feel that there is something really illicit about the DI, and by extension, something wrong with *herself*.

Psychological and genetic research also suffers. Manuel feels that by avoiding any follow-up the DI practitioners' "refusal to know" what kind of children are born relates to defenses against feelings of guilt and/or omnipotence because they are responsible for creating children.

Social workers have pointed out that emotional energy is better expended in facing and resolving the problems inherent in adoption and DI. We must learn from the adoption mistakes and not repeat them for another generation of children—as would be done if we avoided confronting the issues in DI.

12

The Disclosure of Biological Identity

Truth has no special time of its own. Its hour is now . . . always.

—*Albert Schweitzer*

WE HAVE SEEN how medical procedures separate genetic, gestational, and rearing parents and how this confuses family lineage and blurs the very meaning of "family." Whatever the type of assisted conception, the sperm and egg form an embryo that grows up to be an adult wanting to make sense out of its heritage. Media attention about reproductive technology has raised society's awareness of infertile persons, but the needs and rights of the child who results from an assisted conception have for too long gone unrecognized. When adoption practices were first legislated, it was thought best to protect the child from the complications of belonging to two families at the same time, and it was believed that severing the links would suppress the past. Betty Jean Lifton observed that "social workers said that without the facts, the child won't fantasize. Such were the fantasies social workers projected onto adoptive parents just a few years ago" (and onto DI parents today).

Western society is experiencing more and more blended families where kinship goes beyond blood relationships. Successful parenting is not dependent on a biological tie, but on a relationship of love and openness. However, where there is not the usual biological tie, it is in the best interests of the child and all family members that these circumstances be disclosed to the child.

Unlike most adopted children, DI children will at least grow up with half of their genealogical history, but one half does not make a whole. *Genealogical bewilderment* occurs when any important information regarding lineage is lacking from a family, and stress results from not being able to cope with the confusion. Betty Jean Lifton (1987) suggests new terms, "technological bewilderment" and "conception stress." She warns that the confusion experienced by "brave new babies" will result in many of the symptoms of adoptees—"low self-esteem, lack of trust, and a preoccupation with fantasy." DI parents, like adoptive parents, will probably experience some psychological problems explaining the conception, but unlike adoptive parents, there is no pressure on them to tell the child. Therefore, most DI couples do not.

Achilles's (1986) research into the participants in DI revealed that the respondents would express contradictory views that she conceptualized as "opposite poles with acknowledgment of the social significance of biological ties at one end and denial at the other. Because the parent-child relationship is among the most powerful of human bonds, clarity about the meaning of biological and social parenting roles is essential." Yet she observes that "confusion and uncertainty about parental roles arising through DI indicate the social ambiguity about the status of these unique family constellations." While parenting skills are not dependent on biological ties, the persistence of these links as socially significant is evident by the proliferation of genealogical societies, the increase in adoptees and birthparents searching for each other, and the popularity of the series "Roots."

Snowden (1983) wrote:

> Although these fathers had accepted their children, the concept of paternity still caused confusion. It was noticeable that in trying to explain their feelings about fatherhood, very many of the husbands referred to the donor as the "real father" although they were in no doubt that the child was "their" child. Husband 878 tried to describe his confusion: "The fact it was not mine—they are, I know they are mine—but it was in the back of my mind that it was never mine, never my child. I wasn't the one, but father—but I mean I know they are mine now, they will always be mine."

Achilles concludes:

As long as biological ties are culturally understood as a significant component of identity, the link between sperm donors and their biological offspring cannot be eliminated through law or medical procedure. Redefinition of biological parenthood as meaningful but not necessarily primary or central to the quality of parent-child relationship, is a social process essential to the health of both the individuals and the families involved. To do otherwise is to undermine the life-long commitment undertaken by those who rear nonbiological offspring.

Couples who may not have thought of adoption from the point of view of the adoptee as an adult person, quickly are able to understand that legal and emotional parenting does not exclude the adoptee from the fundamental right to know his natural heritage. Couples are not deterred from applying for adoption when the rights of the child are highlighted. As DI becomes more accepted into social life, there will be more communication on the subject and vice versa. Then DI parents will lessen their preoccupation with the concept of the child as a possession, whose love they fear may be lost or diminished through informing her of her origins. In the meantime, this is a transition phase for DI parents who have the courage to share the truth.

The Anguish of Missing Links

A characteristic of individuals suffering genealogical bewilderment, according to Sants, is the relentless pursuit of the facts of their origins, particularly from adolescence onward. The Greek tragedy *Oedipus Rex* tells the story of an adoptee who unknowingly kills his natural father, and also unknowingly commits incest with his mother, finally putting out his own eyes in torment when the truth is disclosed.

> I ask to be no other man than that I am, and I will know who I am. . . . I must pursue the trail to the end, till I have unravelled the mystery of my birth.
>
> —*Sophocles, 6th century* B.C.

It is a common experience for both parents and children who suffer from genealogical bewilderment to scan strangers in public and wonder if they see someone to whom they could perhaps be related. Likewise, it is frustrating for them when people comment, for example, that they look like someone in another town and ask if relatives live there. One of Shakespeare's famous quotations is, "It is a wise child who knows his own father."

Norma McCorvey, the woman in the famous *Roe v. Wade* decision of the U.S. Supreme Court that legalized abortion (too late for her), described her feelings to *Parade* magazine, May 8, 1983, about the child she gave up thirteen years before. She grieves:

> I must tell you that almost every day, when I drive to the job and see kids in a playground or walking to school, I can't help wondering if maybe one of them isn't the one I gave away.

Suzanne Ariel found out the truth about her DI conception when she was thirty-one. Her response then was understandably angry.

> I was glad to know the truth because it is at least based on what's real. But it is a painful issue that will affect me for the rest of my life. I find myself grieving for a father I never knew was there. I need to know that he was something more than an animal who procreated for money. My father felt very ashamed of his infertility and had never come to terms with it.

> Simply because I exist, I have a right to know who my father is. I want to find my father even if it's only to discover what kind of man sells his sperm and his own flesh and blood for $25 and then walks away whistling a happy tune without any of the life he may have created. How is a child produced this way supposed to feel about a father who sold the essence of his life so cheaply and to a total stranger?

Updating the story in 1986, she relates:

> I searched for my birthfather because I could not bear the pain of not knowing who my own flesh and blood was. I could not go through the rest of my life not knowing. I had to follow the search wherever it led me. I did not know if I could ever have the answers to my questions, but the only way I could cope with the pain and

shock of the information was to begin a search for my own answers.

Ariel was advised by physician friends interested in the search to look at photos of students at the only medical school in Los Angeles at the time she was conceived and then to look at a photo of the doctor who inseminated her mother. At the time she was conceived, freezing of sperm had not been perfected and since the inseminations took place over a period of more than a year, it was suggested that there was a 15 to 20 percent chance that the doctor was in fact the donor. After two years of search and investigation, Ariel concluded that the gynecologist who inseminated her mother is her birthfather: "His photo looks just like me, aged about thirty years older." Since he is not Jewish and Ariel's parents had been promised a Jewish donor, she was shocked that her parents too were deceived.

> I take pride in my Jewish heritage, and feel a strong, lifelong identification and responsibility as a Jew in this world. I consider my paternal origins a blight on my background.

> My birthfather may have very well read about my search or heard about it on television, but he has not been directly confronted by me about his being my birthfather. I feel by telling him what I think and how I feel will help me achieve closure on this issue. I believe that within the next year or so I will write to him. I feel certain that he will not wish to meet me, and I don't feel I will push it. I have pictures of him and know his heritage. However, I feel deeply ashamed of him and wish heartily that he was not my birthfather.

The late Peter Sellers admitted in an interview with the *Boston Globe* that he had an illegitimate daughter who was put up for adoption by her mother.

> She doesn't know I'm her dad. Her mother decided to put her in a home, one of those places where they take your name away and people adopt you and they never tell you who your real parents are. And yet sometimes I really, somehow, feel her presence. And the awful thing is that I think she might feel mine, too. I just don't know where to begin to find her, and I've made several attempts.

Go back to your self. For nothing can begin from nothing, and it is from your past, and from what you are at this moment, that what you are going to be must spring.

—André Gide

Formation of Identity Through Others

As the parent-child relationship is among the most powerful of human bonds, clarity about the meaning of biological and social parenting roles is essential.

—Rona Achilles, The Social Meanings of Biological Ties

Sants has explored the psychodynamics of genealogical bewilderment:

> Persons outside ourselves are essential for the development of our complete body-image. The most important people in this respect are our real parents and other members of our family. Knowledge of and definite relationship to his genealogy is therefore necessary for a child to build up his complete body image and world picture. It is an inalienable and entitled right of every person. There is an urge, a call in everybody to follow and fulfill the tradition of his family, race, nation, and the religious community into which he was born. The loss of this tradition is a privation which may result in the stunting of emotional development.

Most readers will be familiar with Hans Christian Andersen's story of the Ugly Duckling who was deprived of his true genealogy as a swan, which paralleled the author's own life as an adoptee.

An adoptee expressed her deep concern about genealogical bewilderment:

> I can't help believing that our natural mother and father are the most important people in our life. A tie that cannot be broken—that's what life is all about—life and death.

Another adult commented that although his father's visits to him when he was a foster child were very erratic, they were "extremely valuable."

> I "know" who my father was, and by knowing him I come to know myself.

A child comes into the world with a genetic heritage that is a real part of her, and to pretend that those parts don't exist is to deny the child a central part of herself. Being a DI child is an added piece of identity that needs to be integrated into the personality. The difficulty, however, is the lack of information about the donor that would round out that dimension. Just as some parents have curiosity about the donor, so the child has the same natural and normal curiosity to learn about herself and her roots. The child must feel that it is acceptable to ask about these things. If the child is given the message that one's origins are a taboo subject, a whole range of feelings and questions about the state of not-knowing cannot be raised and discussed.

Children missing some part of their genetic identity thus have additional factors connected with their status that makes any rejection, loss, or disruption in the family more difficult for them. They may feel different from other children and fear that some people will reject them because of their status. Perhaps some parents who chose to have children with assistance are more prone to experience difficulties in providing for their child's needs than parents of naturally conceived children who will not need to disclose special information. Psychiatrists point out that when adults are confronted with the needs of children, they react with their own unresolved needs. Similarly, many couples are unable to cope with the overwhelming feelings that they experience during their crisis of infertility and cannot see beyond this to the needs of the child. Parents of DI children may still be suffering conflicts and fantasies over the mode of conception and have lingering concerns about unresolved legal and ethical issues. The crux of the problem is that DI professionals themselves do not even address these issues.

As a parallel with adoption, Betty Jean Lifton (1981) says:

> The good adoptee doesn't ask too many questions and is sensitive to his parents' need to make believe he wasn't adopted . . . holding

back curiosity about oneself for the sake of others makes one hold back in other things, too. Adoptees tend to feel rootless, temporarily disconnected, shy, withdrawn, loners, afraid of rejection or conflict, anxious to please, submissive, but filled with rage.

Fantasies about the origins of one's father, while common in children, create a frame of reference for assimilating clues about the truth in family relations. But when the truth is withheld, this further alienates the child from the father.

If the child looks like the mother or members of her family, it certainly is easier to disguise the DI than it is with adoption. Adopted people whose characteristics are never likened to "Grandpa's temper" or "Aunt Amy's nose" are highly aware of the frequency of such genetic references in families. The DI child may grow up noticing that likenesses are seen only on the maternal side of the family, leaving a mysterious gap in her life with regard to the paternal genes.

> It's hard to explain what you never had, much less explain why you need it.
>
> —*Betty Jean Lifton, American Adoption Congress, 1987*

Triseliotis quotes a woman who found out about her adoption when she was studying to become a teacher.

> I feel I am a person not in my own right. I feel I have lived a lie. . . . I stand before the mirror and ask, "Who am I? Who do I belong to?" There are times when I wish I had not been born. . . . I feel I need a whole new life, as if everything has been a huge deception. Soon after I found I was adopted I realized that adopted people are a race apart. When I told my fiancé, his reaction was, "I do not know what my father and mother will feel." You see his mother was very family-tree conscious and very class-conscious. When my boy was born and my mother-in-law visited me in hospital she exclaimed, "Thank God he has taken from our side of the family." I know what she was getting at and it hurt.

Some adoptees see their children as more part of their husband's family and less a part of themselves. Since there is no blood connection with the adoptive family, there is a strong need to find one's natural parents in order to go further back. Another adoptee commented:

> My first child was a boy and my husband's relatives kept saying, Oh! he is so much like his father or grandfather. . . . and I felt very alone because I have nobody of my own to say, Oh! he is like my father or like my mother and this is a terrible thing. Unless you have experienced this you do not realize how deep this feeling is . . . so I have been thinking of finding more about my natural father, especially since I became a parent.

Telling the Truth—The Parents' Responsibility

All persons have a moral right to information that concerns themselves and the circumstances of their birth. The truth does not belong to the parents to withhold—*it is the child's birthright.* Parents *must* develop the wisdom and courage to squarely face the whole issue. It is their responsibility to tell the truth, no matter how difficult or painful that task may be. Certainly it is less painful than in adoption or fostering where there may have been a history of child abuse, rape, murder, or worse. Nevertheless, one can never know too much about one's heritage, whatever the truth may be. Good parents will help the child master the truth about her reality.

> Rumor is more terrifying than assault, ignorance more nerve-racking than knowledge, however bad reality may be.
>
> —*Grantly Dick-Read*

Norman Vincent Peale wrote:

Kids—all kids—whether adopted or children of divorced or deceased parents have a right to know their origins. They should not be penalized by the way they were conceived. The issue here is the child's right to know his own history.

Initially, adoptive parents were reluctant to disclose the circumstances to their children, and thus social workers made it a point of emphasis. Today, adoptive parents no longer ask "should" I tell my child, but how and when? Adoption is no longer regarded as something to hide, instead it is a source of family pride. Society is beginning to mature and recognize the rights of the adoptee. In contrast, couples or donors who want more information about each other are considered unsuitable for DI.

Pauline Ley counsels adoptive parents that

> there is pain in life for everyone, and not to acknowledge it only lays the child open to being ambushed by revelations for which he will be unprepared. Wishful thinking that denying the child the truth of his heritage would help solidify his bond with his parents has been proven wrong.

There is nothing parents can ever say, continues Ley, that will erase the child's existential fate. The truth concerning the conception and the special relationship between the child and her father "should be lovingly shared by the parents, not whispered in the schoolyard by peers or revealed in the heat of a family argument." It gets down to a basic attitude of honesty that should run through the parent-child relationship at all times. Children are aware when something is being withheld, and it is typical of how little adults know about children that they imagine they can get away with lies. Not all children will ask or discuss their birth circumstances, so parents need to feel comfortable doing so when the child seems ready. Being honest and frank with a child does not jeopardize her relationship with the parents. On the contrary, conscious acceptance of known facts, however unsavory, tends to improve rather than worsen relationships. Children are less upset by strange and unpalatable facts than any form of deception. The DI child will mature feeling free to ask questions, and this shows that she feels secure and reassured that such questions will not mean rejection or loss of love. A 1980 article in the Swedish medical journal *Lakartidningen* concluded:

> If the child for some reason or other gets suspicious concerning its origin, the truth ought not to be concealed. This question makes us think about the conflicts and difficulties which perhaps will arise sooner or later for the child and the parents, especially the mother. We must therefore give up egotistical feelings and spare the inno-

cent little ones confessions leading to bitter consequences throughout later life.

Adoptees at least know that the birthmother did not intend to
deceive them. Ley says she would feel great outrage and anguish
if she were a DI child and had to accept that it was a deliberate
choice by "caring professionals" to deny her knowledge of her origins. "It is immoral to ease the pain of one person by causing pain
for another." Our daughter Julia, aged five, expressed remorse at
the thought of unknown sperm coming from a "refrigerator." In
such a situation, she said she would be "very sad and disappointed." When I told her that some couples obtain sperm from a
stranger through their doctor, she said, "Why don't they use a
friend like you did?"

In DI the mother is the biological parent; she goes to great
lengths to have her child. By satisfying her need she sacrifices half
her child's heritage when the donor is anonymous. Is not the child
bound to wonder why? She may be angry at the parents at their
inability to conceive normally. She may resent payment to the donor and destruction of the records that pertain to her conception.
The child could well ask "Didn't you even enquire about the donor . . . didn't you demand to know?"

Lifton (1987) points out that the DI child, like the adoptee, will
be "assured how much she was wanted—how far superior she is
to a baby conceived in the natural way. But, like the adoptee, she
will have secrets of her own: she will know that rather than having been first choice, she was second best to the child who might
have been had her parents been able to conceive naturally." Lifton
continues:

> Can a child endure having an anonymous father? Would that child
> feel anonymous or unborn, as many adoptees do? . . . Like so many
> adoptees, she may act out her anger or grief in her adolescence or
> young adulthood.

Many couples don't discuss secrecy even between themselves, a
fact that has come to light when counseling is offered during the
process of DI. Likewise, even after the birth, a great many couples
will deny that any issues around the DI are ever brought up.

Despite the vow to secrecy, there are at least five people typically involved in DI. The father, mother, doctor, donor/sperm bank, and the child—to say nothing of secretaries, nurses, insurance agents, and computers who may also know.

Manuel (1973) in France found that 77 percent of couples chose absolute secrecy for everybody, including the child. In fact, 80 percent of the couples in the DI program chose DI because of its secrecy. However, 48 percent of these did confide in at least one other person (apart from the physician). In fact, only half of the couples wanting complete secrecy actually kept it. The French study concluded that the higher the sociocultural class, the easier it was for couples to contemplate sharing the DI secret. Infertile couples who assist in recruiting donors (for the program; not reciprocally for their own DI) are then placed at the top of the waiting list. However, for 31 percent of couples, the need to maintain secrecy made donor recruitment by them impossible. Sixteen percent viewed sharing the DI information as a positive event that helped them to handle the secrecy and cope with the stresses.

A 1979 study in Nottingham, England found that only 4 out of 147 couples considered telling the DI child. Thirty-one couples had discussed the DI with one or other parents, and all but one couple were willing to have follow-up. Their greatest concern was how outsiders would react to the information. Another study in 1982 found that 84 percent did not tell their parents and 70 percent planned not to tell the child.

Some physicians are aware of the consequences. A professor of Obstetrics and Gynecology in Athens, Greece, Louros (1973) observes:

> But there is always the possibility that the child may find out the truth and then demand to know his father's identity. Is there a single person among us who would not be shocked to learn that his father was a sperm bank? What court of law would condemn the child for hating, even for using violence against, those who brought him into the world, an unknown father's fruit?

I wouldn't care to owe my origins to a liquid nitrogen tank.

—DI gynecologist, Australia

In Sweden, a 1982 study by Milsom found that only 15 percent had informed relatives or friends, and that 49 percent "never discussed" the inseminations even with each other. Ninety-one out of ninety-two DI couples planned to keep the secret from the child. The authors stated that in the *only* case where the parents planned to inform the child, they had experienced the DI as

> a completely natural solution to their problem and there was therefore no reason to hide the fact. Relatives and friends were aware of their problem and the couple had gained mental support by being able to discuss the matter openly. However, the parents in question pointed out that the child may have greater difficulties in accepting insemination as an explanation of his or her origin compared to the similar situation where a child is adopted. The parents had not decided when to inform the child, but were in agreement that this should be performed as soon as the child is sufficiently mature to understand their explanation.

Two couples were prepared to reveal the truth to the child if she became a doctor or a geneticist, as they believed then their DI decision would be understood. Five couples intended to withhold the truth from the child but wished to make reservations about the future. They were uncertain how they would answer a child's question regarding origins and felt that this would only happen on account of a breach of secrecy within the hospital.

A 1981 Danish survey by Rosenkvist found that 27 percent of the men and 17 percent of the women would tell the child. It is interesting that women tend to be more protective of their spouse.

Social workers at the Royal Women's Hospital in Melbourne, Australia, found that 34 percent of couples in 1976 had talked to others and by 1981 that number had increased to 44 percent. In 1976 thirty percent of the couples intended to inform the child; this increased to 52 percent in 1981. It was noted that couples who share details about their infertility with family and friends have greater confidence and less fear and anxiety than those who conceal it. They don't have the stress of making excuses about the visits to the clinic or are afraid of being seen in the clinic by others. They feel less alone and better able to bear the burden of infertility and the strain of inseminations.

A study in the United States by Ledward et al. in 1979 found that 143 of 147 DI couples clearly stated that they definitely would not inform the child. Of the other couples, 2 had received DI on genetic grounds, so they had already decided to disclose the DI to the child. In a 1982 study, they found that 3.8 percent (14) couples were not prepared to tell the child about DI, whereas 6 percent were, with 22 couples undecided.

In a Canadian survey Berger (1986) reports that only 14 percent of the men and 18 percent of the women were willing to talk about DI with a close friend; 22 percent of the men and 28 percent of the women with a close relative. Only 8 percent of the husbands and 9 percent of the wives felt free to discuss DI with the child.

> Telling the child is not going to relieve any feelings because I don't have feelings to begin with.

> Part of the stress about telling our family is not knowing how they will react.

One of Achilles's respondents told her son at age seven and now feels that if she had to do it all over again she probably would not tell him. "He never asks, but out of curiosity some day, I suppose he might. I hate having this hanging over my head now ... wondering if when he's twenty years old, he doesn't want to say to me, now look, I'm angered because I don't know who my father is."

> I wouldn't have wanted to explain it to a child the year I had her ... but I am counting on the fact that we'll have a lot more liberal society by the time she's old enough to understand.

One woman, whose estranged husband had been sexually abusing the DI daughter, felt that admitting the DI status of the child might mean a lighter judgment by a court because "it's easier to rationalize because it isn't his own flesh and blood."

In Leiblum's 1983 study, forty-nine percent of medical students and 36 percent of infertile couples thought that DI children should be informed of their status when mature. But 78 percent of infertiles and 72 percent of medical students felt that ideally DI should be kept secret from everyone but the couple and their physician.

We have seen how couples try to deny the donor who gave the child half her genes, and will thus live through that child. On the other hand, there is always the potential for the parents to develop a "bad seed" or "bad blood" theory about the origins of the child, stimulated by fears and fantasies about the unknown donor. The temptation to blame any of the child's difficulties on her genetic origins is always present.

Burton Sokoloff, a Los Angeles pediatrician, is adamant that despite all the arguments (e.g., fear of ridicule, lack of record keeping, unsatisfactory legislation, etc.), "the child *should* be told about [her] background," as he stressed in his 1987 article.

I personally found it very easy to discuss with Julia, when she was aged five to six, a whole range of moral and social issues, such as contraception, rape, teenage pregnancy, drugs, and the like. I hope my influence will hold up through the teenage years!

Until the rights of the child to know her heritage outweigh the right of the donor to privacy, there is no way to give children this right if parents seek conventional, closed DI. While we await heightened community awareness and pressure on the legal and medical professions, only DI with a known donor will resolve these problems.

Arguments Against Disclosure

> If DI is so dreadful that no one must know, then frankly it is also too dreadful to be practised or endured.
>
> *—Joseph Blizzard*

Let us examine some common arguments against telling the child.

1. *The child has no right to know.* We have discussed this violation of the child's rights at length already. The decision to go for DI seems very abstract, at the level of coded straws of semen, as the couple sit in the doctor's office and ponder their yet-to-be-conceived child. (This is why couples also need to sit in a counselor's office too, or join group discussions with other infertile couples.) The secrecy issue continues to rear its head, however, and it becomes harder and harder for parents to conspire against an actual

child, who grows up. DI adults, like adoptees, are typically referred to as "the child," which avoids recognizing their adult rights.

2. Some parents justify withholding the truth on the grounds that *the truth is too traumatic or disturbing for the child* to hear . . . that it might "worry" the child to be different from other children. Usually such parents are protecting their own unresolved feelings about their infertility and their choice of DI. If the DI is such a painful and shameful subject, then it is hard to understand how they went ahead with it. Couples may also fear rejection by the child—"she might bear a grudge toward us"—or the child may be seen as a threat to the marriage, because of the one-sided biological link to the mother (which is no different from step-parenting). Anyway, the child usually senses that there is an intense family secret that somehow involves her and has to do with the father.

3. A common excuse is the belief that *it's simpler to "forget" the child's biological origins,* just like the doctor said. This way the father's biological incapacity does not have to be acknowledged. (Birthmothers were also told that they would forget they had ever birthed and relinquished a baby!) *No one forgets such life events.* Also, DI is becoming more and more common. It is discussed in documentaries about reproductive technologies on television and in magazines, and even in fictional dramas. I turned on the television one night at the end of an episode of "Trapper John M.D.," and there was a "humorous" suit against a physician-donor, which was resolved when the records showed that his sperm actually had been rejected. Adolescents commonly ask if they were adopted, and this coming generation will ask the same kind of questions about the new conceptions through reproductive technology.

4. A real dilemma couples often feel is that *there is no point in telling the child about her DI conception if they cannot supply any more information.* They have no knowledge of the donor, or perhaps mixed donors were used. If there really was "no point in telling" there would be no investment in secrecy. Suzanne Ariel has shared her anguish in learning that her biological father was an anonymous donor, but she was relieved to learn the truth and know why she never fit into her family.

5. The conception was artificial and *the child may resent knowing she was conceived in a clinical setting.* After all, the stork story was invented because parents had difficulty sharing information about natural conception. Many parents today, not just DI couples, did not receive early sex education from their parents and so have difficulty offering it to their offspring. Unfortunately, DI parents rarely receive counseling or support to help them explain the facts in a loving way to the child. The practitioners have not dealt with this issue; the couple is left to handle the consequences on their own.

6. Some couples expressed *a need to protect the donor* who under the agreement was guaranteed anonymity. It is strange that parents could care more about the privacy of the donor than the rights of their child, but this is probably a rationalization of their ambivalence. As Achilles observed, there is an "absence of a shared language to describe the familial roles created by DI (like step or foster parent, etc., in other family configurations), revealing the lack of 'cultural legitimacy' for DI." In the case of a heterosexual couple, it is a challenge to decide who is the "real" father . . . and whether the infertile husband should be termed "social," "legal," "rearing," "custodial" or "adoptive parent," which are all "second best" terms." Lifton also notes that there is no commonly accepted terminology and that a new vocabulary is needed to deal with these assisted conceptions.

7. *The child will spread the secret.* This fear is often expressed by DI couples who would otherwise consider telling the child. The community is not sensitized to the issues of DI, as the subject is not openly discussed.

The Timing of the Disclosure

Unlike adoption, there are no traditional guidelines, no scripts for telling the DI child about her origins. Each family is unique and will have to figure out how and when to tell the child. The worst time is during adolescence when almost all children have crises of identity. Adoption studies have shown that the child who learns between the ages of three and five adjusts better to her situation.

As the child grows and learns, her origins will mean new and different things. Parents need to help the child at the various stages of growth, helping her to interpret and assimilate the facts into her self-image. It is a continual, dynamic, lifelong process. As Triseliotis emphasizes, the child should be told by her parents at an early age, and this is not only because "it is impossible to maintain secrecy, but also because it is dishonest to the child not to do so."

Psychologically and emotionally, even well-educated couples may find it difficult to explain the DI decision to the child, family, relatives, and friends. Parents of a DI child may not feel different from any other parent, rather it is a question of how they think others may feel about them that is different.

> Occasionally I wonder whether I should tell some of our friends the story. Things have happened which merited better explanations than we gave. But, of course, when I want to tell them I cannot and when I do not need to, there's no need, so I don't.
>
> —*Joseph Blizzard*

The problem is not only how and when to tell the child, but also how the child may relate it to others, and the reaction the child will experience from members of the community.

In DI, the child may learn the wrong way at the wrong time. As with adoption, disclosure may be avoided, postponed, or mishandled by too much information too soon. Sometimes a stalemate results with the parents waiting for the child to ask and the child waiting for the parents to volunteer information. It is not so much the timing of the disclosure as the way parents present it. Even more important than the phrases used is the totality of the relationship and the underlying feelings between parent and child. No matter what the age, the child will sense the parents' discomfort or ease with the topic. If they are uptight and secretive, she will be too; if they are open and accepting, so will she be. If they act as if DI is shameful, she will regard it that way too. If they act as if it is a natural condition, which they can accept and deal with, she will feel more at home with herself and her father. Only four of the seventy adoptees whom Triseliotis interviewed wished they had never learned about the adoption.

Many adoptees, recognizing their own and their parents' difficulty in raising the subject, would have appreciated help from those who arranged the adoption. The typical stresses of adolescence, being the period when most adoptees first think of searching, adds to the burden for many adoptive parents. Some adoptees felt that the disclosure of origins and any relevant information should not be left to the adoptive parents, as there is never any guarantee that they will retain or share it. (Likewise the birth certificates should be a truthful genetic register.) Birthparents are usually eager to supply information; it is not their cooperation that is lacking but rather that of the agency and its neglect in storing vital information.

The child should be told as early as possible in a deeply loving way, so she can feel and appreciate the emotion around her parents' desire for a baby. Yet often the DI offspring is simply told "Your father is not your father." Many adoptees regret that the adoption disclosure was not used as an opportunity to develop and cement family relationships. While adoptees were aware that the parents withheld or distorted truths to protect them, they still maintained that truth and honesty would have enhanced their respect for them.

The Art of Disclosure

1. *Discuss only as much as the child can absorb.* Preschool children need only simple answers to their questions, not an elaborate biology lesson. Begin with the topic of how the child was conceived, without explaining where the sperm came from. You can consider saying, as I did, that Daddy didn't have any seeds so we got some from X or "a friend," depending on whether you do or do not know the donor, or wish to disclose the friend's name. Julia, who was about three at the time, was much more concerned with understanding why the seeds were absent, and although we

still don't know the medical reason, I explained that we thought it was a childhood illness.

The theme was followed up in the vegetable garden, when we observed infertile seeds that she helped to plant and which did not come up.

2. On a later occasion, *the desire for a child and the source of sperm can be discussed.* Parents have rationalized this as "adopting sperm," although the concept of adoption is too obtuse for young children compared with simple analogies such as "growing you with seed from a friend."

At age four and a half, Julia announced that "the father gets the sperm from his penis and puts it in the mother's hand and then she puts it in her 'gina." At this time I was working on a book with Graham Farrant, an Australian psychiatrist, about prenatal memory, so there was plenty of talk in the house about sperm, eggs, conception, and pregnancy. We were quite amazed by her literal description, especially since there was no possibility she would have ever overheard any of us describing DI in that way. Later that day I asked her if she remembered what she had said about her conception. She said, "Yes, Geoff took the sperm from his pee-pee and put it in your hand so you could put it in your 'gina." I took this opportunity to remind her that Geoff didn't have any sperm, that we had been given some from a very close friend, a very special person, and did she have any idea who this person was? She couldn't guess, so I told her. "Oh," she said, "X got the sperm from *his* pee-pee." End of conversation!

I purposely said no more, to avoid giving the impression that this was anything unusual, nor did I suggest in any way that it was private or secret information. I figured we would deal with community feedback if and when we got any, and I informed Geoff and the donor of this conversation. I certainly didn't want to jeopardize her self-esteem by speculating about the reactions of others. She clearly seemed to understand the facts, as indicated by another exchange a week or so later. Julia often asks when she is going to have a brother or sister, or when I am going to have my next baby. I took the opportunity to check her comprehension. I explained to her how I just had the egg, and that sperm were necessary to create a baby. "Oh, don't worry about that," she replied, "X will give you some more sperm!" Since that time she has also suggested other male friends as potential donors, although she has stated that she would like a sibling to be created with sperm from X "so we can be twins"!

A humorous exchange occurred when she was four, and asked how the little cap of sperm "stayed there." I explained that it was held by suction against the cervix and she said, "No, how does the *cat* keep it on her paw?" The thought of our pregnant cat, doing artificial insemination, was quite hilarious! Since that time she has squarely understood that natural insemination is the usual procedure for both humans and animals.

Language is very important—take care especially with words like "real father" or "natural father." One couple said they would answer that DI was the only possible way to have the child they so keenly wanted. Geoff was put in a corner one night when Julia asked him point blank, "Are you my *real* father?" She persistently reiterated her original question after his explanations. She finally seemed to accept that X gave the sperm, but Geoff was her Daddy in everyday life. As we had so carefully avoided that term, we figured the issue must have arisen with her pregnant babysitter. Julia probably asked where the sitter's sperm came from, or said something about her being made by X's sperm, and the babysitter "reassured" her by emphasizing that Geoff was her "real father."

3. *Share any information you have about the donor,* even if you only know he was a medical student. Although this is about all DI couples are ever told, Professor Bernard Dickens of the Toronto Law School thinks that children should get a "gene map" ("but not a street map"), which is another way of saying information that rounds out an impression of the donor but is not sufficient to identify him. A letter and/or photo from the donor is a nice idea if possible, like birthmothers sometimes write when relinquishing a child for adoption. Of course, if the donor is a family friend, there is already a relationship with the child.

Rather than emphasizing the irregularity of the conception, stress your mutual love and commitment to have this gift, this extra life brought into your family.

4. Be prepared to *answer ongoing questions as the child devel-*

ops her identity. Julia has an amazing understanding of reproduction and her vocabulary is such that she is quite at ease discussing sperm and eggs, having more comments than questions these days. A teenager will ask more searching questions, and may want to investigate records of the DI and even search for the donor. However, as with adoption, it may be the case that the more information given in childhood, the less need the adolescent or adult will have to search for the donor.

If the child has never asked any questions, let her know that at some time when she is ready you are available to talk about how she came to be created. Also, DI is not always done for childless couples. If there are adopted or step-children in the family, then a precedent for discussing origins already exists.

Searching for the Missing Genealogy

Robert Jay Lifton, a Yale psychiatrist, explains that when children ask where they came from, they are really asking for the origin of their lives and the origins of life itself. Freudians see it as sexual curiosity, but the children are actually expressing a need to be connected with those who have gone before them and those who will come after. The need for establishing one's identity is a healthy expression of individuality and independence, stresses Lifton. It is *not* an emotional disturbance but indicates the deep existential interest in one's forebears and the sense of responsibility toward the future continuation of the genetic past. Those who take up the popular pastime of compiling a family tree and tracing the ancestry may, according to an editorial in the Melbourne *Age*,

> emerge from the exercise as a wise and better person with a new evaluation of themselves and an exhilarating sense of the privilege of living, to see the odds so stacked against their being born.

The television series "Roots" epitomized the fascination with family genealogy that has been part of the human condition since ancestor worship. These searches for birth families have been looked upon as merely sentimental journeys, says biologist Elizabeth Omand of the Adoption Forum of Philadelphia. "But believe me, these needs run very deep indeed. Otherwise, why should adopted children be overrepresented by sevenfold, yes sevenfold, in the psychiatric patient population?"

It is a common misunderstanding that only unhappy adoptees search, just as some feel that only the mentally ill seek psychotherapy, whereas therapists would say these are the healthiest members of society. This makes those who search feel that they are betraying their parents, and likewise adoptive parents feel threatened that this behavior indicates a lack of bonding. Carole Anderson observes that adoptive parents of new searchers often fear that finding the birth family will damage relationships in the adoptive family, but she has never known that to happen. However, the parents' refusal to recognize and support the need to search has marred relationships. At the bottom line, searching has to do with knowing the truth about oneself, not finding another set of parents. Triseliotis found, however, that the more unsatisfactory the family relationships, the greater the desire for the adoptee to search—particularly in adolescence.

It is important that DI and adoptive parents realize that the need to search arises from genealogical curiosity rather than from a lack of appreciation or love for the parents in the home. DI parents will be reassured by those parents who can accept this, as told in some letters in *The Adoption Triangle*.

> Even if our son should some day meet his birthparents, why should we feel threatened? If he should become friends with them, or grow to love them, it would not diminish the relationship that we share with him. Love for one individual does not diminish because we also love another individual. If knowing and loving his birthparents would give our son more security and happiness, we would welcome the opportunity for him. We love him—his happiness will make us happy.

> I hope I shall never have to share Lisa with her birthmother. I can't pretend that if she should prefer her natural mother to me, I won't feel heartbroken and bereft. But when I weigh my sense of loss against her peace of mind, if I love her as I do, I really haven't any choice.

It is not only the child's need and right to know her full heritage, but surely the DI parents, who will raise the child, need as much information as they can about the donor too. This also helps them share meaningfully in the paternal identity of the child. Yet they are thwarted in their attempts.

> The doctor gave us *no* information about the donor. Next time we want a better understanding of what characteristics we consider minimum information—height, eye, skin, and hair color. But we were so passive and nervous that we weren't assertive enough.
>
> I even wrote the doctor partway through my pregnancy to ask for more information but never received an answer.

A woman in Canada wrote, "Next time I want to find a doctor who is willing to share selection information with us."

Only a few DI adults have tried to find the donor, but many thousands of adoptees have searched successfully. Of course, in adoption there is a legal trail, whereas in DI the records are usually destroyed. As the need to search and the relief and exhilaration that can arise from making contact with a birthparent become more appreciated, perhaps records will be maintained (as well as for scientific reasons). Birthmothers search for the children they relinquished, just as those children often want to find them. Donors also may want to search or maintain contact (there have been a couple of court cases about this issue) as well as their offspring, who might be searching for them.

Current trends indicate that most adoptees will attempt a search at some point in their life. Triadoption Library polled every search and support group in the United States in 1982 and found that 250,000 searches were begun during that year. The percentage of birthparents initiating the contacts has been steadily rising, and is now about 50 percent. About 5 percent of adoptees never attempt to find out their heritage, or else are satisfied with some knowledge without actually tracing the birthparent(s).

Triseliotis quotes an adoptee:

> You have no one to compare yourself with or to say, "I took a bit after my father or after my grandmother. . . ." If I could just have a glimpse of my mother from a distance I would be satisfied. I don't want to disturb her, but just to look at her. Otherwise I will remain a stranger to myself.

Another confessed to him:

> I am more interested in what she looks like than what I am going to ask her. It's funny but I want to see me in her. It is important to me to find out who I took after.

The motto of an adoptees' search organization is: "It's not what you find, but that you find it." Some adoptees leave phone numbers by the phone for a year before actually plucking up the courage to make the call. As one adoptee said, "Just seeing the record settled me for a while. It is as though I had been born again." It takes a lot of time to process the information and move from one psychological stage to the next. Another adoptee described periods of disappointment and powerlessness as she floated between hope and disappointment, never knowing if she would be successful. Many adoptees find they have to do a lot of "sleuthing and lying and cheating" to find out clues to help them search.

One thirty-year-old adoptee commented to Triseliotis after all the members of his immediate adoptive family had died:

> I feel I have nobody . . . I must do something and find out. If my mother and father had told me about this at ten or eleven or even younger, I might have forgotten all about it—but all this secrecy and no trusting has made me wonder more and more; but it is my brother's death that has really decided me.

Marrying and raising a family did not resolve the need to search. On the contrary, pregnancy, especially for women, made them feel a powerful need to trace their birthmothers. Fear about passing on unknown genetic defects and embarrassment at the void in their medical history made these transitions trying.

Candace Turner wrote to the gynecologist in Los Angeles who inseminated her mother, but he had destroyed records that had accumulated beyond fifteen years. He replied to her:

> Actually, you are only the third one out of some 500 who has ever inquired. The only thing I can assure you of is that the health background was excellent. We have never informed the donor if the DI was successful. *As you may have learned the male practically never concerns himself with paternity when he gets an erection and performs coitus, the Russians claim that the blood goes from the brain to his penis and he becomes senseless.* A study we did some twenty

years ago, showed that the average husband whose wife had DI to become pregnant had forgotten all about it by the time the child was three to five years old (the rate was over 90 percent). [Italics mine]

(This must be one of the most amazing pieces of correspondence ever to be sent out on a physician's letterhead. Had I not seen it with my own eyes, I would never have believed that *anyone* could write such rubbish.)

Afton Blake, a single mother whose child Doron was conceived from Donor #28 at the Repository for Germinal Choice, would like to meet her baby's father. As she told me, she signed a contract not to search for the donor, "but Doron didn't." She knows that Doron is his first conception through the sperm bank and that he must be aware of his existence from all the media publicity she has received.

> Oh, I won't go looking for him because I promised I wouldn't. But I hope he comes looking for me and Doron. I really would like to share Doron with him. (From his photo) he looked like a bubbling, joyous, gentle man. And all of the personal stuff about—he's well liked by his colleagues, he loves all kinds of outdoor sports. So from all that you must get a picture of a man who is pretty well adjusted, a pretty rounded individual. It gives me a feeling about him, a fantasy I've created, based on what I know, that this is a man I would like very much. I have thought more and more about him since I had my baby, because Doron is so wonderful and such a real person. I look at him and I can't help thinking and wondering about the 50 percent of his qualities that came from someone I only know by a number. What is this man really like? I would love him to see Doron and discover how terrific he is.

The parents of a DI child can help by preparing in advance. Get as much information as you can *now* from the doctor or clinic or sperm bank, before records are destroyed—if any were kept. In the absence of records, talk to nurses and secretaries who may remember the donor if fresh semen was used. Otherwise talk to the screening technicians at the sperm bank before they move away or die. One DI mother told me that the clinic she had attended used only fresh semen from residents. I advised her to get a list of those residents before more time was lost.

Although the age of majority is traditionally considered the time to give a child access to such information, what if the child or the donor dies prematurely in an accident? Whose interests are being served by waiting?

One middle-aged DI offspring recently related to me how his conception was disclosed:

> My mother sat me down on my thirty-fifth birthday and said: "I have a secret to tell you and you mustn't tell anyone." I never thought it would be anything to do with me, but that she was going to let me know she had cancer or something. The last thought in my mind was that my Dad was sterile and I was a product of artificial insemination. It hit me like a ton of bricks.

This man's mother was not prepared for his intense curiosity about his paternal origins, and he sat with a notebook and questioned her at length. Subsequently, he traveled to the city where the DI was done, but the doctor, and his nurse, had both died. His social father, who divorced his mother and remarried, had also died. He tried looking through yearbooks and other sources of photographs of medical students and residents around the time of his conception for some resemblance to himself. While his mother told one of his brothers, before he moved abroad, she still insists that the "massive secret" be kept from several other siblings, to whom she does not feel so close. He has honored her request for nearly a decade, but feels the strain of coconspiracy. When he consulted an attorney to draw up a medical release from his mother so he could have access to her records, he was advised to seek psychiatric help. But a psychologist reassured him that his feelings were perfectly normal. Interestingly, he later heard on the grapevine that this particular attorney had DI offspring, which explains his attitude.

In these changing times we can only experiment—lovingly and openly—and share our successes and failures with others in the same situation. Guidelines will perhaps emerge as there are more books, articles, interviews, and discussions on resolving the identity problems of the DI child.

The Search Sequence

The sequence usually includes a desperate, intense search; exhilaration and deep satisfaction at finding one's natural mother (or father); and then a profound letdown, a sense of disillusionment and sometimes depression, as one painfully surrenders the fantasies of a lifetime and absorbs the realization that the found parent is an ordinary human being, sometimes a troubled one, and that neither party knows quite what to do with this relationship. The long-range sense, however, is that the search and reunion have been profoundly valuable and necessary, the source of the adoptee's newly experienced sense of being grounded in reality, no longer a phantom or a replacement but a renewed human being who has reentered the world on a different plane. What these emotions suggest is that everyday feelings of connection and self-definition depend upon being able to locate oneself in the larger human continuity.

What is at stake for each in the reunion, is . . . the re-establishment of connection, the filling-in of a vital biological and historical story, the emergence of the self from a half-life to something approaching full existence.

—*Betty Jean Lifton,*
Lost and Found

The NBC film *Find a Stranger, Say Goodbye* based on the book by Lois Lowry portrayed some typical conversational exchanges.

PARENT: I don't want to see you get hurt. What good can come out of it?
CHILD: At least the secrets will be gone.
PARENT: I never think about the fact that she was adopted, why does she?
FRIEND: Why would you want to do this, you have great parents.
CHILD: It is as if I don't have a past, I don't know who I am.
PARENT: You have a future, the past doesn't count.

Nancy Ayres, an adoptee, states that

I bitterly regret the time I let pass without searching because of other people's feelings. Since locating my mother and resolving the mystery I find that I have opened up so much as a human being, and am experiencing such a richness and depth of feelings that I hadn't thought possible, in all areas of my life. The lines of communication are suddenly open with almost everyone I know, and I have felt such a change in my life since the weight I've carried around so long has been lifted. It has truly been almost a rebirth.

Suzanne Ariel says, after her one brief meeting with her relinquished daughter, then aged fifteen:

> You want to sit and look at the other person, how the fingernails are shaped, how their eyes look, how the hair is. For somebody who has spent her entire life looking for somebody who looks like her, it is a very powerful moment.

> I've come to terms with the loss of her and who she is as a human being. If I never see her again, I have fulfilled her obligations, I have given her back her history and told her the truth about her conception and relinquishment. If she chooses to know me when she gets older, then that would be like icing on the cake.

Adoptee organizations such as WARM, in Washington, report successful reunions (meaning that all parties agreed to meet) in 97 percent of cases. However even in a failed reunion, there can be positive aspects. One adoptee listened to her mother's cold denial on an extension phone while an intermediary made the contact.

> Instead of the grief one would expect, I felt so tremendously relieved and somehow released that I went home, pulled the phone jack, and slept for two days. I had an inner peace and knowing I had never felt before.

At least in this case there was closure, an end to the feeling of having one's birthparents "missing-in-action."

Ganson and Cook, in their 1986 paper, "The Open Records Controversy in Adoption: A Woman's Issue?" conclude that "the gender of an individual appears to be the major influence on attitudes and opinions about adoption." A much greater number of women respond to surveys, and their comments indicate the status of adoptee is very salient to their identity. Gilligan has pointed out the importance to females of attachment to the mother in identity development but for males separation has primacy. One could postulate that as women place such importance on relationships and connections, that likewise the DI issue is of more concern to them. Perhaps female DI offspring, who may experience pregnancy themselves, have more intense feelings about their mother's choice of conception than male offspring. Ganson and Cook conclude that their research has several indications for social policy, as it is men who make the laws in our society. They observe that adoption practices were built on separation, and this reflects the male view that absence of biological ties will facilitate the child's bond with adoptive parents. Future policies, they suggest, may need to "acknowledge the existence of continued attachment between birthparents . . . and to develop institutional remedies to accommodate this attachment."

Because of records, birthmothers are easier to trace than birthfathers. In fact, it is usually only through the birthmother that the father's identity can be known. According to Anderson, nearly all adoptees, after finding the birthmother, discover that they have "just as intense a need to know the other half of their heritage."

Carol Gustavson of Adoptive Parents for Open Records counsels:

> Neither family knows what they will find at the end of a search. We have a responsibility to prepare ourselves and our children for the possibility of eventual contact, as well as other members of the extended family.

DI parents, like adoptive parents, may fear rejection if the child finds the biological parent. However, experience with adoption has shown this is absolutely not the case, and often the converse is true. It is not an either/or situation. As one adoptee put it, "I don't want to leave my home and family. I just want to ask a million questions."

The Adoption Triangle discusses the positive effects of reunions and how solving the mysteries helped the adoptee to accept and appreciate his relationship with his adoptive parents.

> One of the striking aftereffects of reunions was the enhancement of the relationship between the adoptees and their adoptive parents. When the relationship was essentially warm and healthy, it in-

creased in depth and meaning. When it had been a poor parent-child experience, the adoptee was able to view it from a new perspective and to feel for the first time that the adoptive parents were truly the psychological parents.

For many adoptive parents, learning of their child's search was a shock, a trauma, and gave them a sense of failure as parents. However, within a relatively short time, these adoptive parents became reassured that instead of losing the love of their child, they had gained a new, less troubled affection.

An adoptee wrote to the authors:

Perhaps the most surprising change of all has been the growing awareness that I am, for better or worse, the child of my adoptive parents. . . . I see them in me in a way I never could when I spent so much time wondering.

Search Assistance

In recent years a multitude of search organizations have sprung up across the country. International Search Consultants (ISC) in Costa Mesa, California, has publications for many states. The Tri-adoption Library in Westminster, California, publishes an adoption search book called *Techniques for Tracing People.* It has an international referral computerized service to put individuals in touch with over 270 search and support organizations in many countries. There are classes, seminars, lectures, and other educational programs some of which can be ordered on audiocassettes, as well as individual search consultants. The library's programs and publications focus on search, research, contact, reunion, and postreunion experiences. There are audiovisual presentations that can be hired for educational purposes.

As noted earlier, Candace Turner has founded an organization in Missouri called Donors' Offspring for those conceived by DI, their relatives, and others who are concerned. The organization's goals are as follows:

Worldwide goal: To bring the problems of Donors' Offspring and the abuse of artificial insemination to the attention of the world.

Purpose: To let Donors' Offspring have the opportunity to meet someone like themselves and find a support group for their own unique problems.

Outreach: To make ourselves available to infertile couples and those with DI children so that they may make better informed decisions.

Contacts: To promote the use of the International Soundex Reunion Registry so that all the brothers and sisters and other relatives may find each other and eliminate incest.

The International Soundex Reunion Registry, founded in 1975 in Carson City, Nevada, does not search or offer search assistance. It is a free, confidential registry for adults over the age of eighteen who desire a reunion with a next of kin by birth.

Further information about search and support organizations can be found in the Resources.

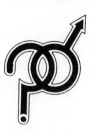

Conclusion

WRITING THIS BOOK has been a deep learning experience for us in the DI triangle. Leaving no stone unturned in my search for truth and knowledge in this field has created a wealth of information that I hope will assist those who provide and receive DI. A book such as this on the subject would have been invaluable to us when we embarked on the process of becoming parents through DI.

The final chapter to our story will never be written, of course, and certainly not in our lifetime. Future generations will be the final evaluators of our actions. However, what we did was in good faith, as forearmed and forewarned as we could be.

Dilemmas that may arise will at least not be those of lost identity or irretrievable information. Whatever sense of mastery we may have enjoyed over the DI procedure, conflict will never be entirely conquered and life unfolds always as a journey into the unknown. Participants in open DI, like those in cooperative adoption, in the words of Rillera and Kaplan are "traveling footpaths rather than paved highways. They may seem unfamiliar. They may seem untraveled. But this does not make the highway better. There would be no highways if footpaths and buggy paths had not preceded them."

In the years that I have been writing this book, events have forced me, initially with reluctance and skepticism, to delve into metaphysics and seriously examine such doctrines as karma and reincarnation. If one believes—as a great many people do—that each soul chooses its parents for its spiritual development in that lifetime, how is this reconciled with the different reproductive technologies? How are the spiritual and physiological dimensions in assisted conceptions integrated? Is it beneficial for the development of the souls of perhaps one million DI offspring around the world never to know their paternal origins? Is it perhaps their karma to have chosen their DI parents rather than their biological ones? Is it right for science to do what nature cannot at the primal level of creating life? Is it karmic destiny when a woman and a man create a child together outside their own marriages? When ovaries malfunction or tubes are blocked or sperm are deficient, are doctors bringing together reluctant gametes? These are questions now raised by recent research into cellular consciousness, and at this time we can only ponder them and consult our intuition on such matters.

My personal belief is that our thoughts create energy fields that affect our bodies, especially gametes. Psychiatric research with adults under various forms of facilitated regression (primal therapy, hypnosis, drugs) has shown that people can reach back to their preverbal organic memories. That is, memories and feelings of conception and implantation, which are experienced and stored in the body long before the brain develops its computer-type of memory. Thus, the emotional and spiritual attitudes of the male and female providing the gametes in conception, whether artificial or natural, are extremely influential. They are just as important as the physical environment of hormones and mucus. Australian psychiatrist Graham Farrant has explored the influence of these early primal events on personality development as well as the implications of reproductive technology at the cellular level of human experience.

The tide of "progress" cannot be turned back. But as technology races forward at a dizzying pace, a strong humanistic wave is affirming the instinctual wisdom, as well as the intellectual knowledge, of our species. I would urge all those involved in DI and other collaborative conceptions to put themselves in the position of the child-to-be with all her vulnerabilities. Recipients need to question the "experts" and take care that professional assistance does not intimidate and disempower them as they struggle to be true to themselves and their offspring.

Despite being a committed feminist, my research has pushed me beyond what Rona Achilles has termed "residual biologism" in families. I spent three very moving days at the 1987 American Adoption Congress in Boston. Hearing the joy, anguish, and other powerful emotions expressed by adults who have searched and are searching for offspring, parents, and siblings further convinced me of the primacy of biological ties in most individuals. In contrast, the huge bibliography in this book testifies to the paucity of interest in the long-term psychology of the DI offspring, and the preoccupation with DI as a transient "medical treatment."

True freedom means no internal choice; equivocation is unnecessary. The child's genetic, medical, and genealogical past—and thus her future—must be protected. We must pledge this birthright to the children born from collaborative reproduction. We are guardians of their future, and we must never fail to acknowledge the privilege of creating and nurturing a new life. In alternative reproduction and blended families, caring means sharing—the truth and the relationships.

May the times change so that the child's right to know her heritage will one day become as unquestioned as the secrecy that presently surrounds the use of donor gametes.

*Bill of Rights and
Responsibilities
Appendixes
Resources
Index*

Bill of Rights and Responsibilities

The Child

The DI child has the right to:

1. Know that she was conceived through donor insemination.
2. A birth certificate that lists both biological father, and social father, if the mother is married.
3. Legal access to medical records concerning the donor and conception procedures.
4. Regular updated information about the donor.
5. Support in contacting the donor at the age of majority, or before, if mutually agreeable.
6. The status of legitimacy.

The DI child has the responsibility to:

1. Acknowledge the DI father as her legal parent.
2. Respect the privacy of the donor and his natural family and not to intrude unless invited.
3. Refrain from lawsuits and inheritance claims against the donor or DI physician.
4. File regularly updated medical reports for the benefit of half-siblings, if requested.
5. Permit contact from the donor, donor's parents and children after reaching majority, or before, if mutually agreeable.
6. Consider requests for research into the DI experience.
7. Press for legislative change that would mandate thorough do-

nor screening, permanent records on donors, recipients and offspring, and guarantee the child's right to know the donor's identity.

The Legal Parents

The DI parents have the right to detailed information about the donor if they have not chosen him through open DI.

The DI father has the right to be regarded by the child and society as the social and legal father.

The DI parents have the responsibility to:

1. Advise the child of her DI status during the preschool years and to keep open communication on the subject.
2. Obtain as much information as possible about the donor and relay it to the child when she enquires.
3. Respect the child's need to know her heritage and to help the child integrate it into her growing self-identity.
4. Never disown the DI child and her children, even if the parents divorce.
5. Communicate with a donor who requests it, either directly or through an intermediary.
6. Acknowledge that the child may want to search for and meet the donor, and to support that search.
7. Respect the privacy of the donor and his family.
8. Press for legislative change that would mandate thorough donor screening, permanent records on donors, recipients, and offspring, and guarantee the child's right to know the identity of the donor.

The Donor

Donors have the right to:

1. Information about the use and outcome of their sperm donations.

2. Information about or contact with the prospective mother or couple.
3. Privacy.
4. Protection from suits for custody and maintenance.
5. Periodic details about the child's development.
6. Contact with the child at the age of majority, or before, if mutually agreeable.

Donors have the responsibility to:

1. Supply a complete medical and social history and to update this at regular intervals.
2. Respect the privacy of the DI parent(s) and child.
3. Contact the parents, or an intermediary, rather than approaching the child directly.
4. Be available for contact with the child when she reaches the age of majority, or before, if mutually agreeable.
5. Reveal the identity of any half-siblings of the DI child.

DI Practitioners

Physicians and other intermediaries have the responsibility to:

1. Be aware of the social and personal aspects of infertility.
2. Obtain a thorough medical history, and do genetic and laboratory screening on the donor.
3. Select the donor in consultation with the woman/couple or arrange for contact, directly or through an intermediary, with the donor.
4. Maintain permanent records on the recipients, donor, and child.
5. Use the sperm of only one donor at any time and to inform the woman/couple of any change in the donor.
6. Arrange for the exchange of regular updated information between the parties involved, and support contact at any time if mutually desired.
7. Facilitate the development of support groups, which include

DI parents and offspring, to educate and counsel those undergoing DI.

8. Press for legislative change that would mandate thorough donor screening, permanent records on donors, recipients and offspring, and guarantee the child's right to know the donor's identity.

Appendix 1

Causes and Treatment of Male Infertility

Infertility is on the increase, afflicting one in five couples according to a 1984 *Newsweek* cover story. While much of unwanted female infertility results from birth control interventions, male infertility is related to environmental pollution, radiation, and other hazards of industrialized societies. Vasectomy is a sterilization procedure for men, and there are over 10 million men with vasectomies in the United States and over 100 million worldwide. In California vasectomy—and then a new marriage—is a more common reason to turn to donor insemination than primary male infertility. Both sexes, of course, are becoming increasingly infertile from the epidemic in sexually transmitted diseases.

According to Howard A. Zacur and John Rock (1983), physicians at Johns Hopkins in Baltimore, in 90 percent of cases the cause could be found within three months—although it may in fact take years. In 35 percent of cases there will be a male factor, in another 35 percent of cases there will be a female factor, and in the remaining 30 percent it will be a combined problem. For 10 percent of infertile couples, no cause will ever be found.

Physician membership in the American Fertility Society doubled between 1974 and 1984, and infertility accounted for more than one and a half million visits to the doctor in 1983. There is more physician interest in fertility problems, more individuals seeking their services, together with greater social and media support for access to such treatment. Most of the impetus is directed to curing infertility rather than to understanding its causes and prevention. Nevertheless, the infertile couple usually grapples with the crisis in a psychosocial vacuum.

Though for most couples who read this book the infertility problem already will have been diagnosed as being with the male, this chapter is nevertheless helpful for family members and others who do not understand "male plumbing." In fact, most nonmedical professionals concerned

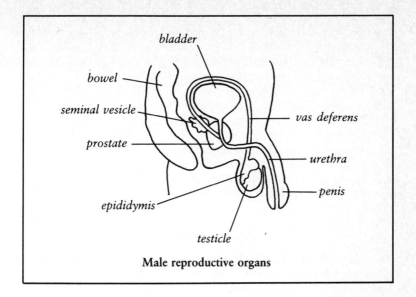

Male reproductive organs

with the practice of DI do not understand male reproductive structure and function, so this will assist them too. Some infertile men also did not really have their problem explained to them in detail.

Overview of Male Anatomy and Physiology

Sperm production takes place in the two testicles, which lie in the scrotum. The testicles hang outside the body in order for the sperm to be kept at a cooler temperature. The scrotal sac changes its position with the weather and thus acts as a natural thermostat to regulate the temperature for sperm production. The male sex hormone, testosterone, is produced by cells in the testes and is responsible for the development of the male hair patterns and deeper voice. At death, the last bodily function to cease is sperm production.

The epididymis sits on the back of each testicle and contains a long, very convoluted, fine tube. This tubule is only 0.4 mm in diameter, but it is about eighteen to twenty feet long. It is here that sperm maturation takes place. The duct of the epididymis becomes continuous with a larger duct, the vas deferens, which is the tube that is cut during vasectomy.

Behind the bladder are two seminal vesicles (or semen sacs), which secrete fluid to transport the sperm. The vas deferens joins with the ducts from these vesicles within the prostate gland to form the ejaculatory duct. Both right and left ejaculatory ducts open into the urethra within the prostate gland. The prostate gland surrounds the base of the urethra and contributes a milky, alkaline fluid to the semen. The final product is reflexly ejaculated following stimulation and engorgement of the penis.

The amount of fluid in a single seminal emission is about 3 ml and the average number of sperm in a single seminal emission is around one hundred and twenty million. Spermatozoa take sixty-four days to form and then another twelve to twenty days to travel via the epididymis before they appear in the ejaculate. They can move very fast up through the uterus and Fallopian tubes and may be viable for a few days.

Male Infertility

The accepted definition of infertility is the inability to conceive a pregnancy after unprotected intercourse for twelve months. Eighty-five percent of couples trying for pregnancy succeed within a year, 60 percent in the first three months. To put it another way, if 100 eggs were exposed to sperm, 35 would become fertilized. Normal fertility is defined as a sperm count of at least 20 million per ml (the American Fertility Society has recommended 40 million per ml as a minimal standard, although this has been criticized as unrealistic), not less than 60 percent of sperm with normal structure, and not less than 60 percent showing normal progressive activity at 30 minutes after ejaculation. Sperm count was considered the most important aspect until the fifties when it was noted that if only sperm density was considered, when the count went above 20 million per ml no increase in the fertility potential was seen. The vitality and morphology (normal forms) of the sperm are actually more important than numbers. The combination of motility and a high number of normal forms compensate for lesser sperm density.

The term infertility, rather than sterility, is used these days as it sounds less final and carries less stigma. With sterility there is no hope of conception, as when there are no sperm at all. It is difficult to draw the line between absolute fertility and relative infertility, so these divisions are rather arbitrary. The term subfertility is used if there are more than a million sperm per ml, and if there are fewer then the term is infertility. Some men have a failure of sperm transport (not facilitated by the female reproductive tract) or deficient sperm-fertilizing capacity, or both. This cannot be predicted by conventional semen analysis or even assessment of sperm quantity and motility. In addition, an in vitro zona-free hamster egg-penetration test has been developed, but the validity of using nonhuman material has been questioned. Also, as the zona pellucida surrounding the female egg has the power to inhibit fertilization in many ways, I find it difficult to understand how a zona-free test can be valid. Another test is done with hen's egg white. There is an outer liquid part and a highly viscous inner part surrounding the yolk. Researchers have found a significant correlation between sperm penetration ability in cervical mucus at ovulation and this intermediate part of the egg white, although this, of course, is a nonhuman tissue too.

Causes of Male Infertility

Impairment in the quality or quantity of sperm may result from functional or structural causes. I. C. Fisher, M.D., at the First World Congress on Fertility claimed that the quality and quantity of sperm is greatly influenced by a man's emotional outlook. It is well known that stress interferes with sperm production and that prisoners, and students at exam time, show decreased sperm counts. It is possible for a normally fertile male to deplete his semen entirely of sperm with excessive ejaculations. This is why several semen samples, taken after three or four days' abstinence, should be examined in an infertility workup.

Azoospermia is the term for complete lack of sperm in the semen—what Dr. Sherman Silber likes to call, in his characteristic military terminology, "shooting blanks." Sperm may or may not be manufactured in the testicles. If surgical biopsy confirms that it is, then clearly the problem is a blockage somewhere. Guerin (1981) found that an enzyme (alpha-glucosidonase, possibly produced by the lining of the epididymis) was regularly absent from the semen of men with an inflammatory obstruction of the reproductive tract. When there is no sperm in the semen, it is important also to check the urine in case a defect in the nervous control of the bladder neck permits "retrograde ejaculation" into the bladder. While azoospermia sounds like the most final diagnosis of sterility, it is important to distinguish pathological from functional azoospermia. There are at least six cases in the literature where despite a diagnosis of azoospermia there have apparently been subsequent natural conceptions.

Oligospermia refers to a diminished number of sperm, less than 10 million per ml. *Necrospermia* means that the sperm are dead, and *athenospermia* describes a severe degree of low motility. *Dyspermia* means substandard seminal fluid and *aspermia* is the term for no ejaculate, as in retrograde ejaculation or in nervous system disorders such as paraplegia or syringomyelia. The sperm is available at its origin but cannot reach a fertile destination physiologically.

Decreased production of sperm is the most common symptom in male infertility. Causes of this include variocele (swelling of the veins in the testicle), testicular failure, endocrine disorders, and cryptorchidism (undescended testicles). *Variocele* is the most frequent cause of male infertility and leads to fewer sperm, decreased motility, and tapered head forms. A study of medical students found that 80 percent of those with variocele had abnormal sperm findings. (In cases with variocele on just one side, it was always on the left, which results from the way the veins are joined on that side.)

Sometimes, when the male is subfertile, the woman can be treated with hormones to favor conception by improving her fertility.

Testicular failure includes germinal cell aplasia, (no development of the sperm-producing cells; this is the most common cause), Klinefelter's syndrome (a genetic defect), infantile or undescended testes, mumps orchitis (inflammation of the testicles), tumor, surgical or other injury, and radiation. Hormones such as gonadotropins, clomiphene citrate, and testosterone have been tried with mixed results.

The most common endocrine problem results from low gonadotropin levels, which can be treated with hormones such as human menopausal gonadotropin and chorionic gonadotropin if the sperm count is at least 10 million. Where there is adrenogenital syndrome (involving the adrenal glands), treatment with glucocorticoids (steroids) appears to be effective. Hypothyroidism may be a rare cause of infertility. Vitamins and dietary changes have been recommended too, probably more to satisfy the physician and couple that everything has been tried.

Smoking, systemic infections such as a viral illness, and stress also play a role in infertility. Sometimes the effects are only temporary. The tight clothing that is popular these days and the use of briefs may also affect sperm production. Personal advice columnists have published several letters from couples who had been considering DI or adoption and went on to successfully conceive after the husband changed to wearing boxer shorts.

The second most common type of male infertility results from *obstruction of the ducts* through surgery or infection. This may be caused by an infection in the epididymis, or ejaculatory duct, commonly from gonorrhea or TB, which leads to an enlarged obstructed epididymis. Epididymitis interferes with sperm maturation. Organisms responsible for the infection include Mycoplasma and chlamydia, which can be treated with antibiotics such as Dovacyclin or Vibramycin.

In *autoimmune conditions,* the sperm becomes clumped. This agglutination results because the man produces an antibody to his own sperm.

Dear Abby:
May I comment on your men's underwear debate? We in our brief-type "Fruit-of-the-Loom's" remain fruitless, while our brothers in their boxer shorts remain "heir-conditioned."

Robert W. in Walterboro, S.C.

Dear Abby:
The fact that too-tight jeans may cause male sterility is nothing new. I wrote this little jingle back in 1970.

"If your jeans are too tight in the crotch
Your parental potential is bad
Better let out your seams just a notch
If you hope to be somebody's dad!"

(BMS)

Although antibody testing is still in its infancy, corticosteroids have helped this condition. The drug Dexamethasone has a 40 percent success rate, but there are many side effects.

Cytotoxic drugs (which kill cancer cells, as in Hodgkin's disease, for example) can cause azoospermia.

There may be a *congenital absence of the vas deferens* (which also means low semen volume).

Infertility may also result from a *failure to deliver the semen* into the vagina. These disturbances include impotence (inability to sustain an erection) or hypospadias (condition that causes retrograde ejaculation, where the semen is lost from a urethral opening in the underside of the penis).

The Infertility Workup

A woman's regular gynecologist is usually the first physician consulted about any delays in conception. Some gynecologists do extensive, and expensive, workups before suggesting a semen analysis, which is a quick, simple, cheap test. A poor semen analysis then leads to urology consultations, biopsies, maybe surgery, and then perhaps back to the woman's gynecologist for DI. Not all gynecologists perform DI, so further delays may ensue as the couple are referred to another specialist or to a hospital that may have a waiting list of months or even years.

If you suspect male infertility, you can find a urologist yourself by looking in the *Dictionary of Medical Specialists* in your local library or by calling the American Fertility Society. (See Resources.) Family planning agencies may be a source of referrals too, although they are more concerned with preventing pregnancy than achieving it. It is important that you find an open and thorough physician with whom you feel comfortable, so shop around if necessary.

First, there is an interview and history taken of both sexual partners. Couples can anticipate questions about frequency of intercourse, techniques, pain, use of lubricants, menstrual history, drugs, systemic and sexually transmitted diseases. Sometimes a diagnosis may be made, but the cause of the condition may remain unknown. It is frustrating if there is no discernible reason *why* a man or a woman's tubes are blocked, for example.

A urological evaluation involves examination of the penis and scrotum, and a detailed history about exposure to substances that may impair fertility. *Semen analysis* looks at several parameters: the number of sperm, motility and forward progression, normal structure, and quantity of ejaculate.

A *vasogram* involves placing a dye within the tubes of the male reproductive system and taking x-rays to check for any blockages. This is a controversial procedure because many urologists feel that the dye itself may damage or further obstruct the very fine tubes involved.

Biopsy of the testicles is the surgical removal of a small part of the tissue of each testicle to check for sperm production. Both the above procedures are done under general or regional anesthesia.

Surgical Treatment of Male Infertility

Removal of variocele. According to New York urologists Lawrence Dubin and Richard Amelar (1971) surgical removal of the varicosity improves the quality of the sperm in 80 percent of cases with a pregnancy rate of approximately 50 percent. The size of the variocele apparently does not influence the outcome of the treatment.

Vasectomy reversals (vasovasostomy) have improved with the advent of microsurgery, and about 50 percent of men can subsequently achieve pregnancy. It takes about six months for sperm production to return to normal after surgery, as long as the vasectomy was done within ten years. After that time, the male often develops antibodies to his own sperm.

Epididymovasostomy is another surgical procedure which bypasses a blockage and reunites the vas with a healthy section of the epididymis.

This surgery does not have a good record of success, as sperm is found in the semen of only 20–25 percent of men a couple of months after the operation, and only a quarter of such men will actually get their partners pregnant.

There are two cases in the literature where sperm was taken directly from the testicle for fertilization. One conception described by Adler and Makris (1951), where testicular tissue was biopsied from the husband, macerated by mortar and pestle, and introduced into the wife's vagina. With that single attempt the woman became pregnant and subsequently delivered a normal child. The baby from the second case was born in April 1985 in Melbourne, Australia, as a result of an IVF conception using sperm from the father's right testicle.

IVF (in vitro fertilization) is also sometimes tried where there is low sperm count or motility.

GIFT (gametes intra-Fallopian tube transfer) is a new surgical procedure where the egg and sperm are placed in the Fallopian tube (where fertilization always occurs). This technique, which was developed by Ricardo Asch at the Texas Medical School, eliminates the hazards for the sperm en route from vagina to the tube.

In many cases, the surgery involved, plus the low chance of success, let alone pregnancy, make donor insemination a more appealing proposition—if the man can resolve his emotional response to his infertility.

Appendix 2

Self-Insemination

In this appendix we will examine the changes in the menstrual cycle that enable women to determine ovulation and will discuss different insemination procedures. These instructions will be helpful for both women doing donor insemination or insemination with a partner's semen. We will also look at some profiles of single and lesbian women who have done their own DI. However, the following pages are not intended to replace personal medical advice, particularly in cases of reproductive difficulty.

The Menstrual Cycle

A woman's monthly reproductive cycle is regulated by hormones secreted by the hypothalamus (a part of the brain) and two endocrine glands, the pituitary (near the brain) and the ovaries in the pelvis. Estrogen, produced by the ovaries, is the dominant hormone during the first part of the cycle. When estrogen output falls beneath a certain level, the hypothalamus releases a hormone, FSHRF (follicle-stimulating hormone-release factor), which stimulates the pituitary gland to release FSH, a hormone that stimulates the growth of about a dozen ovarian follicles. When the level of FSH is sufficient to promote follicular development, together with a consequent rise in the circulating level of estrogen, this hormonal phenomenon is reflected in the production of mucus from glands in the cervix.

As the follicles grow, they secrete increasing amounts of estrogen, which causes the lining of the uterus to proliferate. Usually only one of these follicles reaches full maturity, the others degenerate. The estrogen influences the hypothalamus to suppress FSH production, which decreases the stimulation of the other follicles. When the egg becomes mature in the dominant follicle, this follicle secretes a burst of progesterone along with the estrogen. It is thought that this combination of both female sex hormones stimulates the hypothalamus to secrete FSH-RF and LH-RF, a luteinizing hormone-releasing factor. As a result, the pituitary is signaled to secrete FSH and LH simultaneously. The combined peak of these hormones probably triggers the follicle to release the egg (ovulation) within a day or so after that peak.

Now under the influence of the LH, the follicle is called a corpus luteum and changes its function. It secretes increasing amounts of progesterone and decreasing amounts of estrogen. The progesterone inhibits the production of cervical mucus. It also influences the uterine lining to secrete fluids that will sustain the egg if it is fertilized. When fertilization occurs, the corpus luteum is stimulated by a hormone HCG (human chorionic gonadotropin), secreted by the developing placenta, to continue producing both estrogen and progesterone which will maintain the pregnancy.

If the egg is not fertilized, the corpus luteum degenerates and the levels of hormones from it decline. These dwindling hormone levels fail to maintain the uterine lining, which results in menstruation. When the levels of estrogen fall to a low enough level, the hypothalamus releases FSH-RF and the cycle starts again. Menstruation occurs approximately two weeks after ovulation, the range being usually eleven to sixteen days.

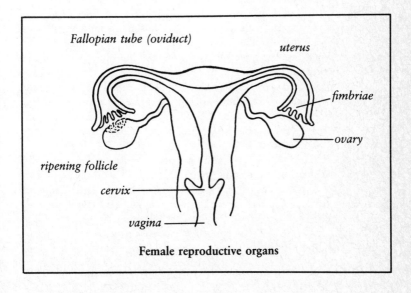

Female reproductive organs

Fertility Awareness

In order for conception to occur, there has to be viable mucus, as well as sperm and an egg. In self-insemination, it is assumed that you are using a donor of known fertility and good health, or that the semen has been screened for good sperm quality. The next step is to determine the woman's time of maximum fertility, which can be assessed through several different observable signs.

Basal Body Temperature (BBT) Charts

These graphs plot the woman's temperature on awakening, prior to any activity, after at least three hours of uninterrupted sleep. The temperature can be taken orally, rectally, or vaginally, but the location should be consistent as well as the time that the temperature is taken. A special basal body thermometer that is marked in large units for easy reading is available from most drugstores. Always use the same thermometer in a cycle, and shake it down after recording the reading so you won't have to perform that physical activity the next time you take your temperature.

Normal cycles during which ovulation occurs are biphasic. This means there are two different temperature levels with a rise occurring at ovulation. The temperature usually drops (the nadir) prior to ovulation and then peaks (the thermal shift) about three to six tenths of a degree at ovulation, staying high until the end of the cycle. In some women the peak is a sharp, obvious rise; in other women it may take two or three days. If you are in doubt, a ruler placed between the high and low points of the graph will indicate a biphasic graph. The rise in body temperature is generally considered a more reliable sign of ovulation than the fall. It also shows that adequate progesterone is being secreted by the corpus luteum.

If pregnancy has not occurred, the temperature begins to drop again. If pregnancy has occurred, the temperature remains high beyond the anticipated time of menstruation.

Occasional cycles without ovulation happen to most women, especially if there is the stress of monitoring them. However, a workup may be in order if several such cycles occur. Anovulatory cycles can be treated with clomiphene citrate (Clomid or Serophene), an anti-estrogen drug that stimulates ovulation. Dr. John Billings claims that infertility is seldom due to a failure to ovulate and that almost all women complaining of infertility have ovulatory cycles. However, almost every woman under great stress—and DI is stressful—will experience an occasional anovulatory cycle.

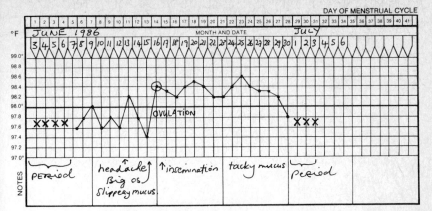

Basal body temperature chart—normal cycle

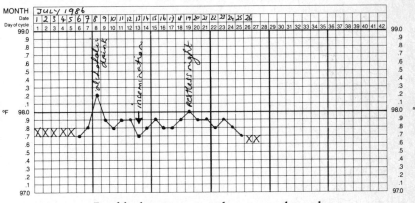

Basal body temperature chart—anovular cycle

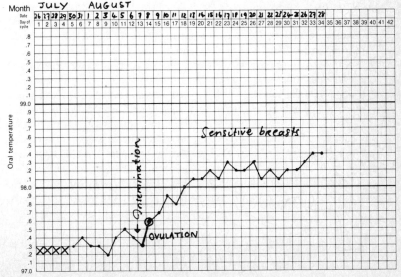

Basal body temperature chart—pregnancy

With the BBT method, ovulation is confirmed only after it has happened. If a woman's cycles are regular, the pattern may be acceptable for estimating peak fertility. When multiple inseminations are done, they are usually performed three times: two days before the anticipated day of ovulation, the day of ovulation, and two days after this day. The dip that occurs prior to the rise in a woman with regular cycles may help predicting ovulation. Several cycles need to be charted so a woman can determine her hormonal pattern.

The Mucus Method

This method is also known as the Billings Method after the husband and wife team of physicians, Evelyn and John Billings, who pioneered this approach more than twenty-five years ago in Australia. The method involves daily observation of the cervical mucus that forms the normal vaginal discharge at the labia. The characteristics of this mucus vary throughout the menstrual cycle and can be compared and charted to determine the time of peak fertility.

The Billingses are adamant that only the *external* mucus should be evaluated. Exploring your vaginal mucus with your finger and palpating the cervix can make it more difficult to assess the qualities of the mucus and to recognize the most fertile time. Thus, internal mucus can confuse the timing if it is taken from the cervix and examined before it flows to the outside.

The Sympto-thermal Method

The Sympto-thermal method combines the above two methods, plus other bodily changes that might occur around the fertile time of the cycle. These include lower abdominal pain or low back pain (called mittelschmerz and believed due to the action of prostaglandins released at ovulation), pelvic pressure, bloating, changes in the elevation and opening of the cervix, increased sexual drive, breast tenderness, vulvar swelling, changes in skin, mood, appetite and energy levels, headaches, and fatigue. One woman told me that she knew when she ovulated because her fingernails would split!

Most women trying to become pregnant conscientiously note every possible sign. However, as Dr. Billings writes in defense of his own mucus method, "When multiple indices of greater or less accuracy are employed, confusion and discouragement are likely when they fail to exhibit congruity."

It is thus both tempting, yet often defeating, to insist on uniformity among the signs. When the signs do not synchronize, a woman tends to give more weight to one sign than to another. And these signs can vary from cycle to cycle. From my own experience, I agree that this can be very confusing. One month I would think, Well, there's no real mucus, but my cervix *is* high, or the os is really wide open, and the next month I might focus on yet another sign. I believe now that there must be enough mucus for it to be observed externally—which was the case only during the month that I conceived. Although each woman has to explore her own cycle and decide which indicators are most reliable for her, I personally feel that the mucus is the cardinal sign.

Cervical mucus is essential for sperm transport and survival. While the egg lives for less than twenty-four hours, sperm may live up to five days in optimal mucus. Features of the mucus vary greatly from woman to woman, and it is the change in quality rather than the quantity which is significant.

During the early part of the cycle, after menstruation, there is commonly a feeling of dryness, with no external mucus, or if any is present, it is tacky or sticky. Other terms to describe the mucus at this time include, "dry, crumbly, adhesive, flaky, claggy, thick." As ovulation approaches, the mucus becomes more moist and more abundant. Around the time of ovulation, the mucus changes from opaque to clear, like raw egg-white. This mucus may also be described as "stretchy, slick, slippery, lubricative, and thin, in sensation, and shiny, clear, glistening," in appearance. This is the most favorable kind of mucus for conception, as the sperm can swim upward through clear channels. Nonfertile mucus is more acidic, whereas fertile mucus is alkaline, which protects and nourishes the sperm. The glucose and saline content of the mucus also increase at this time, and some women and their partners may notice the change by the sweeter or saltier taste of the mucus. It also functions as a filter to screen out abnormal spermatozoa and promotes migration of normal sperm.

Ovulation may be up to twenty-four hours away from the peak mucus, so it is the *last* day of peak mucus which is considered the time of maximum fertility.

Following ovulation the mucus resumes its infertile characteristics, and the increased cell content forms a net that acts as a barrier to sperm migration.

Charting her changing mucus allows a woman to predict ovulation despite the fact that there is variation between her cycles. Colds, alcoholic drinks, insomnia, electric blankets, for example, can alter the BBT, so the mucus is a more reliable guide if you have enough of it and can assess it accurately.

Tests for Ovulation

Tes-Tape, sold over the counter to check the sugar content in urine, can show the increased glucose production in the cervical mucus around ovulation. You can also use *pH* tape to show the range from 8.00 (acid) to 8.4 (alkaline), which is actually a greater change than it appears because the pH scale is logarithmic.

Other features of cervical mucus can be examined under a microscope. Around ovulation there are fewer cells present, and the potassium and sodium salts will crystallize into a *fern pattern* when the mucus dries on a slide.

A *Burn* test involves allowing some mucus to dry at room temperature on a glass slide, and then heating it over an alcohol lamp for about a minute. When observed over a light bulb, any color at all indicates nonfertile mucus, whereas fertile mucus remains clear.

Ultrasound images allow the developing follicle to be measured as a way of predicting ovulation. *Lab tests* include examination of the mucus for an increase in the mucin level, or a decrease in albumen and globulens. Serum LH and FSH (blood tests) and urine LH, FSH, estrogen, and pregnandiol are also available. An *OvuSTICK* urine test was developed in 1984 for home use, but it is very costly, about fifty dollars a cycle. A CUE monitor is expensive to buy but some ob-gyns rent them to their patients. This device measures electrolyte changes in saliva and cervical mucus. Recently, saliva and vaginal mucus tests have also become available. Most women can determine their ovulation without elaborate investigation, so these expensive tests are usually used after long delays in achieving conception. However, for self-insemination, where physician and clinic fees are not incurred, and there is a delay in conceiving, such tests may be worth the expense and the time saved.

Charting

You can rule up your own chart or use graph paper, with large squares of ten. It may be easier to use your own charts—there is more room to write and you can design them with space for the characteristics that are important for you. Only two of the following twelve steps require any internal examination of your organs or mucus.

1. The date and month of the first day of your menstrual cycle.
2. The day of the week (helps to cross reference any omissions and to identify patterns according to your different activities).
3. The day of the cycle. Always note the first day of your period as Day 1.
4. The days of your period, or any spotting in between periods.
5. The days when intercourse occurs. (Seminal fluid obscures cervical mucus. Even penetration without ejaculation will cause lubrication.)
6. The external sensation you feel on your vulva (dry, wet, slippery).
7. The appearance of the mucus (white, clear, thick).
8. Unusual factors in your life, such as colds, stress, exercise, alcohol.
9. Other body changes affecting skin, breast tenderness, headaches.
10. Psychological changes such as mood alterations, headaches, energy levels, sexual desire. You can further investigate your cycle by exploring your cervix with your finger. Then you could note in addition:
11. The height of the cervix (it becomes higher and more difficult to touch around ovulation).
12. Softening around the opening (cervical os). You can also observe the changes in your cervix with a speculum and mirror. A disposable plastic speculum can be obtained from women's health clinics, or from your gynecologist or family physician. Next time you have an internal examination with a speculum, ask to keep it.

Using a Speculum

When you insert the speculum, make sure the duckbills are closed. You can slide it in upwards, or else sideways, turning it when it has been pushed all the way into your vagina. When the handles are above your pubic bone, squeeze them together, which will open your vaginal walls. Press down on the part of the handle that has the finger depression while you are pulling up on the longer handle. You will hear a click when the speculum is locked open. Hold a mirror in front of the speculum and shine a light so that it reflects into your vagina. You should be able to see your cervix, which is round and pink with an opening (the os) in the middle. If you don't see your cervix, and this may be difficult around the time of ovulation when it is higher, or if your uterus is tipped backward (retroverted), move the speculum around or re-insert it. Make sure that you release the handles and collapse the blades before removing it from your vagina. Wash the speculum with soap and warm water.

With a speculum you can observe additional signs:

1. Color changes (around ovulation the cervix is shiny and rosy).

2. Opening of the os (it is at its largest around ovulation, sometimes described as "pouting," with soft edges).
3. Appearance of the mucus (sometimes seen as a clear bubble around ovulation, or a thread like raw egg-white).

It may be helpful to join a group offering instruction in these methods, where women learn the variability and the interpretation of the mucus from each other. Sometimes these groups go by names such as "Fertility Consciousness," "Women-Controlled Birth Control," or "Natural Family Planning," but even if the group is set up primarily to educate about contraception, the information can be just as applicable to promoting conception.

It is recommended that you establish your fertile time for two or three cycles before attempting insemination.

Techniques of Self-Insemination

There are many ways to artificially introduce semen into the female reproductive tract. It can be deposited into the vagina with a syringe (minus the needle), test tube, or even a turkey baster, which has become a legendary symbol in the lesbian community. (However, the small amount of semen does not require such a large instrument. Also it is important not to injure the cervix when using a turkey baster.)

Usually, the woman remains with her hips elevated for fifteen to twenty minutes, or a cervical sponge (Fertilopak) may be inserted to prevent semen leakage. This has a string and can be removed later in the day. However, a 1978 study by Sulweski and colleagues found no difference in pregnancy rates between women who remained on their backs for ten minutes after DI and those who left the clinic directly afterward.

Another common item used in DI is the cervical cup or cap. Rubber cervical caps are designed for contraception (hence the name "cap") but they can be used for insemination. There is also a cervical cup especially designed for insemination by Milex in Chicago, which is slightly larger and more shallow, the name "cup" indicating that it serves as a semen receptacle. This cup is made of Lucite, a rigid opaque plastic, and clings by suction to the cervix. Another similar cervical cup is available, which is placed over the cervix first, and then the semen is introduced through an attached plastic tube. This may be easier if someone else is doing the insemination, but like using a syringe, the sperm is transferred from the receptacle in which it was collected. This extra step can lead to spillage, which can be avoided by using the basic cup.

Inserting the Cervical Cup or Cap

You simply squat down, check the position of your cervix, and insert the cap in that direction, holding it upright at all times. It may be easier to do it in two stages, to insert it midway into the vagina and hold it in place with the muscles of your pelvic floor. Next, you can position it exactly on your cervix. Check all around the top of your vagina to make sure that you didn't miss your cervix.

Some practice beforehand makes this easier—but avoid practicing on the day of insemination as you may dislodge some of the precious mucus. The cup and cap can be removed after several hours. Take care to break the suction by hooking a finger over the edge of it before trying to pull it out.

Handling the Semen

If you are using a known donor, the semen will invariably be fresh and thus perishable. It should be collected either in the cervical cup or cap, or else a clean, dry glass container. (A diaphragm is more flimsy and difficult to insert without spilling the semen.) Avoid metal as it is toxic to sperm. If kept at body temperature, the sperm will be viable for up to a couple of hours. Fresh semen is much more effective than frozen, so one insemination a month should be enough, especially if you feel it is an imposition to bother your donor more often.

Frozen semen may be used when a friend or partner is out of the country, or obtained from a sperm bank. You may want to use two straws each time and try twice or three times in a cycle to compensate for the reduced motility of the sperm after freezing (see Chapter 6). Of course, each sperm bank specimen costs money, plus there are usually only six to nine vials in a portable liquid nitrogen tank. It may be simpler and cheaper to transport and store the sperm in a picnic cooler of dry ice (solid carbon dioxide, $-78.5°$ C). Dry ice lasts about forty-eight hours, and will need to be replenished as it evaporates. Wear gloves to protect your hands from sticking to it. The sperm should be thawed at room temperature and it helps to rotate the straw around in warm water at body temperature to ensure even thawing. Carefully follow the sperm bank's directions for thawing semen.

Gender Selection

Although some people are happy simply to have a healthy baby, many others have a marked preference for either a boy or a girl for many reasons. Sometimes there is a preference because the woman is single or lesbian, or because she is married and her DI offspring to date have all been the same sex. More important, there may be a serious sex-linked genetic condition to avoid. The sperm decide the gender of the offspring as they carry both X and Y chromosomes, whereas the female egg is always XX. A Y-bearing sperm that fertilizes the egg will result in an XY combination—a male. The X-bearing sperm will mean XX, a female. The two types of sperm have different characteristics, which can be observed under the microscope. Trying to facilitate conception by one type of sperm rather than another can be done by home remedies as well as by laboratory techniques. Simple measures that can be tried at home to favor the desired gender are douching and timing of the insemination. However, these measures may also diminish the chance of conception at all in that cycle by depleting the mucus.

Girl

Early insemination is recommended (up to thirty-six hours before the anticipated time of ovulation) and the semen should be deposited low in the vagina. Because the Y sperm is more susceptible to an acidic environment, this allows the Y sperm more chance of drying from contact with the acidic vaginal environment, thus giving the X sperm more opportunity. A douche of two tablespoons of vinegar to a quart of water creates a more hostile acid environment so that the Y sperm have less chance of survival.

Boy

Insemination should be timed as closely as possible to ovulation and the semen should be placed against the cervix to give the faster male sperm the advantage of a shorter distance to swim. A douche with a half-teaspoon of baking soda (sodium bicarbonate) creates a more alkaline environment in the vagina. Orgasm has been said to increase the chances of a boy, as the uterine contractions encourage the faster Y sperm.

Laboratory techniques that separate the two types of sperm cost several hundred dollars per ejaculate with an overall loss of from 10 to 20 percent of sperm. The cost is well worth it in cases of hemophilia, for example (an X-linked genetic condition), and is preferable to amniocentesis and abortion.

Convection Counter Streaming Galvanization was developed at Hahnemann Hospital, in Philadelphia, and allows collection of either type. Y sperm have a negative charge on their cell surface and can be drawn to a positive pole (anode), whereas the X sperm have a positive charge and can be drawn to the negative pole (cathode).

Serum Albumin Sediment screens out the Y sperm as they swim faster through the albumen. Although there is a 15 percent loss, this has made no difference, apparently, because only the fittest have survived. About 75 percent of the Y sperm can be collected; this test is not for those who want a girl.

Immunologic Binding is under development. This test involves antibodies recognizing the antigens in the different sperm.

General Health

A holistic view of health and conception is also necessary. You should make sure that your diet is nutritious, avoid alcohol, caffeine, white sugars, and any kind of drug and medication. This is especially important prior to conception, as the most vulnerable time for the embryo is the first few weeks when many women don't even know they are pregnant.

Psychologically, it is beneficial if you are in a "nesting" phase, that is, enjoying reasonable economic and emotional security. Mental attitude, such as the practice of meditation, and/or visualization of successful conception and pregnancy, affirmations (written statements of positive thoughts), and prayer can be helpful. Clearing past blocks (such as abortion, giving up a baby for adoption) and ambivalence toward parenthood is important. *Conscious Conception* by Jeannine and Frederick Baker is a comprehensive resource guide.

The Anxiety of Waiting

Women in a relationship with a sterile man have generally experienced months of the emotional stress related to failure to conceive. Single or lesbian women may just be starting out with the process of monitoring their cycles and anticipated pregnancy. Some very fortunate women conceive on the first or second attempt. However, for the great number, the monthly rituals are repeated again and again and take their toll. The first two weeks of the cycle are busy with taking temperatures, charting mucus, assessing and organizing the time around the insemination(s). During the last two weeks, at least those decisions have been made and the woman can let up on her biological vigilance, but perhaps the period of waiting is more stressful. During that time a woman can imagine every possible symptom of pregnancy, and if one's period is a day or two late—what a cruel hoax!

Doing insemination yourself with a known donor removes some of the stresses, such as the cost, the length of time allowed on the program, the clinic's routine and its limited days of operation. However, cooperating with a known donor has other stresses. He may be out of town or sick during your fertile time. There is always the sense of imposition on his time and generosity. Visits to his house or his office have to be arranged, and donating semen also affects his sexual life and that of his wife or partner. A period of abstinence is desirable because there should be an interval of about seventy-two hours between ejaculations for the highest sperm count. This means anticipating "the day" so that you can call the donor and give him some notice.

With each unsuccessful cycle it gets harder for both. Even with the most supportive donor, it is disheartening to call up each month with no good news. Second time around it is not any easier, especially as the woman is older and it may take even longer. All the donations add up! I wonder if anyone could press the same donor for more than two children, unless they were lucky enough to conceive very promptly.

Single Women

Women contemplating single motherhood need to evaluate their emotional strengths, financial security, parenting skills, and support network before voluntarily assuming the responsibility of a child. Even with a known donor and a contract, a single woman needs to consider how the child may affect future relationships—with her family, the donor, and male partners. It is helpful to look ahead five, ten, or fifteen years and explore one's life goals. Of course, the "biological time clock" forces the issue for women in their late thirties and early forties.

Lisa Radcliffe of the Oakland Feminist Women's Health Center explains that "there are many different kinds of families, and one kind of family can be as good or as bad as any other. What is at stake here is the kind of nurturing, good parenting that a child receives. . . . Who is to say that a child could not be born because she doesn't have a father in the home?" As we noted in Chapter 9, women become single mothers in great numbers by divorce, desertion, and death as well as by choice.

Lesbian Insemination

Lesbians favor donor insemination because they can avoid both sexual intercourse and a potential paternity suit in a homophobic society that feels threatened by women who don't need men—not even for making babies (directly). Nevertheless it takes courage for single women and lesbians to actually take the step. For lesbian couples, there are few role models in the world to show how two women can have a family together. Raising the child in a world that is not yet comfortable with lesbians is another problem. Lesbians generally face much disapproval from one or both of their parents, although a family who disowns the daughter's lesbianism often becomes supportive when she becomes pregnant. Some parents even play a grandparent role to a DI child of the daughter's partner.

In general, gay men support the rights of lesbians to have children, both verbally and with sperm donations. Many gay men also satisfy their urge to reproduce in this way.

Several booklets on self-insemination have been written by lesbians. *Artificial Insemination: An Alternative Conception for the Lesbian and Gay Community* not only gives practical information but has lists of responsibilities for each party, including the liaison go-between. A sample medical form is also included.

The Oakland Feminist Women's Health Center was the first formal clinic assisting lesbians to have babies. "Yet even more people have been upset about the money issue, about who will support these babies, than the lesbianism," says Laura Brown. She continues:

> The fact is the children may go through a hard time about it. They may get ostracized. But that's life. . . . I hate the word *counseling* because I think it implies that we are all cripples. I think it suggests to a woman that somehow we're going to make it all OK for her.

In recent years, however, the Center has increasingly offered counseling to their clients. Lesbians also have to face their disenchantment with the necessary handling of the semen.

> When you get up, gravity will cause the sperm to drip out. Use a pad or toilet paper so it doesn't drip down your leg. This, plus the unfamiliar or well-forgotten smell and consistency, might take some getting used to.

Lesbian Health Matters! published by the Santa Cruz Women's Health Collective has a cartoon, "Conception Comix," depicting DI on the San Francisco Bridge, with running commentary such as "PEE-EWW! This stuff is gross," "Smells like Clorox," "Hey, don't get any of that on me," and "There's hardly any in there!"

Although some lesbians insist on anonymous donors, others use their partner's relatives, gay friends, or go-betweens. Some lesbians have telephone conversations with the donors even if they never actually meet. Sometimes lesbian pairs will conceive a child with the same donor, making the children half-siblings. Others fear that this would mean too much donor involvement with their family. Interestingly, lesbians who use a known donor refer to him as the "father" whereas those who go for anonymity use the term "donor."

> For me, an anonymous donor was the right way to go. My partner was planning on being extremely involved. She was feeling that if there was a known father and a known mother, what would that make her?

Another pair with an anonymous donor said:

> We will tell the child there are two types of fathers. One type just donates the seed and the other type who raises the child as well.

Still, a lesbian named Maidi, quoted in a Boston *Phoenix* article, concedes that she feels a connection with the father of her child, even though she has no idea of his identity.

> I just had this spiritual feeling about him because he was doing something for someone he didn't even know, something that was important to me.

As I have frequently stated throughout this book, the donor may be invariably invisible but he is nevertheless essential, not only for the conception but also for the genealogical context of the child. It bears repeating that those who seek to exercise their own rights to bear a child by DI should not take away the child's rights to know her paternal origins. Changing the name to AI (alternative insemination) skirts the central issue of the donor; it doesn't resolve it. As happened in a lawsuit, the court held that the (known) donor had the same right to visitation as if the child had been conceived by intercourse. We need honesty in the field of assisted conceptions—not doubletalk.

For example, Susan Robinson, M.D., writing with Hank Pizer in *Having a Baby Without a Man*, states:

> We will use the term alternative insemination or alternative fertilization because there is nothing artificial about the ova, sperm, or offspring involved in artificial insemination. Alternative fertilization is, thus, a natural means of reproduction. It is different from the more commonly employed means of conceiving only in that sexual relations are not involved.

But elsewhere in the book, she contradicts herself:

> While women who become pregnant via sexual intercourse are doing what comes naturally for them, AI mothers are charting new territory. . . . it is

normal to have many questions about a medical procedure, particularly something new and different.

The authors also warn of society's reaction to single women and lesbians who make a "deliberate decision" for "unconventional behavior."

Self-insemination is clearly here to stay and on the increase. By its nature, it lies outside regulation. All that can be hoped for is a more open society that encourages and protects the identity of those involved.

Appendix 3

Guidelines for Evaluating a Donor

This appendix contains information for investigating a donor in addition to the general health screening listed in Chapter 8.

Fraser and Forse (1981) present a set of criteria, also adopted by the American Fertility Society, which I have summarized as simply as possible. As they point out, many of us have close relatives who suffer from diseases that have a major genetic component so it is important to understand which are the serious conditions to avoid.

1. There should be no history for the donor, or his first-degree relatives (parents, siblings, or children) of "nontrivial malformation of complex cause," such as cleft lip or palate, spina bifida cystica, congenital heart malformation, congenital hip dislocation, club foot or hypospadias. There is a 1 percent to 5 percent chance of recurrence in the offspring of a man who is so affected.

2. The donor and his first-degree relatives should be free of nontrivial Mendelian disorders such as albinism (general or ocular-eyes), hemophilia, hemoglobin disorder, hereditary hypercholesterolemia, neurofibromatosis, or tuberosa sclerosis. The risk to the offspring is 50 percent of such autosomal dominant disorders and for the daughter's sons in X-linked recessive disorders. Autosomal recessive diseases are of concern where the disorder is fairly common, such as cystic fibrosis.

3. Family history is especially important with genetic disorders that may appear beyond the age of the donor, such as Huntington's chorea, facioscapulohumeral muscular dystrophy, retinitis pigmentosa, and multiple polyposis of the colon.

4. The donor should be free of familiar disease with a major genetic component, for example, asthma, juvenile diabetes mellitus, epilepsy, hypertension, psychosis, rheumatoid arthritis or severe refractive (visual) disorder. The risk of these occurring for the offspring ranges from 5 percent to 15 percent. Major psychoses, epileptic disorders, juvenile diabetes,

and early coronary disease present a risk to second-degree relatives that ranges from about 1 percent to 5 percent.

5. The donor should not carry an autosomal recessive gene for any disease that is prevalent in the donor's racial group such as sickle-cell disease in blacks, Tay-Sachs disease in Ashkenazi Jews or certain French Canadians, or thalassemia and glucose-6-phosphate dehyrogenase deficiency in Mediterranean races.

6. According to Fraser and Forse, the chances of a healthy young adult male having a chromosome problem that could be deleterious to his offspring are usually small. They conclude that routine karyotyping of donors is not justified. However, if one has any doubt about a prospective donor's personal or family history, consultation with a medical geneticist can be sought.

A very detailed medical history questionnaire follows in the Donor Personal History Form compiled by the Repository of Germinal Choice in Escondido, California.

I would also recommend that a prospective donor study the Bill of Rights and Responsibilities in this book, and that women and couples arranging their own DI consult an attorney in their jurisdiction.

Donor Personal History Form
Repository for Germinal Choice, Escondido, California

Year of birth _____ Married _____, Single _____, Widowed _____,
Height _____ Weight at age 25 ___ Divorced _____, Separated _____
Hair Color at age 25 _____ Hair Type: Straight _____, Wavy _____,
Curly _____, Kinky _____
Present Hair loss: None _____, Thinning _____,
                 Moderate Balding _____, Extensive Balding _____
Eye Color _____ Skin Color _____ Race _____ Ancestry _____

Occupation: _____
Education: _____
_____
_____

Give the country of origin of most of your ancestors and yourself: (i.e., Germany, Ireland, etc.) _____
List any special interests or hobbies: _____
_____

Which best describes you at age 20?
    Athletic _____

Donor Personal History Form (Cont.)

Active _____
Average _____
Inactive _____
Which best describes your musical ability?
Sing or play instrument proficiently _____
Evidence of good ability but untrained _____
Ability unknown but enjoy listening _____
Tone deaf _____
Do you have skills in any of the other fine arts? _____
_____

How would you rate your manual dexterity?
Excellent _____, Good _____, Average _____, Poor _____
How often do you lose your temper?
Frequently: _____, Seldom: _____, Never: _____
Allowing for your age, how would you rate your physical stamina?
Above Average: _____
Average: _____
Below Average: _____
Have you ever excelled in any physical activity: _____
Which best describes you?
Extrovert: _____,   Slight Extrovert: _____
Average: _____,
Introvert: _____,   Slight Introvert: _____
If you have ever taken an intelligence test, state which test if known, your
score, and your age at the time: _____
Are you tactful and work well with your associates?
Above Average: _____
Average: _____
Below Average: _____
How many children do you have? _____   Please give brief description
of their health, intelligence, and abilities.

Describe any significant intellectual, artistic, or academic achievement of
your parents or siblings.

Donor Personal History Form (Cont.)

Donor's Genetic Health

Please try to answer the following questions as accurately and completely as possible. However, if you have not heard of a disorder you probably do not have it. Remember that no one is perfect.

1. Have you *ever* had any of the following:

Yes No

( ) ( ) Hay fever
( ) ( ) Asthma
( ) ( ) Drug allergies (Specify)
( ) ( ) Food allergies (Specify)
( ) ( ) Insect allergies
( ) ( ) Skin Photosensitivity
( ) ( ) Eczema
( ) ( ) Psoriasis (scaly elbows)
( ) ( ) Birthmark
( ) ( ) Vitiligo (areas of depigmentation)
( ) ( ) Other chronic skin disease (Specify)
( ) ( ) Serious dental malocclusion
( ) ( ) Cataract
( ) ( ) Strabismus (crossed eyes; one eye turned out)
( ) ( ) Glaucoma
( ) ( ) Color blindness
( ) ( ) Night blindness
( ) ( ) Eyesight deficiency not correctable with glasses
( ) ( ) Blindness (Specify cause or diagnosis)
( ) ( ) Deafness
( ) ( ) Other hearing loss (Specify cause or diagnosis)
( ) ( ) Congenital hip dislocation

Yes No

( ) ( ) Myotonia
( ) ( ) Abnormal postural positions
( ) ( ) Malignant hyperthermia
( ) ( ) Myasthenia gravis
( ) ( ) Huntington's chorea
( ) ( ) Parkinson's disease
( ) ( ) Epilepsy
( ) ( ) Multiple sclerosis
( ) ( ) Have you ever suffered paralysis of a limb for an extended period of time?
( ) ( ) Familial spastic paralysis
( ) ( ) Ataxia
( ) ( ) Tremor
( ) ( ) Sensory disturbance (for example, increased pain perception, unprovoked tingling, etc.)
( ) ( ) Muscle wasting
( ) ( ) Tic
( ) ( ) Stuttering or stammering or other speech impediment
( ) ( ) Sickle Cell Anemia or trait
( ) ( ) Cooley's Anemia or thalassemia
( ) ( ) Other anemia (for exam-

Donor Personal History Form (Cont.)

( ) ( ) Club foot (talipes equi-
   novarus)
( ) ( ) Cleft lip and/or palate
( ) ( ) Dwarfism
( ) ( ) Arthritis
( ) ( ) Abnormalities of bone
   growth and develop-
   ment (Specify)
( ) ( ) Other chronic skeletal
   system disease
( ) ( ) Muscular dystrophy
   (Specify type)

( ) ( ) ple, pernicious, spher-
   ocytosis, etc.)
( ) ( ) Other hemoglobinopathy
( ) ( ) Hemophilia
( ) ( ) Lupus (Systemic Lupus
   Erythematosis)
( ) ( ) Cystic Fibrosis
( ) ( ) Gaucher's disease or
   other lipid storage dis-
   ease
( ) ( ) PKU (phenylkatonuria)

Have you *ever* had any of the following:

Yes No
( ) ( ) Alcaptonuria
( ) ( ) Any other inherited met-
   abolic disorder
   (Specify)
( ) ( ) Marfan's syndrome
( ) ( ) Ehlers-Danlos syndrome
( ) ( ) Neurofibromatosis
( ) ( ) Any coffee-colored spots
   of skin about the size
   of a nickel or lumps
   under the skin. If so,
   how many?
( ) ( ) Chromosomal transloca-
   tion
( ) ( ) Other chromosomal ab-
   normality
( ) ( ) Brain defect or damage
( ) ( ) Homosexual tendency
( ) ( ) Exposure to mutagenic
   agents (for example
( ) ( ) radiation,
( ) ( ) chemotherapy,
( ) ( ) other
( ) ( ) Leukemia

Yes No
( ) ( ) Congenital malformation
   of gastrointestinal
   tract
( ) ( ) Chronic malabsorption
   syndrome
( ) ( ) Ulcerative colitis
( ) ( ) Crohn's disease (regional
   enteritis)
( ) ( ) Porphyria
( ) ( ) Amyioidosis
( ) ( ) Wilson's disease
( ) ( ) Migraine headaches
( ) ( ) Other severe or disabling
   headaches
( ) ( ) Learning disability
( ) ( ) Retinoblastoma
( ) ( ) Dupuytren's Contracture
( ) ( ) Ankylosing spondylitis
( ) ( ) Depression
( ) ( ) Nervous breakdown or
   extreme nervousness
( ) ( ) Spells of unprovoked
   anxiety
( ) ( ) Hysteria

Donor Personal History Form (Cont.)

( ) ( ) Lymphoma
( ) ( ) Other cancer
( ) ( ) Congenital heart disease
     or defect
( ) ( ) Atherosclerosis
( ) ( ) Blood lipid abnormality
     (cholesterol, triglycer-
     ide, etc.)
( ) ( ) Insulin-dependent
     diabetes
( ) ( ) Insulin-nondependent
     diabetes
( ) ( ) Progressive kidney dis-
     ease
( ) ( ) Polycystic kidneys
( ) ( ) Born with solitary kidney
( ) ( ) Gout, kidney stones, or
     hyperuricemia
( ) ( ) Pyloric stenosis
( ) ( ) Colon polyps (polyps of
     gastrointestinal tract)

( ) ( ) Inability to function due
     to emotional upset
( ) ( ) Phobias
( ) ( ) Suicidal tendency or
     attempts
( ) ( ) Hot or violent temper
( ) ( ) Hallucinations
( ) ( ) Failing memory
( ) ( ) Great swings of mood
     from extreme euphoria
     to deep depression
( ) ( ) Delusions of greatness or
     omnipotence

2. Give details of any psychosis or other mental disorder you have suffered. Specifically, state if you ever received a diagnosis of Schizophrenia,
Manic-depression, or Chronic recurrent depression_____

Have you ever received any psychiatric treatment for other than
above? ( )Yes ( )No If yes, give details_____

3. Are you at risk for any other physical or psychological condition, or
disease that is thought to "run in your family"? ( )Yes ( )No
If yes, please elaborate_____

Donor's Family History
(Parents, Grandparents, Sibling, or Child)

1. Mark "yes" if *any* one of your relatives has had the following conditions. For every "yes" answer, state which family member was/is affected,

Donor Personal History Form (Cont.)

and the *age of onset*, as well as the exact diagnosis. (Use space at bottom of next page for additional information.)

Yes No

( ) ( ) Hay fever
( ) ( ) Asthma
( ) ( ) Eczema
( ) ( ) Drug allergy (Specify)
( ) ( ) Food allergy (Specify)
( ) ( ) Skin photosensitivity
( ) ( ) Psoriasis
( ) ( ) Birthmark
( ) ( ) Vitiligo (areas of depig-
           mentation)
( ) ( ) Other chronic skin dis-
           ease (Specify)
( ) ( ) Serious dental malocclu-
           sion
( ) ( ) Cataract
( ) ( ) Strabismus
( ) ( ) Glaucoma
( ) ( ) Color blindness
( ) ( ) Night blindness
( ) ( ) Eyesight deficiency not
           correctable with
           glasses
( ) ( ) Blindness (Specify cause
           or diagnosis)
( ) ( ) Deafness or hearing loss
           (Specify cause or diag-
           nosis)
( ) ( ) Congenital hip disloca-
           tion
( ) ( ) Club foot (talipes equi-
           novarus)
( ) ( ) Cleft lip and/or palate
( ) ( ) Arthritis
( ) ( ) Ankylosing spondylitis
( ) ( ) Abnormalities of bone
           growth and develop-
           ment

Yes No

( ) ( ) Seizure disorders
( ) ( ) Multiple sclerosis
( ) ( ) Paralysis of a limb for an
           extended period of
           time
( ) ( ) Familial spastic paralysis
( ) ( ) Ataxia
( ) ( ) Tremor
( ) ( ) Muscle wasting
( ) ( ) Tic (habit spasm)
( ) ( ) Stuttering or other
           speech impediment
( ) ( ) Sickle cell anemia/trait
( ) ( ) Thalassemia
( ) ( ) Other anemia
( ) ( ) Other hemoglobinopathy
( ) ( ) Hemophilia
( ) ( ) Nieman-Pick disease
( ) ( ) Histiocytosis
( ) ( ) Tay-Sachs disease
( ) ( ) Failing memory
( ) ( ) Drinking problem
( ) ( ) Psychiatric treatment
( ) ( ) Hallucinations
( ) ( ) Early senility or diagno-
           sis of Alzheimer's
           disease
( ) ( ) Delusions of grandeur
( ) ( ) Other serious illness
( ) ( ) Lupus (Systemic Lupus
           Erythematosis)
( ) ( ) Cystic Fibrosis
( ) ( ) Gaucher's disease or
           other lipid storage
           disease
( ) ( ) Mucopolysaccharidoses
( ) ( ) PKU (phenylketonuria)

Donor Personal History Form (Cont.)

( ) ( ) Chronic skeletal system disease
( ) ( ) Muscular dystrophy
( ) ( ) Myotonia
( ) ( ) Abnormal postural positions
( ) ( ) Loss of muscle coordination
( ) ( ) Malignant hyperthermia
( ) ( ) Myasthenia gravis
( ) ( ) Retinoblastoma
( ) ( ) Dupuytren's Contracture
( ) ( ) Thyroid disorders
( ) ( ) Huntington's chorea
( ) ( ) Parkinson's disease

( ) ( ) Alcaptonuria
( ) ( ) Homocystinuria
( ) ( ) Any other inherited metabolic disorder
( ) ( ) Marfan's syndrome
( ) ( ) Ehlers-Danlos Syndrome
( ) ( ) Neurofibromatosis
( ) ( ) Anyone have coffee-colored spots of the skin about the size of a nickel; and if so, how many? Or lumps under the skin.

Yes No

( ) ( ) Chromosomal translocation
( ) ( ) Down's syndrome (mongolism)
( ) ( ) Other chromosomal abnormality
( ) ( ) Any form of mental retardation, intellectual dullness
( ) ( ) Brain defect or damage
( ) ( ) Cretinism (Congenital hypothyroidism)
( ) ( ) Turner's syndrome
( ) ( ) Neural tube defects, (spina bifida, meningocele, etc.)
( ) ( ) Klinefelter's syndrome
( ) ( ) Testicular feminization syndrome
( ) ( ) Transvestism
( ) ( ) Sex change operation
( ) ( ) Homosexuality or Lesbianism
( ) ( ) Hydrocephaly

Yes No

( ) ( ) Insulin-dependent diabetes
( ) ( ) Insulin-nondependent diabetes
( ) ( ) Progressive kidney disease
( ) ( ) Polycystic kidneys
( ) ( ) Born with solitary kidney
( ) ( ) Born without either kidney (bilateral renal agenesis)
( ) ( ) Gout, kidney stones, or hyperuricemia
( ) ( ) Pyloric stenosis
( ) ( ) Colon polyps (polyps of gastrointestinal tract)
( ) ( ) Congenital malformation of gastrointestinal tract
( ) ( ) Chronic malabsorption syndrome
( ) ( ) Ulcerative colitis
( ) ( ) Crohn's disease (regional enteritis)

Donor Personal History Form (Cont.)

( ) ( ) Anencephaly
( ) ( ) High levels of exposure
         to mutagenic agents
         (for example
( ) ( ) radiation,
( ) ( ) chemotherapy,
( ) ( ) other
( ) ( ) Breast cancer
( ) ( ) Leukemia
( ) ( ) Lymphoma
( ) ( ) Other cancer
( ) ( ) Congenital heart disease
         or defect
( ) ( ) Cardiovascular disease
( ) ( ) High blood pressure
( ) ( ) Atherosclerosis
( ) ( ) Stroke
( ) ( ) Blood lipid abnormality
         (cholesterol, triglycer-
         ide, etc.)

( ) ( ) Porphyria
( ) ( ) Amyloidosis
( ) ( ) Wilson's disease
( ) ( ) Migraine headaches
( ) ( ) Other severe or disabling
         headaches
( ) ( ) Depression
( ) ( ) "Nervous breakdown"
         or extreme nervous-
         ness
( ) ( ) Hysteria
( ) ( ) Phobias (list them)
( ) ( ) Suicidal tendency or
         attempts (Specify)
( ) ( ) Learning disability
( ) ( ) Lung disorders

_____

_____

_____

_____

2. Have any of your relatives been diagnosed as having any psychosis or other mental disorder? Specifically, has a diagnosis of Schizophrenia, Manic-Depression, or Depression ever been made? ( )Yes ( )No

Relative Affected	Diagnosis	Ever Hospitalized	Chronic Disorder Yes/No	Age of Onset
_____	_____	_____	_____	_____
_____	_____	_____	_____	_____

3. Is there a history of early deaths in your family (for example, heart attack)?
( )Yes ( )No
If yes, give details _____
4. Has any female relative had more than two unexplained miscarriages?
( )Yes ( )No
5. Has any member of your family had one or more children with serious birth defects? ( )Yes ( )No

Donor Personal History Form (Cont.)

Relation to you	Number of Children	Nature of defect(s)
_____	_____	_____

6. Has any member of your family had any children who died in infancy or childhood? ( )Yes ( )No
Who? _____ How many children? _____
Causes of death if known (other than accidental death) _____
Age and health data on all blood relatives. Be specific and as accurate as possible. If you are not sure, put a question mark. Include stillborns and infant deaths.

		If deceased,	
Relation to you	Age if living	Age at death	Cause of death
a. maternal grandmother:			
b. maternal grandfather:			
c. paternal grandmother:			
d. paternal grandfather:			
e. mother			
f. father			
g. brothers			
h. sisters			
i. children			
j. mother's sisters/brothers			
k. father's sisters/brothers			

Donor Health History

Have you ever been found to be a carrier of:

Tay-Sachs disease (if Jewish)	Yes _____	No _____
Sickle cell disease (if black)	Yes _____	No _____
B-Thalassemia	Yes _____	No _____
G6PD Deficiency	Yes _____	No _____

Donor Personal History Form (Cont.)

Specify any occupation-related illness/disability_____

List all drugs, prescription and nonprescription, that you have taken during the past 12 months.

_____

Did you wear contact lenses or glasses before age 45? Yes ___ No ___
If yes, please give present prescription:

Have you ever used any mind altering drugs such as marijuana, LSD, heroin or neuroleptic agents (tranquilizers, valium, thorazine, etc.) or chemotherapeutic agents? If yes, give details.

_____

List any serious trauma to yourself.
   Nature of trauma_____
   Post traumatic disorder: seizures _____ learning disability _____
   memory lapse _____ paralysis _____ other_____
List all medical hospitalizations: List all operations:
   Date   Problem   Date   Operation

_____
_____
_____

Did you have any complications ensuing from the surgery (bleeding, embolism, coma) from the anesthetic?

Within the past 5 years have you had an abnormal electrocardiogram, x-ray, or other diagnostic test?

Been advised to have any diagnostic test, hospitalization or surgery which was not completed?

Have you ever had military service deferment, rejection or discharge because of a physical or mental condition?

CHILDHOOD DISEASES   Yes No
HAVE YOU EVER HAD: ( ) ( ) Fungus
Yes No   ( ) ( ) Skin Tumors
( ) ( ) Chicken Pox   ( ) ( ) Moles (Nevi)
( ) ( ) Chorea (St. Vitus Dance) ( ) ( ) Pilonidal Cyst—Spine

Donor Personal History Form (Cont.)

( ) ( ) Diphtheria
( ) ( ) Measles - Regular
( ) ( ) Measles - German
       (Rubella)
( ) ( ) Mumps
( ) ( ) Whooping Cough
( ) ( ) Poliomyelitis (Polio)
( ) ( ) Rheumatic Fever
( ) ( ) Scarlet Fever
( ) ( ) Streptococcal Infection
       (Strep)

HAVE YOU EVER HAD ANY OF
THE FOLLOWING DISEASES
OR DISORDERS:

Yes No

( ) ( ) Amebic Dysentery
( ) ( ) Bronchiectasis (Coughing
       & Spitting)
( ) ( ) Bronchitis (chronic or
       acute cough)
( ) ( ) Bursitis
( ) ( ) Cirrhosis of Liver
( ) ( ) Colitis (kind)
( ) ( ) Diverticulosis or
       Diverticulitis
( ) ( ) Emphysema
( ) ( ) Goitre
( ) ( ) Hepatitis
( ) ( ) Hypoglycemia (low bl.
       sugar)
( ) ( ) Ileitis (Regional)
( ) ( ) Malaria
( ) ( ) Nephritis
( ) ( ) Pancreatitis
( ) ( ) Pleurisy
( ) ( ) Pneumonia
( ) ( ) Pneumothorax
( ) ( ) Polyp
( ) ( ) Rheumatism

( ) ( ) Dizziness (Vertigo)
( ) ( ) Frequent Fainting
( ) ( ) Head Injury
( ) ( ) Guillian-Barre
( ) ( ) Convulsions
( ) ( ) Stroke
( ) ( ) Meningitis
( ) ( ) Encephalitis
( ) ( ) Detached Retina
( ) ( ) Double vision
( ) ( ) Optic Neuritis
( ) ( ) Wear Hearing Aid
( ) ( ) Mastoid Infection
( ) ( ) Polyps of Nose
( ) ( ) Sinus Infection
( ) ( ) Persistent Hoarseness
( ) ( ) Are Your Teeth Good

HAVE YOU EVER HAD:

Yes No

( ) ( ) Underactive Thyroid
( ) ( ) Overactive Thyroid
( ) ( ) Infection of Thyroid
( ) ( ) Tumor of Thyroid
( ) ( ) Shortness of Breath
( ) ( ) Coughing Up Blood
( ) ( ) Embolism of Lungs
( ) ( ) Abscess in Lungs
( ) ( ) Collapsed Lung
( ) ( ) Tumor in Lungs
( ) ( ) High Blood Pressure
( ) ( ) Low Blood Pressure
( ) ( ) Heart Murmur (Leaking
       Valve)
( ) ( ) Chest Pain
( ) ( ) Angina Pectoris
( ) ( ) Heart Failure
( ) ( ) Swelling of Ankles
( ) ( ) Coronary Disease
( ) ( ) Heart Attack

Donor Personal History Form (Cont.)

( ) ( ) Rheumatic Heart Disease
( ) ( ) Tuberculosis
( ) ( ) Tumors
( ) ( ) Typhoid—Paratyphoid
( ) ( ) Ulcers (Stomach or Duodenal)
( ) ( ) Uremia
( ) ( ) Venereal diseases (Syphilis, Gonorrhea, herpes, Chlymedia)
( ) ( ) Chronic Infectious Disease

( ) ( ) Enlarged Heart
( ) ( ) Hiatus Hernia
( ) ( ) Inability to Swallow

Yes No
( ) ( ) Loss of Weight (unexplained)
( ) ( ) Bleeding of Stomach
( ) ( ) Perforation of Stomach
( ) ( ) Gastritis
( ) ( ) Gallstones
( ) ( ) Surgical Removal of Gallbladder
( ) ( ) Jaundice
( ) ( ) Abscess of Liver
( ) ( ) Enlarged Liver
( ) ( ) Neuritis
( ) ( ) Sciatica
( ) ( ) A Disc Problem
( ) ( ) Varicose Veins
( ) ( ) Spinal Curvature
( ) ( ) Back Trouble
( ) ( ) Deformities
( ) ( ) Amputation
( ) ( ) Paralysis
( ) ( ) Fractures
( ) ( ) Phlebitis
( ) ( ) Bones that Break Easily
( ) ( ) Bone or Muscle Tumor
( ) ( ) Bleeding or Clotting Problem

Yes No
( ) ( ) Appendectomy
( ) ( ) Obstruction (kink) of Intestines
( ) ( ) Intestinal Parasites
( ) ( ) Hernia (rupture)
( ) ( ) Hemorrhoids (piles)
( ) ( ) Bleeding from Rectum
( ) ( ) Fistula in Ano
( ) ( ) Infection of Kidneys
( ) ( ) Horseshoe Kidney
( ) ( ) Removal of Kidney
( ) ( ) Bleeding of Kidney
( ) ( ) Tumor of Kidney
( ) ( ) Infection of Bladder
( ) ( ) Stones in Bladder
( ) ( ) Bleeding of Bladder
( ) ( ) Tumor of Bladder
( ) ( ) Sugar in Urine
( ) ( ) Infection of Prostate
( ) ( ) Enlargement of Prostate
( ) ( ) Tumor of Prostate
( ) ( ) Prostate Removed Surgically
( ) ( ) Urethral Stricture
( ) ( ) Testicle Disease or Lumps

Donor Personal History Form (Cont.)

( ) ( ) Infection of Lymph   ( ) ( ) Undescended Testicle
            Glands   ( ) ( ) Discharge from Penis
( ) ( ) Hodgkin's Disease   ( ) ( ) Sore on Penis
( ) ( ) Appendicitis

To what extent have you consumed alcohol in the past?_____
At the present time?_____
Is there any history of alcoholism in your family?_____
Have you ever sought help for an alcoholic problem?_____
Have you had a recent blood test? _____ Date: _____
Chest x-ray?_____ Date:_____
E.K.G.?_____ Date:_____

Do you have any health problems not covered in the previous questions?
Yes _____ No _____
If yes, please explain:
_____
_____
_____
_____

The undersigned states that to the best of his knowledge the information given on these forms is correct. He is aware that the Repository for Germinal Choice does not assume responsibility for the accuracy of the answers provided by him.
Signed _____ Date: _____

Appendix 4

Sample Sperm Bank Contract and Catalog

The following information was supplied by the Southern California Cryobank, Inc., in Los Angeles. Here are copies of their release form, contract, brochure, donor catalog. The protocol is very similar at other sperm banks. Generally, sperm banks do not market directly to consumers but will help clients to find a physician who does DI, or some sperm banks may have their own clinic, such as Idant laboratories in New York. While sperm banks usually keep their own records, they are not yet required by law to do so. The semen, of course, is anonymous and donor tracing would only occur on physician advice after, say, a child was born with a genetic problem. Consumer pressure requesting donors who would adhere to the Bill of Rights and Responsibilities may help to raise consciousness about the rights of the child to know her paternal heritage.

Release Form
Authorization for Release of Semen

I AM REFERRING _____ (name of patient) TO THE CRYOBANK TO OBTAIN SEMEN FOR ARTIFICIAL INSEMINATION. I HAVE INFORMED HER ON THE RISKS AND LIMITATIONS INVOLVED IN ARTIFICIAL INSEMINATION. I AUTHORIZE HER TO PICK UP THE SEMEN DIRECTLY FROM THE CRYOBANK OR TO PHONE ORDER DELIVERIES TO MY OFFICE AS NEEDED FOR INSEMINATION. SHE HAS AGREED THAT ALL SEMEN OBTAINED FROM THE CRYOBANK IS FOR HER PERSONAL USE ONLY. OUR CENTER WILL BE PERFORMING THE INSEMINATION PROCEDURE OR WILL INSTRUCT HER ON HOME INSEMINATION.

DR: _____

DATE: _____

PHONE: _____

Contract

We hereby request and authorize the Southern California Cryobank to select a donor, who in his sole discretion and judgment will meet the qualifications as requested.

We understand that said Southern California Cryobank does not warrant or guarantee the qualifications of said donor, and that in determining whether the said donor meets the aforesaid qualifications the said Southern California Cryobank shall be required to make only such investigations of and concerning such donor as shall in the sole discretion of said Southern California Cryobank seem reasonably necessary.

We further agree that we shall not now, nor at any time, require nor expect the Southern California Cryobank to obtain or divulge to us the name of said donor, nor any other information concerning characteristics, qualities, or any other information whatsoever concerning said donor.

We further agree that following the said insemination the said Southern California Cryobank shall destroy all information and records which they may have as to identity of said donor, it being the intention of all parties that the identity of said donor shall be and forever remain anonymous.

We further covenant and agree to forever refrain from instituting, pressing or in any way aiding any claim, demand, action or cause of action for damages, costs, loss of service expense of compensation for or on account of or hereafter arising out of the premises hereinabove set forth.

We further promise and agree to indemnify and save harmless to said Southern California Cryobank from any loss and/or expenses incurred by them in connection with the defense or payment of any claim or action arising out of the aforesaid premises or agreements herein contained.

We fully understand that such artificial insemination may not be successful.

Compensation for the services of the Southern California Cryobank shall be such as shall be determined by the Southern California Cryobank. These fees shall reflect charges being made by other similar institutions.

This agreement shall be binding upon ourselves, and each of us, our assigns, heirs, executors and administrator.

Dated this _____ day of _____, 19____
Signed _____
_____

NAME: Husband _____Wife _____
HUSBAND'S DESCRIPTION:
  Height _____

Weight _____

Eye Color _____

Hair Color _____

Bone Structure _____

Complexion Type _____   Coloring _____
                       Ruddy, Smooth, etc.   Olive, Fair, etc.

Ethnic Background _____

Religious Preference _____

Other Characteristics Desired _____

_____

Blood Type and RH

Husband's _____   Wife's _____

SIGNED: _____

_____

_____
                                    Witness

Date _____

THE CALIFORNIA CRYOBANK

was founded in 1977 by two physicians, Cappy M. Rothman and Charles A. Sims. Their goal was to provide physicians and their patients a sperm bank and reproductive laboratory that is comprehensive, socially and ethically responsible and committed to the highest standards of care and excellence.

The California Cryobank is now one of the nations largest sperm banks and its services are used by physicians throughout the United States.

A.I.D. DONOR SELECTION AND SCREENING

We adhere to donor screening standards established by the American Association of Tissue Banks which includes independent screening by two physicians for fertility, health, intelligence, and the absence of infectious disease (including AIDS Screening). Each donor is required to have a complete physical examination, medical history and a three generation genetic and family history. Donors are screened for Tay Sachs, sickle cell trait, etc., as is appropriate for the ethnic group of the donor. Chromosome analysis is available on request.

A.I.D. FROZEN SEMEN SPECIMENS

Our frozen semen is packaged in 0.5 ml. vials which contain a minimum of 20 million motile cells when thawed according to instructions. Ordinarily, vials are packed and shipped in sufficient dry ice to keep them frozen for at least 3 days.

There is no container to return. By making special arrangements, the specimens can be shipped in liquid nitrogen. Thawing instructions and an inseminator is included with each vial.

ORDERING A.I.D. SPECIMENS

Select a donor from the catalog which best fits the physical characteristics desired. A 2nd and 3rd choice is advisable. If you cannot find a appropriate match from the catalog please contact us for additional donor information.

Call us at least 48 hours in advance of when you desire delivery. Door to door overnight delivery service is used outside the Los Angeles area. Locally, you may pick up the specimen directly or we will have our courier deliver to you. International shipping can be done with special arrangements.

SPECIAL INSTRUCTIONS

Specimens needed for Monday insemination will be shipped out on Saturday which reduces frozen holding time to 2 days after you receive delivery. You may add additional dry ice to extend the holding time upon receiving the shipment. We do not recommend storing frozen semen in dry ice for more than five to six days. DO NOT STORE SPECIMENS IN STANDARD REFRIGERATOR FREEZER! (If desired you may rent a liquid nitrogen tank for a small monthly fee).

COSTS

Refer to our fee schedule for a listing of our services and charges.

FOR INFORMATION ABOUT OUR FEES AND SERVICES WRITE OR CALL:

California Cryobank, Inc.
2080 Century Park East, Suite 308
Los Angeles, California 90097
(213) 553-9828

FEE SCHEDULE

August 1, 1986

DONOR SEMEN	
1-4 specimens:	$68. ea.
5-9 specimens:	$65. ea.
10-19 specimens:	$60. ea.
20 plus specimens:	$55. ea.
OVERNIGHT DELIVERY:	
Weekday:	$55.
Weekend (Pick up or delivery):	$65.
2-way Tank delivery:	$95.
SEMEN ANALYSIS:	$35.
SEMEN FREEZING:	$40.
SEMEN STORAGE:	$95./year
(reduced rate for multi year prepayment)	
2 years:	$180.
3 years:	$250.
4 years:	$330.
5 years:	$400.
ANTI-SPERM ANTIBODY TESTING:	
Kibrick Method	$40.
Membrane Specific (IgG, IgA, IgM)	$75.
SPERM PENETRATION ASSAY:	
(Hamster Zona-Free Ova)	$250.
SPERM WASHING/MOTILITY ENHANCEMENT: $45.	
SPERM SWIM-UP	$75.
CERVICAL MUCUS PENETRATION TEST:	$40.
SEX SELECTION	$150./treatment
INFERTILITY PROFILE:	$90.
semen analysis	
sperm antibody test, (wife's serum)	
cervical mucus penetration test, (husband's semen)	
TESTICULAR FUNCTION:	
FSH	
LH	$118.
TESTOSTERONE	

DONOR CATALOG   OCT. 1986   CALIFORNIA CRYOBANK, INC.
(213) 5539828
(Please select at least three donors from this list)

Donor ID#	Race/Ethnic Origin	Blood Type	Hair	Eyes	Skin
35	CAUC, GERMAN	A+	BLD/STRT	BLUE	FAIR
84	CAUC, ITALIAN	A+	LT BRN/STRT	BROWN	FAIR
92	CAUC, FRENCH/GERMAN	O−	BRN/STRT	HAZEL	FAIR
97	CAUC, NORWEGIAN	AB+	BLD/STRT	BLUE	FAIR
106	CAUC, GERMAN/IRISH	B+	BRN/WAVY	BLUE	FAIR
111	CAUC, FRENCH/ENGLISH	A+	BRN/STRT	BROWN	FAIR
128	CAUC, GERMAN/ENGLISH	A−	RED/STRT	BLUE	FAIR
133	CAUC, GERMAN/ CANADIAN	A+	BLD/STRT	BLUE	FAIR
138	CAUC, ITALIAN/GERMAN	O+	BLD/STRT	BLUE	FAIR
140	CAUC, ENGLISH/DUTCH	B+	BRN/STRT	BLUE	FAIR
142	CAUC, IRISH	B+	BRN/STRT	BROWN	FAIR
143	CAUC, ENGLISH	A+	BLD/WAVY	BLUE	FAIR
150	CAUC, ENGLISH	B+	BLD/STRT	BLUE	FAIR
169	CAUC, NORWEGIAN	A+	BLD/STRT	HAZEL	FAIR
173	CAUC, FRENCH/GERMAN	O+	BLD/STRT	GREEN	FAIR
179	CAUC, ENGLISH	O−	BLD/STRT	GREEN	FAIR
184	CAUC, ASSYRIAN/ PORTUGL	A+	BRN/STRT	BROWN	OLIVE
195	CAUC, POLISH	A−	BLD/CURLY	BLUE	FAIR
201	CAUC, ENGLISH/SCOTCH	A+	BLD/WAVY	BLUE	FAIR
202	CAUC, SCOTTISH/SWISS	O+	BRN/WAVY	GREEN	FAIR
204	CAUC, IRISH/ENGLISH	O+	BRN/STRT	BROWN	FAIR
205	CAUC, GERM/ENGL/IRISH	A+	BRN/WAVY	BROWN	FAIR
208	CAUC, IRISH	O+	BRN/CURLY	BROWN	FAIR
211	CAUC, GERMAN/POLISH	A+	BRN/WAVY	BROWN	FAIR
223	CAUC, IRISH/WELSH	O+	BRN/WAVY	BLUE	FAIR
227	CAUC, DANISH/ GERM/ENGL	O+	BRN/STRT	BROWN	FAIR
228	CAUC, AUSTRIAN	A+	LT BRN/STRT	BLUE	FAIR
110	CAUC, TURKISH	O+	BLK/STRT	HAZEL	OLIVE
68	CAUC, JEWISH/RUSSIAN	AB+	BRN/STRT	HAZEL	FAIR
82	CAUC, JEWISH/RUSSIAN	A+	BLK/WAVY	GREEN	FAIR
118	CAUC, JEWISH/ENGL/ GERM	A+	BRN/WAVY	BROWN	FAIR
137	CAUC, JEWISH/BELGIAN	A+	BRN/STRT	GREEN	FAIR
148	CAUC, JEWISH/RUSSIAN	A+	BRN/WAVY	BROWN	FAIR
167	CAUC, JEWISH/GERM/ HUNG	O+	BLD/STRT	BLUE	FAIR
193	CAUC, JEWISH/RUSS,CZEC	O+	BLD/STRT	GREEN	FAIR
199	CAUC, JEWISH/AUSTRIA	O−	BRN/WAVY	BROWN	FAIR
203	CAUC, JEWISH	O+	BRN/CURLY	BROWN	FAIR
210	CAUC, JEWISH/ENGLISH	A+	BRN/WAVY	BROWN	OLIVE
53	BLACK, AFRICAN	O+	BLK/WAVY	BROWN	DARK
60	MEXICAN	A+	BRN/WAVY	BROWN	OLIVE
81	MEXICAN	A+	BRN/WAVY	BROWN	OLIVE
163	MEXICAN	O+	BLK/STRT	BROWN	OLIVE
54	JAPANESE	O+	BRN/STRT	BROWN	OLIVE
102	JAPANESE	A+	BRN/STRT	BLACK	OLIVE

DONOR CATALOG   OCT. 1986   CALIFORNIA CRYOBANK, INC.
(213) 5539828

Ht.	Wt.	Yrs. College	Occupation	Special Skills/Interests
5-9	150	5	ACTOR	DANCING, PIANO
5-9	150	6	SOCIAL WORKER/M.A.	SWIMMING, TRACK
5-11	160	4	STUDENT/POL. SCIENCE	WEIGHTS/SOFTBALL/POLITICS
6-0	160	4	STUDENT/FILM & T.V.	WRITING
5-9	160	6	EDITOR	POLITICS, FILM
5-11	175	7	LAW STUDENT	POLITICS/TENNIS
6-0	180	9	PhD. BIOCHEMISTRY	ATHLETICS
6-0	170	6	M.S. CHEM. ENGINEERING	SKIING/SAILING
5-10	155	3	STUDENT/THEATER	SPORTS/ACTING
6-1	185	3	ACTOR	PIANO/COINS
5-11	160	2	STUDENT/MUSIC	PIANO/ASTRONOMY
5-11	160	4	GRAD. STUDENT/ THEATER	ART DESIGN
6-0	171	3	STUDENT/MUSIC & DANCE	MT. CLIMBING, PHILOSOPHY
6-2	165	4	STUDENT/BUSINESS	SKIING, MUSIC, WEIGHT-LIFTING
6-2	155	3	STUDENT/FINANCE	TRAVEL & ART
5-11	150	5	STUDENT/ENGLISH	PHOTOGRAPHY, ART, WRITING
5-10	155	1	STUDENT/PRE-MEDICINE	SWIMMING/SKIING
6-0	165	4	STUDENT/LAW	POLITICS, SPORTS
6-4	180	4	STUDENT/MUSIC	SPORTS, MUSICAL
6-1	165	6	STUDENT/MUSIC	ATHLETIC, WRITING
6-2	205	3	STUDENT/ARCHITECTURE	GUITAR, SWIMMING
6-2	176	1	STUDENT/BUSINESS	SWIMMING, WT. LIFTING
5-10	150	5	GRAD STUDENT/BIOLOGY	RUNNING/BASKETBALL
6-1	175	1	ACTOR	SPORTS/ARTS
6-0	175	3	STUDENT/HISTORY	SWIMMING/WT. LIFTING/ PIANO
6-0	195	6	STUDENT/BUSINESS	SWIMMING, BICYCLING
6-0	170	4	STUDENT/MUSIC	MUSICAL, CAR RACING
5-8	160	9	PhD. ELECTRICAL ENG.	PHOTOGRAPHY, SAILING
5-6	130	5	STUDENT/PSYCHOLOGY	SKIING, SAILING
6-0	185	5	MANAGEMENT	PAINTING, PHOTOGRAPHY
5-9	155	3	STUDENT/LITERATURE	ACTING, ATHLETICS
5-7	130	1	STUDENT/ENGLISH	MUSIC
5-7	140	5	GRAD STUDENT/CHEM.	SPORTS, READING
6-0	175	3	STUDENT/ECON.	TENNIS, SKIING, SAILING
5-11	180	5	ACTOR	ART/FILM/ATHLETIC
5-9	145	7	STUDENT (MFA) CINEMA	WRITER/SCULPTOR
6-1	135	2	STUDENT/ACCOUNTING	WRITER/POETRY/TENNIS
5-10	165	3	MUSICIAN	MUSICAL/SWIMMING
5-9	150	3	STUDENT/BIOLOGY	BASKETBALL, JOGGING
5-8	145	4	WRITER	SPORTS/ACTING
5-9	185	4	STUDENT/PSYCH.	WRITING, SWIMMING
5-6	135	2	STUDENT/BUSINESS	SURFING, JOGGING, BICYCLE
5-8	155	4	STUDENT/ECONOMICS	SKIING/SPORTS
5-8	150	6	STUDENT/LAW	SKIING/THEATER

Resources

Adoptees' Liberty Movement Association (ALMA), P.O. Box 627M, Morristown, NJ 07960.

Adoptees' Rights, P.O. Box 3026, Cleveland, OH 44130.

Adoption Connection, Inc. 11 Peabody Square #6, Peabody, MA 01960.

Adoption Information Exchange, P.O. Box 4153, Chapel Hill, NC 27514.

Adoption Triangle Ministry, P.O. Box 1860, Cape Coral, FL 33912.

Adoptive Parents for Open Records, 9 Marjorie Drive, Hackettstown, NJ 07840.

Alan Guttmacher Institute, 111 Fifth Avenue, New York, NY.

American Adoption Congress, P.O. Box 44040, L'Enfant Plaza Station, Washington, D.C. 20026-0040.

American Association of Tissue Banks, 12,111 Parklawn Drive, Rockland, MD 20852. Phone: (301)738-0600. (Standards for sperm banks)

American College of Obstetricians and Gynecologists, 600 Maryland Avenue, S.E., Suite 300, Washington, DC 20024. (Referrals to infertility specialists)

American Fertility Society, 1608 Thirteenth Avenue South, Suite 101, Birmingham, AL 35205. (Physician referrals, literature, and the journal *Fertility Sterility*)

American Society of Law and Medicine, 765 Commonwealth Ave., Boston, MA 02215.

Association for Voluntary Surgical Contraception, 122 E. 42d Street, New York, NY 10168.

Barren Foundation, 60 East Monroe Street, Chicago, IL 60603. (Resources for the infertile)

Biogenetics Corporation, 950 Sanford Ave., Irvington, NJ 07111. Phone: (1)(800)942-4646 (Sperm bank, infertility testing.)

Boston Women's Health Book Collective, 47 Nichols Avenue, Watertown, MA 02172.

Cape Association for Truth in Adoption, P.O. Box 606, Woods Hole, MA 02543.

Center for Communications in Infertility, Inc., P.O. Box 516, Yorktown Heights, NY 10598.

Center for Reproductive Alternatives, 3333 Vincent Rd., Suite 222, Pleasant Hill, CA 94523. Phone: (415) 930-6220. (Open donor program)

Child Welfare League of America, 440 First St. NW, Washington D.C. 20001. Phone: (202) 638-2952.

Committee Against Reproductive Hazards of the Coalition for the Medical Rights of Women, 1630-B Haight Street, San Francisco, CA 94117.

Committee for Responsible Genetics, 186A South Street, Boston, MA 02111.

Concerned United Birthparents, CUB Inc. 2000 Walker Street, Des Moines, IA 50317.

Concern for the Infertile and Children, P.O. Box 125, Vermont, Victoria, Australia 3133.

Couple-to-Couple League, P.O. Box 11184, Cincinnati, OH 45211 (Natural family planning)

Donors' Offspring, P.O. Box 33, Sarcoxie, MO 64862. Phone: (417)548-3679. (For all associated with reproductive technology, and especially searching DI offspring)

Elizabeth Blackwell Health Center for Women, 1124 Walnut Street, Philadelphia PA 19107. Phone: (215)923-7577.

Emma Goldman Clinic for Women, 715 N. Dodge, Iowa City, IA 52240. Phone: (319)337-2111.

Everywoman's Clinic, 1936 Linda Drive, Pleasant Hill, CA 94523. Phone: (415)825-7900.

Families Adopting Children Everywhere, FACE, P.O. Box 102, Bel Air, MD, 21014. (Adoptive parents support organization, not an agency)

Family of the Americas Foundation, P.O. Box 219, Mandeville, LA 70488. (Billings ovulation method)

Family Connection, 25 Irwin Avenue, Toronto, Ont. M4Y I24 Phone: (416)923-5946. (Counseling, search assistance, speakers)

Farrant, Graham, M.D. 57 Erin Street, Richmond (Melbourne) VIC 3121 Australia. (Psychiatric expert on cellular consciousness, prenatal memories, alternative reproduction)

Feminist International Network to Resist Reproductive and Genetic Engineering (FINNRAGE), Box 441216, West Somerville, MA 02144.

Feminist Women's Health Center, 6411 Hollywood Boulevard, Los Angeles, CA 90028.

Fenway Community Health Center Insemination Project, 16 Haviland Street, Boston, MA 02115. Phone: (617)267-7573.

Fertility Center of California, 1125 E. 17th Street, #120, Santa Ana, CA 92701. Phone: (714)953-4683. (Insemination for married and single women, support groups)

Fertility Selections, 4639 Main Street, Bridgeport, CT 06606. (Ericsson serum albumin technique to favor conception of a male child; also researching techniques for female conception)

Gametrin Ltd., 475 Gates Road, P.O. Box 1507, Sausalito, CA 94966. Phone: (415)332-3141. (Albumin gradient selection for sperm)

Idant Laboratories, 645 Madison Avenue, New York, NY 10022. Phone: (212)935-1430. (Sperm bank; infertility clinic)

Independent Adoption Center, 3313 Vincent Road, Suite 202, Pleasant Hill, CA 94523. Phone: (415)944-4744.

International Search Consultants, P.O. Box 10857, Costa Mega, CA 92627.

International Soundex Reunion Registry, P.O. Box 2312, Carson City, NV 89701. (For those involved in adoption and DI who are searching for offspring or birthparents)

Jigsaw International, 39 Manifold Road, Blackett, Sydney, Australia. (Adoption search agency)

Kennedy, Joseph, M.D., 9834 Genesee Avenue, Suite 300, La Jolla, CA 92037. (Infertility and DI)

Lambert (Dalston) Ltd., Dalston House, Hastings Street, Luton Lui SBW UK. (Rubber cervical caps)

Lesbian Mother National Defense Fund, P.O. Box 21567, Seattle, WA 98111. (Artificial insemination packet available for three dollars)

Lesbian Rights Project, 1370 Mission Street, San Francisco, CA 94103.

Lesbians Choosing Children Network, 46 Pleasant Street, Cambridge, MA 02139. Phone: (617)354-8807.

Linde, Carey. 208-1650 Duranleau, Granville Island, Vancouver, British Columbia, V6H 3S4. Phone: (604)684-7798. (Lawyer involved in DI reform)

Los Angeles Fertility Institute, Donald H. Adler, M.D., 435 N. Bedford Drive, Beverly Hills, CA 90210.

March of Dimes Birth Defects Foundation, 1275 Mamaroneck Avenue, White Plains, NY 10605. (Information and referrals on genetic counseling)

Maternal and Child Health Center, Elizabeth Noble, director, 2464 Massachusetts Avenue, Cambridge, MA 02140. Phone: (617)864-9343. (DI counseling, educational programs for pregnancy and postpartum)

Midwest Adoption Triad, P.O. Box 37262, Omaha, NB 68137.

Milex, 405 N. Wabash Avenue, Chicago, IL 60618. (Plastic cervical cups; Fertilopaks)

My Family Books, c/o Concerned United Birthparents, Inc., P.O. Box 23641, L'Enfant Plaza Station, Washington, DC 20024. (Personal record books of genealogy)

National Committee for Adoption, Suite 512, 2025 M. Street N.W. Washington, DC, 20036. Phone: (202)463-7359.

National Family Planning and Reproductive Health Association, 122 C Street, NW Suite 300, Washington, DC 20001.

National Genetics Foundation, 555 West 57th Street, New York, NY 10019.

National Institute for Occupational Safety and Health (NIOSHA), 4676 Columbia Parkway, Cincinnati, OH 45226. Phone: (313)684-2427.

(Health hazard evaluation program, testing of sperm samples at workplaces with toxic exposure)

National Research Foundation for Fertility, 53 E. 96th St., New York, NY 10128.

National Women's Health Network, 224 Seventh Street S.E., Washington, DC 20003.

The Natural Women's Calendar, Lemon Tree Publishing, 890 Thompson River Road, Marion, MT 59925. (Fertility awareness)

Oakland Feminist Women's Health Center, 2930 McClure Street, Oakland, CA 94609. Phone: (415)444-5676. (Sperm bank and DI)

Open Adoption Resources, P.O. Box 3681, Eugene, OR 97403. Phone: (503)343-4825.

Open Door Society of Massachusetts, Inc., 25 West Street, Boston, MA 02111. (Support group for adoptive families)

Operation Identity, 13101 Blackstone Road NE Albuquerque, NM 87111. (Adoptees' support)

Organized Adoption Search Information Service (OASIS), P.O. Box 53–0761, Miami Shores, FL 33133.

Origins, P.O. Box 44, East Brunswick, NJ 07755. (Adoption search assistance)

Orphan Voyage. c/o Jean Paton, Cedaredge, CO 81443. (Open adoption)

Ovulation Method Newsletter, Ovulation Method Teachers' Association, P.O. Box 14511, Portland, OR 97214.

OvuSTICK, 2319 Charleston Road, Mountain View, CA 94043. Phone: (1)(800)227-8855. (Urine test for ovulation)

Parenting Resources, 250 El Camino Real, Suite 111, Tustin, CA 92680. (Adoption and DI support)

Parents for Private Adoption, P.O. Box 7, Pawlet, VT 05761. (Networking and support—not an agency)

Perspective Press, 905 West Wildwood Avenue, Fort Wayne, IN 46807. (Publisher and distributor of materials related to infertility and adoption)

Planned Parenthood Federation of America, 810 Seventh Ave, New York, NY 10019.

Pratten, Alan and Shirley, 2621 Rosstown Road, Nanaimo, B.C. V9T
3S4, Canada. Phone: (604) 785-0075. (DI support group)

Pre-and Perinatal Psychology Association of North America, 36 Madison
Avenue, Toronto, ONT MSR2S4. (Journal and conferences on pre- and
perinatal psychology including alternative reproduction, cellular consciousness, birth and other preverbal memories)

Repository for Germinal Choice, 450 S. Escondido Boulevard, Escondido,
CA 92025. Phone: (619)743-0772. (Sperm bank)

Reproductive Rights National Network, 17 Murray Street, 5th Floor,
New York, NY 10007.

Resolve, Inc., 5 Water Street, Arlington, MA 02174. Phone: (617)643-
2424. (National self-help group for the infertile)

Reunite, Inc. P.O. Box 694, Reynoldsburgh, OH 43068. (Adoption)

Rights of Adoptees' Parents, Inc. (ROAP), P.O. Box 30326, Cleveland,
OH 44130. Phone: (216)572-1599.

Right to Know, P.O. Box 1409, Grand Prairie, TX 75050. (Adoption)

Royal College of Obstetricians and Gynaecologists, 27 Sussex Place, Regent's Park, London NW1 4RG. Phone: 01-262 5425. (Referrals to infertility specialists)

Search, P.O. Box 1432, Litchfield, AZ 85340. (Adoptee support)

Single Mothers by Choice, Box 7788, FDR Station, New York, NY
10150. (Support group)

Sorger, Leo, M.D., 314 Clifton Street, Malden, MA 02148. Phone:
(617)321-3767. (Infertility, DI)

Southern California CryoBank, Inc. 2080 Century Park East, Suite 308,
Los Angeles, CA 90067. Phone: (213)553-9828. (Sperm bank)

Triadoption Library, P.O. Box 638, Westminster, CA 92683. (Adoption
support)

Tyler Medical Clinic, 921 Westwood Boulevard, West Los Angeles, CA
90024. Phone: (213)272-1905.

Urban Woman and Child Health, 545A Centre Street, Jamaica Plain, MA
02130. Phone: (617)522-2300.

Vercollone, Carol Frost, 257 Ferry St., Malden, MA 02148. Phone:
(617)321-0702. (Social worker and DI counselor)

Vermont Women's Health Center, 336 N Avenue, Burlington, VT 05401.

Vista Del Mar Child Care Service, 3200 Motor Avenue, Los Angeles, CA 90034. Phone: (213)836-1223. (Adoption, counseling, referrals for infertility, DI)

Washington Adoptees Rights Movement (WARM), 305 S. 43rd Street, Renton, WA 98055.

Women's Choice Clinic, 1200 Sonoma Avenue, Santa Rosa, CA 95405.

Xytex Corporation, 1519-A Laney-Walker Boulevard, Augusta, GA 30904. Phone: (1)(800)241-9722. (Sperm bank)

Yesterday's Children, P.O. Box 1554, Evanston, IL 60204. (Open adoption)

Zetek, Inc., 794 Ventura Street, Aurora, CA 80011. Phone: (303)343-2122. (CUE fertility monitor)

Films

Alternative Conceptions by Women Make Movies, 225 Lafayette Street, Suite 212, New York, NY 10012. Phone: (212)925-0606. (Lesbians and donor insemination)

Choosing Children: A Film About Lesbians Becoming Parents. Cambridge Documentary Films, P.O. Box 385, Cambridge, MA 02139. 1985.

Trying Times: Crisis in Fertility. Fanlight Productions, 47 Halifax Street, Boston, MA 02130. 1980.

Videos available from Donors' Offspring (see above).

Bibliography

Books

Achilles, Rona. "The Social Meaning of Biological Ties: A Study of Participants in Artificial Insemination by Donor" (Ph.D. thesis, in process of publication, Department of Education, University of Toronto, 1986).

Airola, Paavo. *Sex and Nutrition*. New York: Award Books, 1975.

Amelar, R. D., et al. *Male Infertility*. Philadelphia: W. B. Saunders, 1977.

Andrews, Lori B. *New Conceptions: A Consumer's Guide to the Newest Infertility Treatments*. New York: St. Martin's Press, 1984.

Annas, George. *The Rights of Hospital Patients*. New York: Avon, 1975.

Anonymous, Mary, and Sarah: Union WAGE members. *Women Controlled Conception*. San Francisco: Womanshore books, 1979.

Ansfield, Joseph G. *Adopted Child*. Springfield, Ill.: Thomas, 1971.

Arditti, Rita, R. D. Klein, and S. Minden. *Test-Tube Women: What Future for Motherhood?* Boston: Routledge and Kegan Paul, 1984.

Arms, Suzanne. *To Love and Let Go*. New York: Knopf, 1984.

Artificial Insemination: An Alternative Conception for the Lesbian and Gay Community. 1979 Lesbian Health Information Project, c/o San Francisco Women's Center, 3543 18th Street, San Francisco, CA 94110.

Ashford, J. I., ed. *The Whole Birth Catalog: A Sourcebook for Choices in Childbirth*. Trumansburg, N.Y.: Crossing Press, 1983.

Baker, Frederick H. and Jeannine P. *Conscious Conception*. Freestone Publishing Co., Monroe, Utah 1986.

Baker, Lynn S. *The Fertility Fallacy*. Philadelphia: W. B. Saunders, 1981.

Banks, Velma. *Adoption: A Self-Discovery Journey*. Irvington, 1986.

Bayles, M. D. *Reproductive Ethics*. Englewood Cliffs, N.J.: Prentice-Hall, 1976.

Becker, H. *Outsiders*. New York: Free Press, 1963.

Behrman, S. J., and R. W. Kister. *Progress in Infertility.* 2d ed. Boston: Little, Brown, 1975.

Benet, Mary. *The Politics of Adoption.* New York: Free Press, 1976.

Berezin, Nancy. *After a Loss in Pregnancy.* New York: Simon and Schuster, 1982.

Billings, Evelyn, and Ann Westmore. *The Billings Method.* New York: Random House, 1980.

Billings, John. *Natural Family Planning: The Ovulation Method.* 3d ed. Collegeville, MN: Liturgical Press, 1975.

Birke, Lynda. *Women, Feminism and Biology: The Feminist Challenge.* Sussex, UK: Harvester Press, 1986.

Biskind, S. *Emergent Concepts in Law and Society.* Philadelphia: Temple University Press, 1973.

Bleier, Ruth. *Science and Gender.* New York: Pergamon, 1984.

Blizzard, J. *Blizzard and the Holy Ghost: Artificial Insemination—A Personal Account.* London: Peter Owen, Ltd., 1977.

Bok, Sissela. *Lying: Moral Choice in Public and Private Life.* New York: Pantheon, 1978.

———. *Secrets: On the Ethics of Concealment and Revelation.* New York: Random House, 1983.

Boston Women's Health Book Collective. *The New Our Bodies Ourselves.* New York: Simon and Schuster, 1985.

Bourne, R. B., et al. *Artificial Insemination.* New York: Irvington, 1972.

Brudenell, M., A. McLaren, R. Short, and M. Symonds. *Artificial Insemination: Proceedings of the Fourth Study Group of the Royal College of Obstetricians and Gynaecologists.* London, 1976.

Campbell, Lee, ed., *Understanding the Birthparent.* Dover, NH: Concerned United Birthparents (CUB), 1975.

Chance, N. A. *The Eskimo of North Alaska.* New York: Holt Rinehart and Winston, 1966.

Cherfas, Jeremy, and John Gribbin. *The Redundant Male.* London: Paladin, 1985.

Church Information Office (CIO). *Artificial Insemination by Donor: Two Contributors to a Christian Judgment.* London, 1960.

———. *Fatherless by Law?* Appendix I. London, 1966.

CIBA Foundation Symposium. *The Family and Its Future #93.* Amsterdam: Elsevier, 1970.

Corea, Gena. *The Mother Machine.* New York: Harper and Row, 1985.

Cox, R., and J. Peel, eds. *Population and Pollution.* London: Academic Press, 1972.

Cushan, A. M., ed. *Proceedings of the Conference Adoption and AID: Access to Information?* Clayton, Victoria, Australia: Monash University Centre for Human Bioethics, 1984.

David, Georges, and Wendel S. Price, eds. *Human Artificial Insemination and Semen Preservation*. New York: Plenum, 1980.

Davitz, L. L. *Baby Hunger: Every Woman's Longing for a Baby*. New York: Harper and Row, 1984.

Dawkins, Richard. *The Selfish Gene*. Oxford: Oxford University Press, 1976.

Dick-Read, Grantly. *Childbirth Without Fear*, rev. ed. New York: Harper and Row, 1979.

Dowrick, Stephanie, and Sibyl Grundberg, eds. *Why Children?* New York: Harcourt Brace Jovanovich, 1981.

Duprau, Jeanne. *Adoption: The Facts, Feelings and Issues of a Double Heritage*. New York: Messner, 1981.

Dusky, Lorraine. *Birthmark*. New York: M. Evans, 1979.

Earnshaw, Averil. *Family Time*. Sydney, Australia: A & K Enterprises, 1983. Cawarrah Rd., Middle Cove, Sydney, N.S.W. 2065, Australia, 1983.

Eichenbaum, L., and S. Orbach. *What Do Women Want? Exploring the Myth of Dependency*. New York: Berkley, 1984.

Elan, D. *Building Better Babies: Preconception Planning for Healthier Children*. Millbrae, CA: Celestial Arts, 1980.

Erichsen, Jean, and E. Heine. *Adoption Kit: U.S. Adoptions*. Los Ninos, 1982.

Erikson, Erik. *Childhood and Society*. New York: Norton, 1964.

―――. *Identity and the Life Cycle. Selected Papers*. New York: International Universities Press, 1959.

Farson, R. *Birthrights*. New York: Macmillan, 1974.

Feminist Self-Insemination Group. *Self Insemination*. London: Feminist Self-Insemination Group, 1979.

Finegold, W. J. *Artificial Insemination*. 2d ed. Springfield, IL: Thomas, 1975.

Fisher, Florence. *The Search for Anna Fisher*. New York: Fawcett, 1983.

Fletcher, John C. *Coping with Genetic Disorders*. New York: Harper and Row, 1984.

Francoer, R. J. *Utopian Motherhood: New Trends in Human Reproduction*. New York: Doubleday, 1973.

Frees, Nita J. *We Have Two Mommies*. 1223 Tico Road, Ojai, CA 93023.

Friedman, Daniel. *Human Sociobiology*. New York: Free Press, 1979.

Fromer, M. J. *Ethic Issues in Sexuality and Reproduction*. St. Louis: C. V. Mosby, 1983.

Gatto, Briseis. *Are You My Father?* (privately published) 1987; *An Underground History of Adoption* (privately published) 1987; *Lost Children* (privately published) 1987. 235 W. Seventy-sixth Street, New York, NY 10023.

Georges, D., and W. S. Price. *Human Artificial Insemination and Semen Preservation.* New York: Plenum, 1980.

Gill, D. *Illegitimacy, Sexuality and the Status of Women.* Oxford: Blackwell, 1977.

Gilligan, C. *In a Different Voice.* Cambridge, Mass.: Harvard University Press, 1982.

Gillette, Nealy, and Guren, D. *The Ovulation Method: Cycles of Fertility.* 4760 Aldrich Road, Bellingham, WA 98225, 1982. (Privately published)

Gilman, Lois. *Adoption Resource Book.* New York: Harper and Row, 1984.

Glass, R. H., and R. J. Ericsson. *Getting Pregnant in the 1980s.* Berkeley: University of California Press, 1982.

Glover, William K. *Artificial Insemination Among Human Beings: Medical, Legal, and Moral Aspects.* Washington, D.C.: Catholic University of America Press, 1948.

Goffman, Irving. *Stigma.* New York: Prentice-Hall, 1963.

Goldstein, J., A. Freud, and A. J. Solnit. *Beyond the Best Interests of the Child.* New York: Free Press, 1973.

Greer, Germaine. *Sex and Destiny: The Politics of Human Fertility.* New York: Harper and Row, 1984.

Guay, Terry. *The Personal Fertility Guide: How to Avoid or Achieve Pregnancy Naturally.* New York: Beaufort Books, 1985.

Haimes, Erica, and Noel Timms. *Adoption, Identity and Social Policy: The Search for Distant Relatives.* New York: Gower, 1985.

Hallenbeck, Carol. *Our Child.* Wayne, PA: Our Child Press, 1984.

Hampshire, Susan. *The Maternal Instinct.* London: Sphere, 1984.

Hanscombe, Gillian E., and Jackie Forster. *Rocking the Cradle: Lesbian Mothers—A Challenge in Family Living.* Boston: Alyson Publications, 1982.

Harper, Patricia, and Jan Aitken, eds. *A Child Is Not the Cure for Infertility.* National workshop on Infertility, September 1981: Report of Proceedings, Institute of Family Studies and Citizen's Welfare Service of Victoria, Australia. 766 Elizabeth Street, Melbourne, 3000, February 1982.

Harrison, John. *Love Your Disease—It's Keeping You Healthy.* Sydney: Angus and Robertson, 1984.

Harrison, Mary. *Infertility.* Boston: Houghton Mifflin Company, 1977.

Hasegawa, T., et al. *Fertility Sterility: Proceedings of the VII World Congress,* Kyoto Japan, October 1973. New York: Elsevier, 1973.

Hitchens, Donna. *Lesbians Choosing Motherhood: Legal Issues in Donor Insemination,* 1984. (Available from Lesbian Rights Project, 1370 Mission Street, 4th fl., San Francisco, CA 94103.

———. *Lesbian Mothers' Litigation Manual,* 1984. (Available from Lesbian Rights Project, 1370 Mission Street, 4th fl., San Francisco, CA 94103.

———. *Lesbian Mothers and Their Children: An Annotated Bibliography of Legal and Psychological Materials.* 2d ed. 1983. (Available from Lesbian Rights Project, 1370 Mission Street, 4th fl., San Francisco, CA 94103.)

Holmes, Helen B., et al. *The Custom-Made Child.* Clifton, NJ: Humana, 1981.

Hormann, Elizabeth. *After the Adoption.* Old Tappan, N.J.: Revell, 1987.

Huxley, Aldous. *Island.* New York: Harper and Row, 1973.

Inglis, Kate. *Living Mistakes.* Boston: George Allen and Unwin, 1984.

Jacobovits, I. *Jewish Medical Ethics.* New York: Bloch, 1966.

Johnston, Patricia Irwin. *Understanding: A Guide to Impaired Fertility for Family and Friends.* Ft. Wayne, IN: Perspectives Press, 1983.

———. *Perspectives of a Grafted Tree: Thoughts for Those Touched by Adoption.* Ft. Wayne, IN: Perspectives Press, 1983.

———. *An Adopter's Advocate.* Ft. Wayne, IN: Perspectives Press, 1984.

Jones, A., and W. F. Bodmer. *Our Future Inheritance: Choice or Chance?* London: Oxford University Press, 1974.

Kaplan, Sharon, and M. J. Rillera. *The Open Adoption Handbook.* Westminster, CA: Triadoption Publications, 1983.

Keller, Helen. *The Story of My Life.* Kutchoge, N.Y.: Buccaneer Books, 1984.

Kippley, John F., and Sheila K. Kippley. *The Art of Natural Family Planning.* 3d ed. Cincinnati: Couple to Couple League, 1984.

Kirk, David. *Adoptive Kinship: A Modern Institution in Need of Reform.* Port Angeles, Wash.: Ben Simon, 1985.

———. *Shared Fate.* New York: Free Press, 1964.

Kistner, R. *Infertility.* Boston: Little, Brown, 1968.

Kleegman, S. J., and S. A. Kaufman. *Infertility in Women.* Philadelphia: F. A. Davis, 1966.

Krementz, Jill. *How It Feels To Be Adopted.* New York: Knopf, 1982.

Kübler-Ross, Elisabeth. *On Death and Dying.* New York: Macmillan, 1969.

Lacey, Louise. *Lunaception: A Feminine Odyssey into Fertility and Contraception.* New York: Warner, 1976.

Laing, R. D. *Knots*. New York: Pantheon, 1970.

Lasnik, R. S. *A Parent's Guide to Adoption*. New York: Sterling, 1979.

Leach, G. *The Biocrats*. London: Jonathan Cape, 1970.

Lewontin, R. C., Steven Rose and Leon J. Kamin. *Not In Our Genes*. New York: Pantheon, 1984.

Lifton, B. J. (foreword), and M. K. Benet. *The Politics of Adoption*. New York: Free Press, 1981.

Lifton, Betty Jean. *Lost and Found*. New York: Harper and Row, 1987.

———. *Twice Born: Memoirs of an Adopted Daughter*. New York: Penguin, 1985.

Livingstone, Carole. *Why Was I Adopted?* Secaucus, NJ: Lyle Stewart, 1978.

Marcus, Clare. *Adopted? A Canadian Guide for Adopted Adults in Search of Their Origins*, Seattle, WA: Vancouver Int. Self-Counsel Press, 1979.

———. *Who Is My Mother?* Toronto, Canada: Macmillan, 1981.

Martin, C. D. *Beating the Adoption Game*. La Jolla, CA: Oak Tree Publications, 1980.

Matthews, C. D., ed. *Current Statutes of Artificial Insemination in Australia*. Melbourne: Monash University Press, 1980.

Mazor, Miriam, ed. *Medical and Psychology Aspects of Infertility*. New York: Human Sciences Press, 1982.

McKuen, R. *Finding My Father: One Man's Search for Identity*. New York: Coward Publishing, 1976.

McNamara, Joan. *Adoption Adviser*. New York: E. P. Dutton, 1975.

McWhinnie, A. *Adopted Children: How They Grow Up*. Boston: Routledge and Kegan Paul, 1967.

Meezan, W., and Sanford Katz. *Adoption Without Agencies: A Study of Independent Adoptions*. New York: Child Welfare League of America, 1977.

Mehl, L. *Mind and Matter: Foundations for Holistic Health* (vol. 1) Berkeley: Mindbody Press, 1981.

Menning, Barbara Eck. *Infertility: A Guide for the Childless Couple*. New York: Prentice-Hall, 1977.

Milunsky, A., and G. Annas. *Genetics and the Law II*. New York: Plenum, 1980.

Nilsson, Leonard. *How Was I Born?* New York: Delacorte, 1975.

Nofziger, M. *The Fertility Question*. Summertown, Tennessee: The Book Publishing Co., 1982.

———. *A Cooperative Method of Natural Birth Control*. 2d ed. Summertown, Tennessee: The Book Publishing Co., 1978.

Notman, M., and C. Nadelson, eds. *The Problem of Infertility.* New York: Plenum Press, 1978.

O'Donnell, Mary, Kate Pollock, Val Leoffler, Deisel Sandert. *Lesbian Health Matters.* Santa Cruz CA: Santa Cruz Women's Health Center Publication, 1985.

Paton, Jean M. *The Adopted Break Silence: Forty Men and Women Describe Their Search for Natural Parents.* Philadelphia: Life History Study Center, 1954.

Peale, Norman Vincent. *The Power of Positive Thinking.* Englewood Cliffs, NJ: Prentice-Hall, 1978.

Perloe, M., L. G. Christie. *Miracle Babies and Other Happy Endings for Couples with Fertility Problems.* New York: Rawson Assoc., 1986.

Perry, Enos J., ed. *The Artificial Insemination of Farm Animals.* New Brunswick, NJ: Rutgers University Press, 1952.

Pfeffer, Naomi, and Anne Woollett. *The Experience of Infertility.* London: Virago, 1983.

Phillips, H., and J. Hilton. *Girl or Boy? Your Chance to Choose.* Rochester, VT: Thorsons, 1985.

Pies, C. *Considering Parenthood: A Workbook for Lesbians.* San Francisco: Spinsters Ink, 1985.

Pukei, M., et al. *Look to the Source.* Honolulu: Hui Hanai, 1972.

Rakusen, J., and N. Davidson. *Out of Our Hands: What Technology Does to Pregnancy.* London: Pan Books 1982.

Richardson, D., et al. *Frozen Human Semen: Proceedings of a Workshop upon the Cryobiology of Human Semen and Its Role in Artificial Insemination by Donor.* London: Royal College of Obstetricians and Gynaecologists, 1979.

Rillera, Mary J. *Adoption Searchbook: Techniques for Tracing People.* Westminster, CA: Triadoption Library, 1983.

―――― and S. Kaplan. *Cooperative Adoption: A Handbook.* Westminster, CA: Triadoption Library, 1985, P.O. Box 638, Westminster CA 92684.

Robinson, Susan, and H. F. Pizer. *Having a Baby Without a Man: The Woman's Guide to Alternative Insemination.* New York: Simon and Schuster, 1985.

Rohleder, Hermann. *Test Tube Babies: A History of Artificial Impregnation in Human Beings.* New York: Panurge Press, 1934.

Rothman, B. Katz. *The Tentative Pregnancy: Prenatal Diagnosis and the Future of Motherhood.* New York: Viking Press, 1986.

Schellen, A. M. *Artificial Insemination in the Human.* Amsterdam: Elsevier, 1957.

Scott, Russell. *The Body as Property.* U.K.: Viking, 1981.

Shawyer, Joss. *Death by Adoption.* Auckland, New Zealand: Cicada Press, 1979.

Shettles, L., and D. Rorvik. *How to Choose the Sex of Your Baby.* New York: Doubleday, 1984.

Silber, Kathleen, and Phylis Speedlin. *Dear Birthmother.* San Antonio, TX: Corona Publishing Co., 1983.

Silber, Sherman J. *Reproductive Infertility and Microsurgery in the Male and Female.* Baltimore, MD: Williams and Wilkins, 1984.

———. *The Male.* New York: Scribner's, 1982.

———. *How to Get Pregnant.* New York: Warner, 1981.

Silverman, Phyllis R. *Helping Women Cope with Grief.* London: Sage Publications, 1981.

Sims, J. M. *Clinical Notes on Uterine Surgery.* New York: William Wood, 1873.

Singer, P., and D. Wells. *The Reproductive Revolution: New Ways of Making Babies.* New York: Oxford University Press, 1986.

———. *Making Babies: The New Science, Ethics of Conception.* New York: Scribner's, 1987.

Snow, Rosie, ed. *Understanding Adoption: A Practical Guide.* Sydney, Australia: Fontana, 1983.

Snowden, Elizabeth, and Robert Snowden. *The Gift of a Child.* Boston: George Allen & Unwin, 1984.

Snowden, Roberet, and G. D. Mitchell. *Artificial Reproduction: A Social Investigation.* London: George Allen & Unwin, 1983.

———. *The Artificial Family: A Consideration of Artificial Insemination by Donor.* London: Allen & Unwin, 1981.

Sorosky, Arthur D., Annette Baran, and Reuben Pannor. *The Adoption Triangle.* New York: Doubleday, 1979.

Souaid, Robert. *Adoption: A Guide for Those Who Want to Adopt.* Coun. NY Law, 1982.

Taylor, G. R. *The Biological Time Bomb.* London: Thames and Hudson, 1968.

Titmuss, R. *The Gift Relationship: From Human Blood to Social Policy.* New York: Pantheon, 1971.

Triseliotis, John. *In Search of Origins.* London: Routledge & Kegan Paul, 1973.

Tziard, Barbara. *Adoption: A Second Chance.* London: Open Books, 1977.

Walters, W., and Peter Singer, eds. *Test-Tube Babies.* Melbourne: Oxford University Press, 1982.

Warnock, Mary. *A Question of Life: The Warnock Report on Human Fertilisation and Embryology.* New York: Blackwell, 1985.

Whelan, Elizabeth. *Boy or Girl?* New York: Pocket Books, 1984.

———. *A Baby? . . . Maybe.* New York: Bobbs-Merrill, 1981.

Williamson, N. *Sons or Daughters: A Cross-Cultural Survey of Parental Preferences.* New York: Russell Sage, Sage Library of Social Research, 1976.

Wimperis, V. *The Unmarried Mother and Her Child.* Boston: Allen & Unwin, 1960.

Wishard, Laurie, and W. Wishard. *Adoption: The Grafted Tree.* New York: Avon, 1979.

Wolstenholme, G. E. W., and D. Fitzsimons. *Law and Ethics of Artificial Insemination by Donor and Embryo Transfer,* North Holland: CIBA Foundation Symposium #17, Elsevier Excerpta Medica, 1975.

Wood, Carl, ed. *Artificial Insemination by Donor.* Melbourne, Australia: Brown, Prior and Anderson, 1980.

Wood, Carl, and Ann Westmore. *Test-Tube Conception.* Melbourne, Australia: Hill of Content, 1983.

Young, Leontine. *Out of Wedlock. A Study of the Problems of the Unmarried Mother and Her Child.* Westport, CT: Greenwood Press, 1978.

Articles

Adler, L., and A. Makris. "Successful Artificial Insemination with Macerated Testicular Tissue." *Fertility & Sterility* 2: (Sept.-Oct. 1951) 459.

Aicken, D. R. "Issues Arising from Artificial Conception Practices," *New Zealand Medical Journal* 98(775) (March 27, 1985): 186–7.

Aimon, J. "Factors Affecting the Success of Donor Insemination." *Fertility & Sterility* 37(15) (Jan. 1982): 94–9.

Albanese, F. "Artificial Insemination—European Legislation," in *Human Artificial Insemination,* Georges David and Wendel S. Prices, eds. New York: Plenum, 1980.

Albrecht, B. H., et al. "Factors Influencing the Success of Artificial Insemination." *Fertility and Sterility* 37(6) (June 1982): 792–7.

Alexandre, Claude. "Infertile Couples Facing AID," in *Human Artificial Insemination and Semen Preservation.* New York: Plenum, 1980.

Alfredsson, J. H. "Artificial Insemination with Frozen Semen: Sex Ratio at Birth." *International Journal of Fertility* 29(3) (1984):152–5.

———, et al. "Artificial Insemination by Donor with Frozen Semen." *Obstetrics and Gynecology Survey* 43(5) (1983):743–7.

AMA Judicial Council Report on "Human Artificial Insemination." *Connecticut Medicine* 38 (1984):481.

Anderson, Carole. "Closed Adoptions Promote Abortions." "Thoughts to Consider for Newly Searching Adoptees." "Surrogates and Other Nontraditional Reproduction." CUB, Inc., 2000 Walker Ave., Des Moines, Iowa, 50317.

Andrews, Lori. "Yours, Mine, Theirs." *Psychology Today* (December 1984).

Annas, George. "Redefining Parenthood and Protecting Embryos: Why We Need New Laws." *Soundings: Hastings Center Report* 14(5) (October 1984):50–2.

———. "Fathers Anonymous: Beyond the Best Interests of the Donor." *Family Law Quarterly* 14(1) (Spring 1980).

———. "Making Babies Without Sex. The Law and the Profits." *American Public Health* 74(1984) 1415.

"Anonymity and Donor Insemination" (letter) *American Journal of Psychiatry* 138(2) (Feb. 1981):262.

Anonymous (A Practitioner). "Artificial Insemination." *Lancet* (May 24, 1958):118–9.

———. "Artificial Insemination: A Critical Review." *Family Planning* 7:1974.

———. "I Search for My Father." *Redbook* March 24, 1953.

Ansbacher, R. "Artificial Insemination with Frozen Spermatozoa." *Fertility & Sterility* 29 (1978):375.

Anscombe, G. E. M. "You Can Have Children Without Sex." Chapter 6 of *Ethics, Religion and Politics*. Minneapolis: University of Minnesota Press, 1981.

Arnold, J. M., and D. N. Joyce. "Artificial Insemination by Donor." *Practitioner* (July 1982):226.

———. "Artificial Insemination Bypasses M.D.s." *Toronto Star* June 29, 1982.

Asche, A. "AID and the Law," in *Artificial Insemination by Donor*, C. Wood, ed. Melbourne: Brown, Prior and Anderson, 1980.

Atallah, Lillian. "Artificial Insemination: A Test-Tube Baby Tells Her Story." *Evening Bulletin*, Philadelphia, April 20, 1976.

———. "Report from a Test-Tube Baby." *The New York Times*, Sunday, April 18, 1976.

Bacon, Doris Klein. "Happy." *People* October 18, 1982.

Banks, A. L. "Aspects of Adoption and Artificial Insemination." Chapter 31 in *Progress in Infertility*, S. J. Behrman and R. W. Kistner, eds. Boston: Little, Brown, 1968.

Baran, Annette, et al. "Open Adoption." *Social Work.* March 1976.

Barton, M., K. Walker, and B. P. Weisner. "Artificial Insemination." *British Medical Journal* 13(1) (Jan. 1945)40–43.

Beck, W. W., Jr. "A Critical Look at the Legal, Ethical and Technical Aspects of Artificial Insemination." *Fertility and Sterility* 27 (1976):1–8.

———. "Artificial Insemination and Semen Preservation." *Clinical Obstetrics and Gynecology* (Dec. 1974) 17:4.

Behrman, S. J. "Artificial Insemination." *International Journal of Fertility* 6 (1961):291.

———. "Artificial Insemination." *Clinical Obstetrics & Gynecology* 22 (1979):245.

———. "Artificial Insemination and Public Policy." *New England Journal of Medicine* 300 (March 15, 1979):619–20.

———. "Artificial Insemination and the Preservation of Semen." *Urology Clinic of North America,* (1978) 5:593.

Behrman, S. J., and Ackerman, R. R. "Freeze Preservation of Human Sperm." *American Journal of Obstetrics & Gynecology* 103 (69):654.

Bender, S. "End Results in Primary Sterility." *British Medical Journal* 2 (1952):409–13.

Benedek, T. "Some Emotional Factors in Infertility." *Psychosomatic Medicine* 15 (1953):485.

Berger, D. M. "Psychological Aspects of Donor Insemination." *International Journal of Psychiatry in Medicine* 12 (1982):49.

———. "Reply on Anonymity and Donor Insemination." *American Journal of Psychiatry* 138(2) (1981):262.

———. "Couples' Reactions to Male Infertility and Donor Insemination." *American Journal of Psychiatry* 13 (Sept. 1980):1047–9.

———. "The Role of the Psychiatrist in a Reproductive Biology Clinic." *Fertility & Sterility* 28 (Feb. 1977):141–5.

———. "Psychological Assessment of Infertile Couples." *Canadian Family Physician* 20 (1975):89–95.

———. "Psychological Patterns in Donor Insemination Couples." *Canadian Journal of Psychiatry* 31(1986) 818.

Bergquist, Carol A., J. A. Rock, J. Miller, D. S. Guzick, A. C. Wentz, G. S. Jones, "Artificial Insemination with Fresh Donor Semen Using the Cervical Cap Technique: A Review of 278 Cases." *Obstetrics & Gynecology* 60 (August 1982):2.

Bernard, V. W. "Adoption" in *Encyclopedia of Mental Health,* Albert Deutsch and Helen Fishman, eds. 1 New York: Watts, 1963.

Berry, W. R., R. L. Gottesfeld, H. J. Alter, et al. "Transmission of Hepatitis B Virus by Artificial Insemination." *Journal of the American Medical Association* 257 (1987): 1079–81.

Bieren, R. "Artificial Insemination." *American Journal of Obstetrics and Gynecology* 71 (1956):212–14.

Billings, J. T. "Cervical Mucus: The Biological Marker of Fertility and Sterility." *International Journal of Fertility* 26(3)(1981):182–195.

Biskind, S. "The Rights of Children." in *Emergent Concepts in Law and Society*. Philadelphia: Temple University Press, 1973.

Blakely, Mary Kay. "Surrogate Mothers: For Whom Are They Working?" *Ms.* March 1983.

Bockle, F. "Insemination from the Ethical Viewpoint." *Munchener Medizinische Wochenschrift* (German) 47 (Nov. 25, 1983):1090–1.

Boetcher, B., et al. "Successful Treatment of Male Infertility Caused by Anti-Spermatozoal Antibodies." *Medical Journal of Australia* 2(10) (Nov. 13, 1982):471–4.

Bok, S. "Lying to Children: The Risks of Paternalism." *Soundings Hastings Center Report* 8(13) (June 1978):10–13.

Bohn, Z. S. "Artificial Insemination: Psychological and Psychiatric Evaluation." *University of Detroit Law Journal* 34 (1957):397.

Bonython, A. S. "Artificial Insemination—An Alternative to Adoption." *Australian Child & Family Welfare* Sept. 1976.

———. "Some Social Aspects of AID." Second National Working Party on AID at the Women's Hospital, Sydney, Australia, August 28, 1978.

Brandon, J., and J. Warner. "AID and Adoption: Some Australian Comparisons." *British Journal of Social Work* 7 (1977):3.

———. "Telling the AID Child." *Adoption and Fostering* 95(1) (1979):13–14.

Bratt, H., et al. "Donor Insemination: The Patient's View of Anonymity." *Tidsskr Nor Laegeforen* (Norwegian) 105(16) (June 10, 1985): 1159–60.

Breakey, Barry A. "Sperm Banks' Status." *University of Michigan Centre Journal* 39(3) (July-Sept. 1973):129.

Bresnick, Ellen. "A Holistic Approach to the Treatment of the Crisis of Infertility." *Journal of Marital and Family Therapy* April 1981.

——— and M. Taymor. "The Role of Counseling in Infertility." *Fertility & Sterility* 32 (August 1978):154–6.

Brewer, C. "Let Lesbians Have a Fecund Choice." *General Practitioner* 20 (Jan. 1978).

Broekhuizen, F. F., et al. "Laparoscopic Findings in 25 Failures of Artificial Insemination." *Fertility & Sterility* 34(4) (Oct. 1980):351–5.

Bromwich, P., and M. Kilpatrick. "Artificial Insemination with Frozen Stored Donor Semen." *British Journal of Obstetrics and Gynecology* 83 (1978):641.

Bunge, R. G., and J. K. Sherman. "Fertilizing Capacity of Frozen Human Sperm." *Nature* 172 (1953):627.

———, et al. "Clinical Use of Frozen Semen." *Fertility & Sterility* 5 (1954):520.

———. "Frozen Human Semen." *Fertility & Sterility* (1954) 5:193.

Bunyard, Peter. "An Alternative to Adoption?" *World Medicine* 7 (May 3, 1972):16.

Cabau, A. "Female Fertility in AID and Psychological Factors," in *Human Artificial Insemination and Semen Production,* Georges David and Wendel S. Price, eds. New York: Plenum, 1980.

Campbell, H. "Infertility: Its Incidence and Hope of Cure." *British Medical Journal* (1958) 429:33.

Canterbury, His Grace the Archbishop of. "Report of a Commission on Artificial Human Insemination." London: Society for the Propagation of Christian Knowledge, 1948.

Capron, A. M. "The New Reproductive Possibilities: Seeking a Moral Basis for Concerted Action in a Pluralistic Society." *Law, Medicine and Health Care* Oct. 1984.

Carr, Joseph E. "Artificial Insemination: Problems, Policies and Proposals." *Alabama Law Association Law Review* 26 (Fall 1973):120–62.

Carruthers, G. B. "Husband and Donor Insemination in Infertility." *Medicine, Gynecology and Sociology* 5(2) (1970):13–15.

Cary, W. H. "Results of Artificial Insemination." *Medical Aspects Human Sexuality* 15 (May 1985):70.

———. "Results of Artificial Insemination with an Extramarital Specimen (semiadoption): Report on 89 Cases." *American Journal of Obstetrics & Gynecology* 56 (1948):727–32.

———. "Experiments with Artificial Impregnation in Treating Sterility: Report of 35 cases." *Journal of the American Medical Association* 14 (1940):2183–7.

Cashion, B. G. "Female-headed Families: Effects on Children and Clinical Implications." *Journal of Marital Family Therapy* 8 (1982):77.

Castleman, Michael. "Why Johnny Can't Have Kids." *Mother Jones* April 1982.

Chesser, E. "Artificial Insemination." (letter) *British Medical Journal* (Jan. 1947).

Chester, R. "Is There a Relationship Between Childlessness and Marriage Breakdown? *Journal of Biosocial Science* 4 (1972):443–54.

Chevret, M. "Problems Related to Requests for AID and Psychological

Assistance Offered to Couples," in *Human Artificial Insemination and Semen Production,* Georges David and Wendel S. Price, eds. New York: Plenum, 1980.

Christiaens, M. "Donor Insemination and the Human Viewpoint." *Nederlandse Tijdschrift Voor Geneeskunde* (Dutch) 128(43) (Oct. 27, 1984):2051–5.

Chong, A. P., and M. L. Taymor. "Sixteen Years' Experience with Therapeutic Donor Insemination." *Fertility & Sterility* 26 (1975):791.

Clamar, A. "Psychological Implications of Donor Insemination." *American Journal of Psychoanalysis* 40 (1980):173–7.

———. "Artificial Insemination by Donor: The Anonymous Pregnancy." *American Journal of Forensic Psychology* (1984) 2:27..

Clark, H. "Fate, the Experts and Individual Choice." *Soundings: Hastings Center Report* 50(4) (1978):331–43.

Clayton, C. E. "AID Offspring: Initial Follow-up Study of 50 Couples." *Medical Journal of Australia* 1(8) (April 17, 1982):338–9.

———, and G. T. Kovacs. "AID—A Pretreatment Social Assessment." *Australian & New Zealand Journal of Obstetrics & Gynaecology* 20 (1980):208.

Cohen, M. R., et al. "Optimal Time for Therapeutic Insemination." *Fertility & Sterility* 7 (1956):141.

Coleman, A. H. "AID and the Illegitimate Child." *Journal of the National Medical Association* 57 (1965):331–2.

Colon, Fernando. "Family Ties and Child Placement." *Family Process* (Sept. 1978):17.

Cooke, R. "Some Single Women Inseminating Themselves Successfully." *The Boston Globe,* April 5, 1984.

Correy, J. F., et al. "The Outcome of Pregnancy Resulting from Clomiphene-induced Ovulation." *Australian and New Zealand Journal of Obstetrics and Gynaecology* (Feb. 1982) 22(1):18.

Corson, S. L., et al. "Sex Selection by Sperm Separation and Insemination." *Fertility & Sterility* 42(5) (Nov. 1984):756–60.

———. "Donor Insemination." *Obstetrics & Gynecology Annual* 12 (1983):283–309.

———. "Factors Affecting Donor Artificial Insemination Success Rate." *Fertility & Sterility* 33 (1980):415.

Curie-Cohen, Martin, et al. "Current Practice of Artificial Insemination by Donor in the USA." *New England Medical Journal* 300 (1979):587.

———. "The Frequency of Consanguinous Matings due to Multiple Use of Donors in Artificial Insemination." *American Journal of Human Genetics* 32 (1980):589–600.

Curran, W. S. "Public Health and The Law: Artificial Insemination." *American Journal of Public Health* 58 (1968):1460–61.

Cusine, D. J. "Developments in Human Reproduction and Their Eugenic, Ethical and Legal Implications." *Proceedings of the Annual Symposium of the Eugenics Society* 19 (1983):227–36.

———. "Legal Aspects of AID," in *Human Artificial Insemination and Semen Production,* Georges David and Wendel S. Price, eds. New York: Plenum, 1980.

Czyba J. C., and M. Chevret. "Psychological Reactions of Couples to Artificial Insemination with Donor Semen." *International Journal of Fertility* 24(4) (1979):240–5.

Dalrymple, J. C., et al. "Reduced Pregnancy Rates in AID Women with Unsuspected Ovulatory Failure." *Clinical Reproduction and Fertility* 2(1) (March 1983):27–32.

D'Andrea, K. G. "The Role of the Nurse-Practitioner in Artificial Insemination." *Journal of Obstetrical Gynecological & Neonatal Nursing* 13(2) (March-April 1984):75–8.

Daniels, K. R. "The Practice of Artificial Insemination of Donor Sperm in New Zealand." *New Zealand Medical Journal* 98 (1985): 235–39.

———. "Artificial Insemination by Donor and Its Implications for Social Work," in *Social Work Issues for the 1980s,* K. R. Daniels, ed. Christchurch, N.Z., University of Canterbury, Dept. of Sociology, 1981.

———. "AID: A Social Work Approach to Researching the Psychosocial Factors." *Social Work in Health Care* (1986) 11(4):49.

David, A., and D. Avidan. "Artificial Insemination Donor: Clinical and Psychological Aspects." *Fertility & Sterility* 27 (1976):528.

Davidson, H. "The Male Factor in the Infertile Marriage." *Practitioner* 169 (1952):126–32.

Davis, Ivor, and Sally O. Davis. "Whose Sperm Is It Anyway?" *Los Angeles* December 1982.

Davis, J. H. "The Pediatric Role in Adoption." *Clinical Pediatrics* 7 (1979)438.

Debrovner, C. H., et al. "Sexual Problems in the Infertile Couple." *Medical Aspects of Human Sexuality* (1975):140–150.

Deckins, D. M. "Artificial Insemination and the Law." *Journal of Legal Medicine* 4 (1976):17–22.

D'Elicio, et al. "Discussions with Couples Requesting AID," in *Human Artificial Insemination and Semen Production,* Georges David and Wendel S. Price, eds. New York: Plenum, 1980.

Denber, H. C. "Psychiatric Aspects of Infertility." *Journal of Reproductive Medicine* 20 (Jan. 1978):23–29.

De Stoop, D. F. "Human Artificial Insemination and the Law in Australia." *Australian Law Journal* 50 (1976):298.

Dixon, R. E., and V. C. Buttram. "Artificial Insemination Using Donor Semen: A Review of 171 Cases." *Fertility & Sterility* 27 (1976):130.

Donovan, P. "New Reproductive Technologies: Some Legal Dilemmas." *Family Planning Perspectives* 18(1986) 2:57.

Dubin, L., and R. D. Amelar. "Etiologic Factors in 1294 Consecutive Cases of Male Infertility." *Fertility & Sterility* 22 (1971):469.

Dunstan, G. R. "Ethical Issues Relating to AID." *Artificial Insemination: Proceedings of the Fourth Study Group of the Royal College of Obstetricians and Gynaecologists* 1976 (27 Sussex Place, Regent's Park, London NW1 4RG).

————. "Ethical Aspects of Donor Insemination." *Journal of Medical Ethics* 1 (1975):42–4.

————. "Moral and Social Issues Arising from Artificial Insemination by Donor," in *The Law and Ethics of AID or Embryo Transfer*, Wolstenholme, G. W. and D. Fitzsimmons, eds. North Holland CIBA Foundation, Symposium #17, Elsevier Excerpta Medica, 1975.

Dusky, Lorraine. "The Daughter I Gave Away." *McCall's* July 1983.

————. "Brave New Babies." *Newsweek* December 6, 1982.

Editorial. "A Natural Birthright." *The Age*, Melbourne, Australia, August 10, 1981.

————. "Artificial Insemination." *Medical Journal of Australia* 1(11) (March 15, 1975):324–5.

————. "Artificial Insemination." *British Medical Journal* 4(5987) (Oct. 4, 1975):2–3.

————. "Artificial Insemination." *New England Journal of Medicine* 294(5) (Jan. 25, 1976):280–81.

————. "Suggested Code of Practice for Artificial Insemination by Donor (AID)." *South African Medical Journal* 58(19) (Nov. 8, 1980): 781–3.

Edmonds, D. K., et al. "Tubal Patency Testing in a Program of Artificial Insemination with Donor Semen." *British Journal of Obstetrics and Gynaecology* 88(7) (July 1981):761–4.

Edvinsson, A., et al. "Characteristics of Donor Semen and Cervical Mucus at the Time of Conception." *Fertility & Sterility* 39(3) (March 1983):327–32.

Edwards, J. H. "A Critical Examination of the Reputed Primary Influence of ABO Phenotypes on Fertility and Sex Ratio." *British Journal of Preventive and Social Medicine* 11 (1957):79–80.

Elias, S., and G. J. Annas. "Social Policy Considerations in Noncoital Reproduction." *Journal of the American Medical Association* 255 (Jan. 3, 1986):162–68.

Ellis, W. H. "The Socio-Legal Problems of Artificial Insemination." *Indiana Law Journal* 28 (1952):620.

Elstein, M. "Effect of Infertility on Psychosexual Functioning." *British Medical Journal* 3 (1975):296–9.

Emperaire, J., et al. "Female Fertility and Donor Insemination." *Lancet* 1 (1980):1423.

Ennis, J. "AID: The Gift of Life." *Nova* (1972):20–22.

Ericsson, R. J., et al. "Isolation of Fractions Rich in Human Y Sperm." *Nature* 246 (1973):421.

Etter, J. "Two Fathers Make Open Adoption Work." *Williamette Valley Observer* (Oregon), June 23, 1982.

Farris, E. J., and M. Garrison. "Emotional Impact of Successful Donor Insemination: Report on 38 Couples." *Obstetrics & Gynecology* 3 (1954):19.

Federation CECOS, H. Mattei, and B. Le Marec. "Genetic Aspects of Artificial Insemination by Donor (AID): Indications, Surveillance and Results." *Clinical Genetics* 23 (1983):132–138.

———, D. Schwartz, and M. J. Mayaux. "Female Fecundity as a Function of Age: Results of Artificial Insemination in 2,193 Nulliparous Women with Azoospermic Husbands." *New England Journal of Medicine* 306 (1982):404–406.

Feldschuh, J. "Artificial Insemination in Clinical Practice." *The Integrity of Frozen Spermatozoa*. National Academy of Sciences, Washington, D.C. 1978.

Feversham Committee, Her Majesty's Stationery Office. "Report of Departmental Committee on Human Artificial Insemination." *British Medical Journal* 2 (1960):379–80.

Fiore, J. P. "Mechanism for Delivery of Sperm to the Fimbria in Oligospermia." (letter) *Fertility & Sterility* 38(1) (July 1982):119.

Fish, S. "Continuing Problems of Artificial Insemination." *Postgraduate Medicine* 38 (Oct. 1965):415–420.

Fiumara, N. J. "Transmission of Gonorrhea by Artificial Insemination." *British Journal of Venereal Disease* 48 (1972):308–9.

Fleming, J. "The Basic Question Not Addressed." *The Advertiser* Adelaide, Australia, April 30, 1984.

Ford, B. E., et al. "A Psychological Approach to the Study of Infertility." *Fertility & Sterility* 54 (1966):456–65.

Forse, R. A., et al. "Possible Teratogenic Effects of Artificial Insemination by Donor." *Clinical Genetics*, 28(1) (July 1985):23–6.

Foss, G. L. "Artificial Insemination by Donor: Review of 12 Years' Experience." *Journal of Biosocial Science* 14(3) (July 1982):253–263.

Foss, G. L., and M. G. R. Hull. "Results of Donor Insemination Related to Specific Male Infertility and Unsuspected Female Infertility. *British Journal of Obstetrics and Gynaecology* 93 (1986): 275–78.

Frankel, M. S. "Artificial Insemination: the Medical Profession and Public Policy." *Connecticut Medicine* 38(9) (Sept. 1974):476–80.

————. "Human Semen Banking: Implications for Medicine and Society." *Connecticut Medicine* 39(1975):313–17.

————. "Cryobanking: Ethical Issues." *Journal of Medical Ethics* 1 (April 1975):36–8.

————. "Semen Cryobanking: Need for a Policy." *British Medical Journal* 3 (Sept. 7, 1974):619–21.

————. "Role of Cryobanking in American Medicine." *British Medical Journal* 3 (1974):619.

Fraser, F. C., and R. A. Forse. "On Genetic Screening of Donors for Artificial Insemination." *American Journal of Medical Genetics* 10 (1981):399.

————. "Heredity Counseling: The Darker Side." *Eugenics Quarterly* 3 (1956):45.

Fried, C. "Ethical Issues in Existing and Emerging Techniques for Improving Human Infertility." CIBA Foundation Symposium #17: *Excerpta Medica*. North Holland: Elsevier, 1973.

Friedman, S. "Artificial Donor Insemination with Frozen Human Semen." *Fertility & Sterility* 28 (1977):1230.

Gallup Poll. "Concern over Donor Sperm." *The Advertiser* (Adelaide, Australia) August 6, 1984.

Ganson, Harriet C., and J. A. Cook. "The Open Record Controversy in Adoption: A Woman's Issue?" New York: American Sociological Association (81st Annual Meeting), 1986.

Garner, P. R. "Artificial Insemination." *Canadian Medical Association Journal* 6 (Jan. 1979):120.

Gerber, W. L., and L. S. Bresau. "Semen Abnormalities in Artificial Insemination Donor Candidates." *Journal of Urology* 130 (August 1983):266.

Gerstel, G. "A Psychoanalytical View of Artificial Donor Insemination." *American Journal of Psychotherapy* 17 (1963):64–77.

Gilbert, Sarita. "Artificial Insemination." *American Journal of Nursing* 76 (Feb. 1976):2.

Glass, D. V. "Human Fertility and Artificial Insemination: The Demographic Background." *Journal of the Royal Statistical Society* (Sec. A) 123 (1960) 171.

Glass, R. H. "Sex Preselection." *Obstetrics and Gynecology* 49 (1977) 122.

Glezerman, M., et al. "The Cervical Factor of Infertility and Intrauterine Insemination." *International Journal of Fertility* 29(1) (1984):16–9.

Glezerman, M., and R. White. "270 Cases of Artificial Donor Insemination: Management and Results." *Fertility and Sterility* 35(2) (Feb. 1981) 180–7.

Godfrey, B. "Sex Ratio of Births Resulting from Artificial Insemination." *British Journal of Obstetrics & Gynaecology* 89(8) (Aug. 1982): 683–4.

Goldenberg, R. L., et al. "Artificial Insemination." *Connecticut Medicine* 40(3) (March 1976):187–8.

———, and R. White. "Artificial Insemination." *Journal of Reproductive Medicine* 18(3) (March 1977):149–54.

Golin, M. "Paternity by Proxy." *New Physician* 1962:425–9.

Golombok, S., et al. "Children in Lesbian and Single-Parent Households: Psychosexual and Psychiatric Appraisal." *Journal of Child Psychology & Psychiatry* 24 (1983):551.

Goodman, Ellen. "Artificial Insemination—Good or Bad?" *The Boston Globe,* March 28, 1979.

Goss, D. A. "Current Status of Artificial Insemination with Donor Semen." *American Journal of Obsterics and Gynecology* 122(2) (May 15, 1975):246–52.

Gradstein, Bonnie D., et al. "Private Adoption." *Fertility & Sterility* 37 (April 1982):548–51.

Green, Richard. "The Best Interests of the Child with a Lesbian Mother." *Bulletin of the American Academy of Psychiatry & Law* 10 (1982):7.

———. "Sexual Identity of Thirty-seven Children Raised by Homosexual or Transsexual Parents." *American Journal of Psychiatry* 135 (1978):692.

Greenblatt, R. M., H. H. Handsfield, M. H. Sayers, et al. "Screening Therapeutic Insemination Donors for Sexually Transmitted Diseases: Overview and Recommendations." *Fertility & Sterility* 46 (1986):351–64.

Greenburg, J. "Social Variables in Acceptance or Rejection in Artificial Insemination." *American Sociological Review* 16 (1951):85.

Greer, Germaine. "The Pain of Protecting Procreation." *Matilda* Canberra, Australia, February 1985.

Gregoire, A. T., and R. C. Mayer. "The Impregnators." *Fertility & Sterility* 16 (January 1965):1.

Guerin, J. F., et al. "Enzymes in the Seminal Plasma from Azoospermic Men Correlated with the Origin of their Azoospermia." *Fertility & Sterility* 36(3) (September 1981):368.

Guerrero, R. "A Statistical Association with the Time and Type of Insemination in the Menstrual Cycle." *International Journal of Fertility* 15 (1970):21.

———. "Association of the Type and Time of Insemination Within the Menstrual Cycle with the Human Sex Ratio at Birth." *New England Journal of Medicine* 291 (Nov. 1974):1056.

Guttmacher, A. F. (editorial) "Artificial insemination," *Fertility & Sterility* 5 (1954) 4–6.

———. "The Role of Artificial Insemination in the Treatment of Sterility." *Obstetrics & Gynecology Survey* 50 (Dec. 1960):767.

———. "Artificial Insemination." *Annals of New York Academy of Sciences* 97 (1962):623.

———. "Physicians' Credo for Artificial Insemination." *Southwestern Journal of Surgery, Obstetrics, and Gynecology* 50 (1942) 357.

Guttmacher, A. F., et al. "The Use of Donors for Artificial Insemination: A Survey of Current Practices." *Fertility & Sterility* 1 (May 1950):264–70.

Guzick, D., et al. "A Parametric Method for Comparing Cumulative Pregnancy Curves Following Infertility Therapy." *Fertility & Sterility* 37(4) (April 1982):503.

Hafez, E. S. E. "Ethical and Moral Aspects of Artificial Insemination by Donor and Embryo Transfer." *Archives of Andrology* 5 (1980):44–52.

Hajnal, J. "Artificial Insemination and the Frequency of Incestuous Marriages." *Journal of the Royal Statistical Society* (Sec. A) 123(1960) 182.

Halbrecht, I. "Artificial Insemination (Report on 80 Cases)." *American Journal of Obstetrics and Gynecology* 51 (1944):526–28.

Haman, J. O. "Results in Artificial Insemination." *Journal of Urology* 2 (1954):557.

———. "Therapeutic Donor Insemination: Review of 440 Cases." *California Medicine* 90 (1959):130–3.

Handelsman, D. J., et al. "Psychological and Attitudinal Profiles in Donors for Artificial Insemination." *Fertility & Sterility* 43(1) (Jan. 1985):95–101.

Hansen, B. K., et al. "Artificial Insemination in Denmark by Frozen Donor Semen Supplied by a Central Bank." *British Journal of Obstetrics and Gynaecology* (1979)86:384.

Hanson, F. W., et al. "A Study of the Relationship Between Motile Sperm Numbers in Cervical Mucus 48 Hours after Artificial Insemination with Subsequent Fertility." *American Journal of Obstetrics and Gynecology* 143(1) (May 1, 1982):85–90.

Hard, A. D. "Artificial Impregnation." *Medical World* 27 (1909):163.

Hargreave, T. B. "Artificial Insemination by Donor." *British Medical Journal* 291(6496) (Sept. 7, 1985):613–4.

———, and R. A. Elton. "Is Conventional Sperm Analysis of Any Use?" *British Journal of Urology* 55 (1983):774–9.

Harlap, S. "Gender of Infants Conceived on Different Days of the Menstrual Cycle." *New England Journal of Medicine* 300(1979)1445.

Harrison, R. F., and G. Wyn-Williams. "Human Artificial Insemination." *British Journal of Hospital Medicine* 96 (June 1973):760–2.

Healey, J. M. "Legal Aspects of Artificial Insemination and Paternity Testing." in *Genetics and Law*, A. Milunsky and G. Annas, eds. New York: Plenum Press, 1976.

Heiman, M., and S. Kleegman. "Insemination, a Psychoanalytic and Infertility Study." *Fertility & Sterility* 17 (Jan.-Feb. 1966):117–25.

———. "Toward a Psychosomatic Concept in Infertility." *International Journal of Fertility* 4 (1959):247.

Henahan J. "Artificial Insemination Has Few Untoward Effects." *Journal of the American Medical Association* (News) 250(10) (Sept. 9, 1983):1256.

Hilgers, J. W. and A. T. Barley. "Basal Body Temperature and Estimated Time of Ovulation." *Obstetrics and Gynecology* 55(1980) 333.

Hill, A. M. "Experience with Artificial Insemination." *Australian & New Zealand Journal of Obstetrics & Gynaecology* 10 (1970):112.

———. "Experience with Artificial Insemination." *Human Fertility* 11 (1946):72–4.

Hillix, W. A., et al. "Secrets." *Psychology Today* Sept. 1970.

Hirsh, B. D. "Parenthood by Proxy." *Journal of the American Association* 249(16) (April 1983):2251.

Hitchens, Donna. "Lesbians Choosing Motherhood: Legal Implications of Donor Insemination." Lesbian Rights Project, 1370 Mission St., San Francisco, CA 94103 1981.

Hoeffer, B. "Children's Acquisition of Sex-role Behavior in Lesbian Mother Families." *American Journal of Orthopsychiatry* 51 (1981):536.

Hoffer, William. "The Legal Limbo of AID—Artificial Insemination by Donor." *Modern Medicine* Nov. 1, 1975.

Holland, Joan. "Adoption and Artificial Insemination: Some Social Implications." *Soundings: Hastings Center Report* 50(4) (1971): 302–7.

Hormann, Elizabeth. "Sharing the Joy." *Today's Christian Woman* Summer 1982.

Horne, H. W., Jr. "Artificial Insemination by Donor: An Issue of Ethical and Moral Values." (editorial) *New England Journal of Medicine* 293(17) (October 23, 1975):873–4.

Hornstein, Francie. "Lesbian Health Care." Feminist Women's Health Center, 6411 Hollywood Boulevard, Los Angeles, CA 90028 1984.

———. "Children by Donor Insemination" in *Test-Tube Women: What Future for Motherhood?* R. Arditti, et al. eds. Boston: Routledge and Kegan Paul, 1984.

Huerre, P. "Psychological Aspects of Semen Donation," in *Human Artificial Insemination and Semen Production,* Georges David and Wendel S. Price, eds. New York: Plenum, 1980.

Hughes, J. B. and P. F. "Psychological Well-Being as an Outcome Variable in the Treatment of Infertility by Chlomiphine." *British Journal of Medical Psychology* (1982):375–77.

Huisingh, D. "Artificial Insemination Donor: A Simple Medical Technique; A Complex Human Problem." *Hastings Center Report* 50(4) (1971).

Hulka, J. F. "Donor Insemination: Guidelines for Uncharted Territory." (editorial) *Fertility & Sterility* 35(5) (May 1981):500–1.

Humphrey, M. E. "Infertility and Adoption: Follow-up of 21 Couples Attending a Hospital Clinic." *British Journal of Preventive & Social Medicine* 21 (1962):90–96.

———, and C. Ounsted. "Adoptive Families Referred for Psychiatric Advice. Part I: The Children." *British Journal of Psychiatry* 109 (1963):399–605.

———. "Part II: The Parents." *British Journal of Psychiatry* 110 (1964).

Humphries, D. "Women Allege Bias over Test-tube Delay." *The Age* Melbourne, Australia, November 10, 1983.

Hunter, N., and N. Polikoff. "Custody Rights of Lesbian Mothers: Legal Theory and Litigation Strategy." *Buffalo Law Review* 25 (1976):691.

Huxley, Julian. "Eugenics in Evolutionary Perspective." *Perspectives in Biology & Medicine* Winter 1963.

Iddenden, D. A., et al. "A Prospective Randomized Study Comparing Fresh Semen and Cryopreserved Semen for Artificial Insemination by Donor." *International Journal of Fertility* 30(1) (1985):55–56.

Iizuka, R., et al. "The Physical and Mental Development of Children Born Following Artificial Insemination." *International Journal of Fertility* 13 (1969):24–32.

"Insemination Procedure: Cervical Cap." (letter) *Fertility & Sterility* 34(4) (Oct. 1980):407–8.

Jackson, M., and D. Richardson. "The Use of Fresh and Frozen Semen and Human Artificial Insemination." *Journal of Biosocial Science* 9 (1977):251–62.

———. "Artificial Insemination (Donor): A Symposium." *Eugenics Review* 48 (1957):203–11.

Jacobsen, E. "Up 400%—Artificial Insemination." *Sexual Medicine Today*, Dec. 6, 1976.

Jakobovits, E. "Artificial Insemination, Birth Control, and Abortion." *Hebrew Medical Journal* 2(1953)183.

James, B., et al. "Psychological Well-being after Outcome Variable in the Treatment of Infertility by Clomiphene." *British Journal of Medical Psychology* 559 (1982)375.

James, W. H. "Results of Donor Insemination Related to Specific Male Infertility and Unsuspected Female Infertility." (letter) *British Journal of Obstetrics and Gynaecology* 93 (October 1986): 1112.

Jennings, R. T., et al. "The Risk and Prevention of *Neisseria* gonorrhea Transfer in Fresh Ejaculate Donor Insemination." *Fertility & Sterility* 28 (1977)556.

Jequier, A. M. "Non-Therapy Related Pregnancies in the Consorts of a Group of Men with Obstructive Azoospermia." *Andrologia* 17(1) (Jan.-Feb. 1985):6–8.

Jeyendrau, R. S. "Concentration of Viable Sperm for Artificial Insemination." *Fertility & Sterility* 45(1) (Jan. 1986):132–4.

Johnson, W. G., et al. "Artificial Insemination by Donors: the Need for Genetic Screening: Late-infantile GM2 Gangliosidosis Resulting from This Technique." *New England Journal of Medicine* 304(13) (March 26, 1981):757–9.

Johnston, Ian. "The Donor," in *Artificial Insemination by Donor*, C. Wood, ed. Melbourne: Brown Prior Anderson, 1980.

Jones, A. "Artificial Insemination by Donor and the Treatment of Infertility," in *Our Future Inheritance: Choice or Chance?* A. Jones and W. F. Bodmer, eds. Oxford: Oxford University Press, 1974.

Jones, W. R., et al. "Artificial Insemination by Donor." (letter) *Medical Journal of Australia* 141(5) (Sept. 1984):317.

Joyce, D. "Sperm-Mucus Interaction and Artificial Insemination." *Clinical Obstetrics and Gynaecology* 8(3) (Dec. 1981):587–610.

Kamlet, Leonard G. "Artificial Insemination—A Model Statute." *Cleveland State Law Review* 24 (1975):341.

Kardimon, S. "Artificial Insemination in the Talmud." *Hebrew Medical Journal* 2 (1942):162–4.

Karow, A. M. "Family Secrets: Who Is To Know About AID?" (letter) *New England Journal of Medicine* 306(6) (Feb. 11, 1982):372.

Karp, L. E. "Artificial Insemination—A Need for Caution." *American Journal of Medical Genetics* 9 (1981):179.

Karpel, M. A. "Family Secrets." *Family Process* 19 (Sept. 1980):3.

Kating, C. E., et al. "Donor Insemination at a Private Infertility Center." *Journal of the South Carolina Medical Association* 80(2) (Feb. 1984) 56–7.

Katz, Sanford N., and M. Inker. "Fathers, Husbands and Lovers: Legal Rights and Responsibilities." *Family Law Quarterly* Fall 1979.

Katzorke, T., et al. "Analysis of Cycle Changes Following AID." *Archives of Andrology* 5 (1980):44–52.

Kelly, G. "Teachings of Pope Pius XII on Artificial Insemination." *Linacre Quarterly* 23 (1956):5–17.

Kerr, M. G., and C. Rogers. "Ethical Aspects of Donor Insemination." *Journal of Medical Ethics* 1 (1975):30–33.

Kiely, Rosemary. "AID—A Child's Right to Know." *The Age* Melbourne, Australia, July 22, 1981.

Kilbrandon, Lord. "Discussion of Biological Aspects." *CIBA Foundation Symposium #17 Law and Ethics of AID and Embryo Transfer. Excerpta Medica.* North Holland: Elsevier, 1973.

King, C. R. and E. Magenis. "Turner Syndrome in the Offspring of Artificial Insemination Pregnancies." *Fertility & Sterility* 30(1978)604.

Kirk, H. D., et al. "Are Adopted Children Especially Vulnerable to Stress?" *Archives of General Psychiatry* 14 (1966):291–8.

Kirkpatrick, M., et al. "Lesbian Mothers and Their Children: A Comparative Survey." *American Journal of Orthopsychiatry* 51 (1978):536.

Klay, L. J. "Clomiphene-regulated Ovulation for Donor Artificial Insemination." *Fertility & Sterility* 27 (1976):383.

Kleegman, S. J. "Therapeutic Donor Insemination." *Fertility & Sterility* 5 (1954):1.

———. "Therapeutic Donor Insemination." *Connecticut Medicine* 31 (1967):705–13.

———, et al. "Roundtable: Artificial Donor Insemination." *Medical Aspects of Human Sexuality* 4 (1970): 85.

Klier, E. "Artificial Insemination: Various Views of the Problems." *Fertility & Sterility,* VII World Congress, 1971. *Fertility Sterility: Proceedings of the VII World Congress,* T. Hasegawa, et al. Kyoto, Japan, October 1973. New York: Elsevier, 1973.

Kolecku, U. "Donor Baby Heartbreak." *The Sun* Melbourne, Australia, Dec. 13, 1983.

Koren, Z., and R. Lieberman. "Fifteen Years' Experience with Artificial Insemination." *International Journal of Fertility* 2(1976)119.

Kovacs, G. T., et al. "Outcome of AID in Initial and Subsequent Courses of Treatment." *Clinical Reproduction and Fertility* 2(4) (Dec. 1983):295–8.

———. "Infertile Couples Use Sperm from Husbands' Relatives." *The Age* Melbourne, Australia, May 11, 1983.

———. "The Attitudes of Semen Donors." *Clinical Reproduction & Fertility* 291 (March 1983):73–5.

———. "Artificial Insemination with Donor Semen: Review of 252 Patients." *Medical Journal of Australia* 2(11) (November 29, 1980):609–12.

Kraft, A. D., et al. "The Psychological Dimension of Infertility." *American Journal of Orthopsychiatry* 50(1980)618.

Kraus, J., and P. E. Quinn. "Human Artificial Insemination: Some Social and Legal Issues." *Medical Journal of Australia* 2(11) (May 7, 1977):609–12.

Kremer, J., et al. "Psychosocial Aspects of Parenthood by Artificial Insemination by Donor." (letter) *Lancet* 1(8377) March 17, 1984:628.

———. "Psychosocial Aspects of Parenthood by AID: The Results of an Anonymous Investigation of 153 Couples." *Archives of Andrology* 5 (1980):44–52.

———. "Pitfalls and Snags in Donor Insemination." (Dutch) *Nederlandse Tijdschrift Voor Geneeskunde* 126(20) (May 15, 1982):889–92.

Kritchevsky, Barbara. "The Unmarried Woman's Right to Artificial Insemination: A Call for an Expanded Definition of Family." *Harvard Women's Law Journal* 4 (1981):1–42.

Lakartidningen 77(38) (September 17, 1980). (Swedish medical journal, issue focusing on Artificial Insemination.)

Lamson, H. D., et al. "Sociological and Psychological Aspects of Artificial Insemination with Donor Semen." *Journal of the American Medical Association* 145 (1951):1062–4.

Lane, T. E. "Artificial Insemination at Home." *Fertility & Sterility* 5 (July–Aug. 1954) 372.

Langer, G., et al. "Artificial Insemination: A Study of 156 Successful Cases." *International Journal of Fertility* 14 (1969).

Lansac, J. "Pregnancy and Labor after Insemination with Frozen Semen from a Donor." *Journal of Gynecology, Obstetrics Biology and Reproduction* (Paris) 12(5) (1983):511–18.

Lauerson, Niels, and E. Ukane. "New Ways of Making Babies: How Science Can Help." *Cosmopolitan* November 1982.

Lauritzen, C. "Insemination Techniques and Ethical Problems." (German) *Munchener Medizinische Wochenschrift* 123(20) (May 15, 1981): 833–6.

Lawton, J. J., and S. Z. Gross. "A Review of the Psychiatric Literature on Adopted Children." *Archives of General Psychiatry* 11 (1964):635–44.

Leach, W. B. "Perspectives in the Atomic Age: the Sperm Bank and the Fertile Descendant." *American Bar Association Journal* 48 (1962):942.

Leader, A., et al. "The Prediction of Ovulation: A Comparison of the Basal Body Temperature Graph, Cervical Mucus Score, and Real-time Pelvic Ultrasonography." *Fertility & Sterility* 43(3) (March 1985):385–8.

Ledward, R. S., et al. "Social and Environmental Factors as Criteria for Success in Artificial Insemination by Donor (AID)." *Journal of Biosocial Science* 14 (1982):263–75.

———. "Social Factors in Patients for Artificial Insemination by Donor (AID)." *Journal of Biosocial Science* 11(4) (1979):473–9.

———. "The Establishment of a Programme of Artificial Insemination by Donor Semen within the National Health Service." *British Journal of Obstetrics and Gynaecology* 83 (1976):917–20.

Leeton J., et al. "A Preliminary Psychosocial Follow-up of Parents and Their Children Conceived by Artificial Insemination by Donor (AID)." *Clinical Reproduction and Fertility* 1(4) (December 1982):307–10.

———, and J. Blackwell. "Artificial Donor Insemination." *Australian & New Zealand Journal of Obstetrics and Gynaecology* 15 (1976):45.

———. "Artificial Donor Insemination: Frozen versus Fresh Semen." *Australian and New Zealand Journal of Obstetrics and Gynaecology* 20 (1980) 205.

———. "Artificial Insemination by Donor: The Main Treatment for Male Infertility." *Australian Family Physician* 10(2) (Feb. 1981):102–4.

Leiblum, S. R., et al. "Artificial Insemination by Donor: A Survey of Attitudes and Knowledge in Medical Students and Infertile Couples." *Journal of Biosocial Science* 15(2) (April 1983):165–72.

Le Lannou, Dominique. "Sperm Banks and Donor Recruitment in France," in *Human Artificial Insemination and Semen Production,* Georges David and Wendel S. Price, eds. New York: Plenum, 1980.

Leridon, H. "Public Opinion on AID and Sterility," in *Human Artificial Insemination and Semen Production,* Georges David and Wendel S. Price, eds. New York: Plenum, 1980.

Leto, S., and F. Frensilli. "Changing Parameters of Donor Semen," *Fertility & Sterility* 36(6) (Dec. 1981).

Levie, L. H. "An Inquiry into the Psychological Effects on Parents of Artificial Insemination with Donor Semen." *Eugenics Review* 59 (1967):91.

———. "Donor Insemination in Holland." *World Medical Bulletin* 19(5) (Sept.-Oct. 1972):90–1.

Lifton, Betty Jean. "Brave New Babies in a Brave New World." *Women and Health* December 1987.

Lim, C. "Artificial Insemination with Donor Semen: An Analysis of 53 Recorded Pregnancies in 50 Patients." *Singapore Medical Journal* 23(4) (August 1982):198–200.

Lourus, N. C. "Against Heterologous Insemination." *International Surgery* 58 (1973):190–1.

Løvset, J. "Artificial Insemination—Attitudes of Patients in Norway." *Fertility & Sterility* (2)5 (1951):415.

MacLean, A. B., et al. "Artificial Insemination by Donor." *New Zealand Medical Journal* 97(760) (July 25, 1984):484–6.

MacLeod, S. C. "Human Male Infertility." *Obstetrics & Gynecology Survey* 26 (1971):335–51.

MacNaughton, M. D. "Artificial Insemination by Donor." *Scottish Medical Journal* 27(2) (1982):109–110.

Macourt, D., and G. R. Jones. "Artificial Insemination with Donor Semen." *Medical Journal of Australia* 1 (1977):693–5.

Mady, T. M. "Surrogate Mothers: The Legal Issues." *American Journal of Law and Medicine* 7(3) (Fall 1981):323–52.

Mahadevan, M. M., et al. "Effect of Factors Related to the Recipient and Insemination Characteristics on the Success of Artificial Insemination with Frozen Semen." *Clinical Reproduction & Fertility* 1(3) (Sept. 1982):195–204.

———. "Influence of Semen and Donor Factors on the Success Rate of Artificial Insemination with Frozen Semen." *Clinical Reproduction and Fertility* 1(3) (Sept. 1982):185–93.

Mai, F., et al. "Psychiatric Interview Comparisons between Infertile and Fertile Couples." *Psychosomatic Medicine* 34 (1972):436.

Mantegazza, D. "Fisiologia sullo Sperma Umano." *Rend Reale 1st Lombardo* 3 (1866): 183.

Manuel C., et al. "Handling of Secrecy by Artificial Insemination Couples," in *Human Artificial Insemination and Semen Production,* Georges David and Wendel S. Price, eds. New York: Plenum, 1980.

———. "A Follow-up Study on Children Born through Artificial Insemination by Donor," in *Human Artificial Insemination and Semen Production,* Georges David and Wendel S. Price, eds. New York: Plenum, 1980.

Marshall, J. "AID: An Occasion for Creative Law-Making." *Soundings* 50(4) (1971):325–30.

Mascola, L., and M. E. Guinan. "Screening to Reduce Transmission of Sexually Transmitted Diseases in Semen Used for Artificial Insemination." *New England Journal of Medicine* 314 (1986): 1354–59.

———. "Banishing AIDS from Donor Semen." *Contemporary Obstetrics and Gynecology* 28 (1986): 27–35.

———. "Semen Donors as the Source of Sexually Transmitted Diseases in Artificially Inseminated Women: The Saga Unfolds." *Journal of the American Medical Association* 257(8) (Feb. 27, 1987) 109–34.

Mason, S. "Abnormal Conception." *Australian Law Journal* 56 (July 1982):347.

Matchan, L. "What It's Like to Be a Lesbian Mother," *The Boston Globe,* September 25, 1980.

Matheson, G. W., et al. "Frozen Human Semen for Artificial Insemination." *American Journal of Obstetrics and Gynecology* 104 (1969):495–501.

Mattei, J. F., et al. "Genetic Aspects of Artificial Insemination by Donor (AID): Indications, Surveillance and Results." *Clinical Genetics* 23(2) (Feb. 1983):132–8.

Matteson, R. L., and G. Terranova. "Social Acceptance of New Techniques of Child Conception." *Journal of Social Psychology* 101 (1977):225–229.

Matthews, C. D., et al. "Screening of Karyotype and Semen Quality in an Artificial Insemination Program: Acceptance and Rejection Criteria." *Fertility & Sterility* 40(5) (Nov. 1983):648–54.

———. "The Influence of Insemination Timing and Semen Characteristics on the Efficacy of a Donor Insemination Program." *Fertility & Sterility* 31 (1979):45.

Mayaux, M. J., et al. "Conception Rate According to Semen Characteristics in a Series of 15,364 Insemination Cycles: Results of a Multivariate Analysis." *Andrologia* 17(1) (Jan.-Feb. 1985):9–15.

Mayo, M. "The Legal Status of the AID Child in Australia." *Australian Law Journal* 50 (1976):562.

Mazor, Miriam. "Barren Couples." *Psychology Today* May 1978.

McCormack, M. K., et al. "Attitudes Regarding the Utilization of Artificial Insemination by Donor in Huntington's Disease." *American Journal of Medical Genetics* 14(1) (Jan. 1983):5–13.

McGowan, M. P. et al. "Selection of High Fertility Donors for Artificial Insemination Programmes." *Clinical Reproduction and Fertility* 2(4) (Dec. 1983):269–74.

McGuire, L. S. "Obstetrics and Gynecology: Psychologic Management of the Infertile Woman." *Postgraduate Medicine* 57 (May 1975):173–76.

McGuire, M., and N. Alexander. "Artificial Insemination of Single Women." *Fertility & Sterility* 43(2) (Feb. 1985):182–84.

McLaren, Anne. "Biological Aspects of Artificial Insemination." CIBA Foundation Symposium #17. New Holland, Amsterdam: Elsevier, 1973.

———, and A. S. Parkes. "Legal and Other Aspects of Artificial Insemination by Donor (AID) and Embryo Transfer." *Journal of Biosocial Science* 5 (1973):205–8.

McLaughlin, E. A., et al. "Use of Home Insemination in Programmes of Artificial Insemination with Donor Semen." *British Medical Journal* 287 (October 15, 1983):1110.

McLeod, J., and Y. Want. "Male Fertility Potential in Terms of Semen Quality: A Review of the Past, a Study of the Present." *Fertility & Sterility* 31 (1979):103.

Mehren, E. "A Controversial Sperm Bank Where the Women Are in Charge," *Los Angeles Times* February 6, 1983.

Menning, Barbara Eck. "The Emotional Needs of Infertile Couples." *Fertility & Sterility* 34(4) (Oct. 1980):313–9.

———. "Counseling Infertility Couples." *Contemporary Obstetrics and Gynecology* February 1979.

———. "Donor Insemination: The Psychosocial Issues." *Contemporary Ob-Gyn* 18(4) (Oct. 1981)155.

———. "The Psychosocial Impact of Infertility." *Nursing Clinics of North America* 17(1) (March 1982) 155–63.

Miller, N. "Family Planning: Artificial Insemination and Single Mothers." *The Boston Phoenix* December 11, 1984.

———. "Artificial Insemination." *Glamour* November 1980.

Miller, Warren B. "Reproduction, Technology and the Behavioral Sciences," *Science* 1974 149.

Milsom I. "A Study of Parental Attitudes after Donor Insemination." *Acta Obstet Gynecol Scandinavia* 61(2) (1982):125–8.

Milunsky, A., and G. Annas. "Legal Aspects of Artificial Insemination by Donor—Paternity Testing." *Genetics and the Law* New York: Plenum, 1976.

Mitchell, G. D., and R. Snowden. "Why AID Is More than a Medical Issue." *World Medicine* (March 8, 1980):85–7.

Miyata, J., et al. "Timing of Ovulation by a Rapid Luteinizing Radioimmunassay." *Fertility & Sterility* 21 (1970):784.

Mochimaru et al. "Physical and Mental Development of Children Born Through AID," in *Human Artificial Insemination and Semen Production*, Georges David and Wendel S. Price, eds. New York: Plenum, 1980.

Moghissi, K. S. "Accuracy of Basal Body Temperature for Ovulation Detection." *Fertility & Sterility* 27 (1976):1415.

Molne K., et al. "Donor Insemination." *Tidsskr Nor Laegeforen* 102(22) (Norwegian) (August 10, 1982):1058–61.

Monoham, T. P. "Is Childlessness Related to Family Stability?" *American Sociological Review* 1055(20):446.

Morgan, J., et al. "Risk of AIDS with Artificial Insemination." (letter) *New England Journal of Medicine* 314(6) (Feb. 6, 1986):386.

Mortimer, D. "Sex Ratio of Births Resulting from Artificial Insemination." *British Journal of Obstetrics and Gynaecology* 89(2) (Feb. 1982):132–5.

Mudge, T. D. "Updates in Brief—The Concept of Fecundity." *Clinical Reproduction & Fertility* 1 (1982):331–40.

Muller, H. J. "Human Evolution by Voluntary Choice of Germ Plasm." *Science* 134 (1961):643–9.

Murdock, R. L., et al. "Trisomy 21 from an AID Pregnancy: Questions Regarding Management." (letter) *American Journal of Medical Genetics* 15(2) (1983):341–2.

Murphy, D. P. "Donor Insemination: a Study of 511 Prospective Donors," *Fertility & Sterility* 15(5) (1964):528–33.

———, and E. Torrano. "A Study of 112 Women." *Fertility & Sterility* 17 (March-April 1966):273–7.

———. "The Day of Conception: A Study of 48 Women Having Two or More Conceptions by Donor Insemination." *Fertility & Sterility* 14 (1963):410.

Nagel, T. C., G. E. Tagatz, and B. F. Campbell. "Transmission of Chlamydia Trichomatis by Artificial Insemination." *Fertility & Sterility* 46 (1986): 959–60.

Nakamura, M. S., et al. "Conception Rate after AIH." *Archives of Andrology* 5 (1980):46.

Nash, D., et al. "The Value of Hysterosalpingograms Prior to Donor Insemination." *Fertility & Sterility* 31 (1979):378–80.

Need, J. A., et al. "Pre-eclampsia in Pregnancies from Donor Inseminations." *Journal of Reproductive Immunology* 5(6) (Nov. 1983):329–38.

Nevill, R., et al. "The Basal Body Temperature Chart in Artificial Insemination by Donor Pregnancy Cycles." *Fertility & Sterility* 38(4) (Oct. 1982):431–8.

Newall, R. G. "AID—Artificial Insemination by Donor—A Review of 200 Cases." *British Journal of Urology* 48 (1976):139–44.

Newton, J. R. "Artificial Insemination with Frozen Stored Donor Semen." *British Journal of Obstetrics and Gynaecology* 85(9) (1978):641–4.

Nicholas, M. K., and J. P. Tyler. "Characteristics, Attitudes and Personalities of Artificial Insemination Donors." *Clinical Reproduction & Fertility* 2 (1983):47.

Nijs, P., et al. "AID Donors: Medical and Psychological Aspects: A Preliminary Report," in *Human Artificial Insemination and Semen Production*, Georges David and Wendel S. Price, eds. New York: Plenum, 1980.

———, and L. Rouffa. "AID Couples' Psychological and Psychopathological Evaluation." *Andrologia* 7(3) (1975):187–194.

———. "AID Couples: Psychological and Psychopathological Evaluation," in *The Family*, H. Hirth, ed. Basel, Switzerland: Karger, 1975.

Norton, R., et al. "Risk Parameters Across Types of Secrets." *Journal of Counselling Psychology* 21 (1974):450–4.

Olshansky, E. F., and L. N. Sammons. "Artificial Insemination: An Overview." *Journal of Obstetrical, Gynecological and Neonatal Nursing* (Supplement) Nov.-Dec. 1985.

O'Neil, J. "Artificial Insemination of Donor Sperm." (letter) *New Zealand Medical Journal* 96(272) (March 9, 1983):183–4.

Ostrom, K. "Psychological Considerations in the Evaluation of AID." *Soundings: Hastings Center Report* 50(4) (1971):290–301.

Parker, P. J. "Psychological Factors for Adults Involved with Reproductive Alternatives and their Input to the Children." Presented at the American Society of Law and Medicine Conference, Cambridge, MA, Oct. 1984.

———. "Motivation of Surrogate Mothers: Initial Findings." *American Journal of Psychiatry* 140(1) (Jan. 1983):107–18.

———. "Surrogate Mothers: The Interaction of Litigation, Legislation and Psychiatry." *International Journal of Law & Psychiatry* (5) (1983):341–51.

Payne, S., and R. F. Skeels. "Fertility as Evaluated by Artificial Insemination." *Fertility & Sterility* 5 (1951):1.

Peckins, D. M. "Artificial Insemination and the Law." *Journal of Legal Medicine* 4 (1976):17–22.

Peek, J. C., et al. "Estimation of Fertility and Fecundity in Women receiving Artificial Insemination by Donor Semen and in Normal Fertile Women." *British Journal of Obstetrics & Gynaecology* 91 (1984):1019–24.

Peel Committee. "Report of the Panel on Human Artificial Insemination." *British Medical Journal* 2 (suppl.) 3 (April 7, 1973):51.

Pennington, G. W. "Artificial Insemination by Donor." *British Medical Journal* 4(5990) (Oct. 25, 1975):225–226.

———, and S. Naik. "Donor Insemination: Report of a 2-Year Study." *British Medical Journal* 2 (1977):132.

Peyser, H. S. "Untoward Effects of Artificial Insemination." *New York State Journal of Medicine* 65 (1965):1876.

Peyser, M. R., et al. "Impact of Stress of AID on the Menstrual Cycle." *International Journal of Fertility* 26(1) (1981):68–70.

———. "Stress-Induced Delay of Ovulation." *Obstetrics and Gynecology* 42 (1973): 667–71.

Philipp, E. E. "Moral, Social, and Ethical Issues," in *Human Artificial Insemination,* Georges David and Wendel S. Price, eds. New York: Plenum, 1980.

Pinkerton, C. R. "Artificial Insemination for the Single Woman." (letter) Lancet 1(8278) (April 24, 1982):968.

Poland, M. L., et al. "Impact of Stress of AID on the Menstrual Cycle." *International Journal of Fertility* 26(1) (1981):68–70.

Pollock, M. "Sex and Its Problems, VIII: Artificial Insemination." *Practitioner* 99 (August 1962):244–52.

Portnoy, L. "AID Experiences with Its Use in 80 Barren Marriages." *Fertility & Sterility* 7 (1956):327.

Portuondo, J. A., et al. "Clomiphene Use for Donor Artificial Insemination." *International Journal of Fertility* 27(3) (1982):171–5.

Potter, R. G. "Artificial Insemination by Donor: Analysis of Fertility Series." *Fertility & Sterility* 9(1958)37.

Poyen, B., et al. "Is There a Right to AID?" in *Human Artificial Insemination and Semen Production,* Georges David and Wendel S. Price, eds. New York: Plenum, 1980.

Propping D., et al. "AID Success Rates: One or More Inseminations Per Cycle? *Archives of Andrology* 5 (1980):44–52.

Quindlen, Anna. "Baby Craving: Facing Widespread Infertility, a Generation Presses the Limits of Medicine and Morality." *Life* June 1987.

Quinlivan, W. L. "Therapeutic Donor Insemination (TDI) versus Artificial Donor Insemination (AID)." *Fertility & Sterility* 40(5) (1983):705.

———. "Therapeutic Donor Inseminations: Results and Causes of Nonfertilization." *Fertility & Sterility* 32 (1972):157.

———, and H. Sullivan. "Spermatozoal Antibodies in Human Seminal Plasma as a Cause of Failed Artificial Donor Insemination." *Fertility & Sterility* 28 (1977):1082–5.

———. "The Immunological Effect of Husband's Semen on Donor Spermatozoa During Mixed Insemination." *Fertility & Sterility* 28(1977) 448.

Raboch, J., and Z. D. Tomaset. "Therapeutic Donor Insemination— Results." *Journal of Reproduction & Fertility* 14 (1967):421–5.

Rajan, R. "Eight Years with Therapeutic Insemination." *Journal of Indian Medical Association* 79(8) (Oct. 16, 1982):112–5.

————. "Laparoscopy and Laparotomy Evaluation of Artificial Donor Insemination Failures." *Journal of Indian Medical Association* 79(4) (August 16, 1982):50–3.

Ramsay, J. "Artificial Insemination Option." *McCall's* August 1975.

Rawson, G. "Human Artificial Insemination by Donor and the Australian Community." *Clinical Reproduction & Fertility* 3(1) (March 1985):1–19.

Rayner, K. "AID" (Artificial Insemination by Donor) Social Responsibilities Commission on Human Artificial Insemination, Anglican Church Office, 44 Currie Street, Adelaide, South Australia 5000.

Reading, A. E., et al. "A Survey of Patient Attitudes toward Artificial Insemination by Donor." *Journal of Psychosomatic Research* 26(4) (1982):428–33.

Renaud, R. "Ultrasound Monitoring of Ovulation." *Lancet* 1 (1979):665.

Report on Panel of Human Artificial Insemination. (Appendix V). *British Medical Journal* April 7, 1973.

Richards, R. P. "Artificial Insemination: Ethical and Theological Aspects." *Soundings: Hastings Center Report* 50:4 (1971) 315–23.

Richards, S. "Open Adoption Can Ease Qualms of Both Families." *The Oregonian* August 9, 1983.

————. "Ethical and Theological Aspects." *Soundings: Hastings Center Report* 50 (1971):4.

Richardson, D. W. "Factors Influencing the Fertility of Frozen Semen," in *Frozen Human Semen: Proceedings of a Workshop Upon the Cryobiology of Human Semen and its Role in Artificial Insemination by Donor*, D. Richardson, et al., eds. London: Royal College of Obstetricians and Gynaecologists, 1979.

————. "Organization of Sperm Banks on a National Basis," in *Human Artificial Insemination and Semen Production*, Georges David and Wendel S. Price, eds. New York: Plenum, 1980.

Richter, M. A., et al. "Artificial Donor Insemination: Fresh versus Frozen Semen: The Patient as Her Own Control." *Fertility & Sterility* 41(2) (Feb. 1984):277–80.

Robertson, John "Procreative Liberty and the Control of Conception, Pregnancy and Childbirth." *Virginia Law Review* 69(3) (April 1983).

Rock, J. A., et al. "AID with Fresh Donor Semen Using the Cervical Cap Technique: A Review of 273 Cases." *Archives of Andrology* 5 (1980):27–33.

Rooyackers, J. M. "Adoption, Sperm Donorship and Confidentiality." *Nederlandse Tijdschrift Geneeskunde* (Dutch) 129 (51) (December 21, 1985):2473–4.

Rorvik, D. N. "Birth Without Sex." *Esquire* 71 (April 1969):110.

Rosenberg, H. "Legal Aspects of Artificial Insemination." *New England Journal of Medicine* 278 (March 7, 1968):552–54.

Rosenfeld, A. "The Adoptees Union." *Science* October 1981.

Rosenkvist, H. "Donor Insemination: A Prospective Socio-Psychiatric Investigation of 48 Couples." *Danish Medical Bulletin* 28 (1981):4.

Rosner, F., and S. P. Deaner. "Artificial Insemination in New Mexico." *National Research Journal* 1(2) (1970):353.

Rothman, B. Katz. "The Meanings of Choice in Reproductive Technology," in *Test-Tube Women: What Future for Motherhood?* R. Arditti, et al., eds. Boston: Routledge and Kegan Paul, 1984.

———. "How Science Is Redefining Parenthood." *Ms.* July-August 1982.

Rowland, R. "Attitudes and Opinions of Donors on an Artificial Insemination by Donor (AID) Programme." *Clinical Reproduction and Fertility* 2(2) (June 1983):151–60.

———. "Social Implications of Reproductive Technology." *International Review of Natural Family Planning* 8(3) (1984):189–205.

Rowland, R., and C. Rufin. "Community Attitudes to Artificial Insemination by Donor Programme." *Clinical Reproduction and Fertility* 2(1983):249–59.

Roy, D. J. "AID: An Overview of Ethical Issues," in *Human Artificial Insemination and Semen Production*, Georges David and Wendel S. Price, eds. New York: Plenum, 1980.

Rubin, B., et al. "Psychological Aspects of Human Artificial Insemination." *Archives of General Psychiatry* 13 (1965):121–32.

Rubin, S. (letter) School Paper, California State University, Northridge, CA, Sept. 1981.

———. "A Sperm-donor Baby Grows Up" in *The Technological Woman*, J. Zimmerman, ed. New York: Praeger, 1983.

Ruiz-Velasco, V., et al. "Role of Laparoscopy in Heterologous Therapeutic Insemination (AID)." *International Journal of Fertility* 27(2) (1982):119–20.

Russell, J. K., and A. P. B. Mitchell. "Clinical Approach to Infertility." *Lancet* 1 (1952):1161–62.

Rutherford, R. N., and L. Banks. "Semiadoption Technics and Results." *Fertility & Sterility* 5 (1954):271.

Sagall, E. "Artificial Insemination." *Trial* 9 (Jan.-Feb. 1973):59–63.

Sampson, J. H., et al. "Gender after Artificial Induction of Ovulation and Artificial Insemination." *Fertility & Sterility* 41 (Jan. 1984):144–5.

Samuels, A. "Artificial Insemination and Genetic Engineering: The Legal Problems." *Medical Science Law*, 22(4) (Oct. 1982):261–8.

Sandler, B. "Artificial Insemination—the Social Implications." *Mental Health* 24 (Feb. 1965):16–18.

———. "Donor Insemination in England." *World Medical Bulletin* 19(5) (Sept.-Oct. 1972):87–89.

Sants, H. J. "Genealogical Bewilderment in Children with Substitute Parents." *British Journal of Medical Psychology* 37 (1964):133–41.

Sargeant, D. A. "The Legal Status of Artificial Insemination: A Need for Policy Formulation." *Drake Law Review* 19 (1970):409–440.

Saunders, M. (letter) "Artificial Insemination with Donor Semen." *New England Journal of Medicine* (Jan. 29, 1976) 294–5.

Sawada, Y. "Heterologous and Homologous Insemination with Human Frozen Semen Frozen and Stored in a Liquid Nitrogen Tank Refrigerator." *Fertility & Sterility* 17(1966)451.

Sawada, Y., et al. "Motility and Respiration of Human Spermatozoa after Cooling to Various Low Temperatures." *Fertility & Sterility* 6 (1979):775.

Schaad, C. "AID and Its Medical and Psychological Indications." *Archives of Andrology* 5 (1980):44–52.

Schacht, L. E., et al. "Frequency of Extra-marital Children as Determined by Blood Groups." in *Second International Conference of Human Genetics*, Brockington, et al. eds. Amsterdam: Excerpta Medica 1961.

Schatkin, Sidney B. "The Legal Aspects of Artificial Insemination." *Fertility & Sterility* 5 (1954):1.

Schiff, I., et al. "HTLV III Antibody Testing in Sperm Donors." *New England Journal of Medicine* 312 (1985):1638.

Sclaff, W. D. "Transmission of Disease During Artificial Insemination." *New England Journal of Medicine* 315 (1986): 1289.

———. "Mode of Evaluation of Results in Artificial Insemination," in *Human Artificial Insemination and Semen Production*, Georges David and Wendel S. Price, eds. New York: Plenum, 1980.

Schoysman, R. "Problems of Selecting Donors for Artificial Insemination." *Journal of Medical Ethics* 1 (1975):34.

Schroeder, L. O. "New Life or Property?" *American Journal of Psychiatry* 131 (May 1974):541–4.

Schwartz, D., et al. "Donor Insemination: Conception Rate According to Cycle Day in a Series of 821 Cycles with a Single Insemination." *Fertility & Sterility* 31 (1979):226.

————. "Female Fecundity as a Function of Age: Results of Artificial Insemination in 2193 Nulliparous Women with Azoospermic Husbands." *New England Journal of Medicine* 306(7) (February 18, 1982):404–6.

Segel, S., and M. Sherer. "The Use of Donor Mucus and Insemination for Cervical Factor." *International Journal of Fertility* 24(4) (1979):291–2.

Seligmann, J. "Life Without Father: AID." *Newsweek* September 22, 1975.

Selwood, T. S., and J. F. Leeton. "Frequency of Insemination for Artificial Insemination by Donor." *Australian and New Zealand Journal of Obstetrics and Gynaecology* 22(2) (May 1982):84–5.

————. "Medical and Psychological Preliminaries for Artificial Insemination." *Fertility & Sterility* VII World Congress, in T. Hasegawa, et al., eds., *Fertility & Sterility: Proceedings of the VII World Congress.* Kyoto, Japan, October 1973. New York: Elsevier, 1973.

Semenov, G., et al. "Attempt at Follow-up of Children Born Through AID," in *Human Artificial Insemination and Semen Production,* Georges David and Wendel S. Price, eds. New York: Plenum, 1980.

Shapiro, D. N., et al. "Familial Histiocytosis in Offspring of Two Pregnancies after Artificial Insemination." *New England Journal of Medicine* 304(1981)757.

Shapiro, S. S. "Induction of Pregnancy in a Woman with Seminal Plasma Allergy." *Fertility & Sterility* 36(3) (1981):405–7.

————. "Some Unresolved Questions about Artificial Insemination." *Contemporary OB-GYN* 17 (Jan. 1981):129.

Shearer, Lloyd. "Father's Identity—the Right to Know." *Parade* July 29, 1984.

————. "This Woman and This Man Made History." *Parade* May 3, 1983.

————. "The Rise of Illegitimate Births." *Parade* Dec. 16, 1984.

Sheikh, H. H., and M. A. Yussman. "Radiation Exposure of Ovaries during Hysterosalpingogram." *American Journal of Obstetrics and Gynecology* 124 (1976):307–10.

Sherman, J. K. "Frozen Semen: Efficiency in Artificial Insemination and Advantage in Testing for Acquired Immune Deficiency Syndrome." *Fertility & Sterility* 47(1) (Jan. 1987):19–21.

————. "Synopsis of the Art of Frozen Human Semen Since 1964: State of the Art of Human Semen Banking." *Fertility & Sterility* 24 (May 5, 1973):397–412.

————. "Research on Frozen Human Semen." *Fertility & Sterility* 15 (1975):487.

————. "Long-Term Cryopreservation of Motility and Fertility of Human Spermatozoa." *Cryobiology* 9 (1972): 332.

————. "Research on Frozen Human Semen: Past, Present, and Future." *Fertility & Sterility* 5 (1964):485.

————. "Improved Methods of Preservation of Human Spermatozoa by Freezing and Freeze-Drying." *Fertility & Sterility* 14 (1963): 49.

————. "Freezing and Freeze-Drying." *Fertility & Sterility* 5 (1954): 357.

Sherwood, H. J. "Some Legal Implications of Frozen Semen Banks." *Journal of Reproductive Medicine* 8 (1972):190.

Shields, Frances E. "Artificial Insemination as Related to the Female." *Fertility & Sterility* 1(3) (1950):271.

Silber, S. "Babies for Infertile Couples: Part 2: For Males," *Saturday Evening Post* April 1982.

Simmons, F. A. "The Role of the Husband in Therapeutic Donor Insemination," *Fertility & Sterility* 8(6) (1957):547–50.

Simpson, J. L. "Genetic Screening for Donors in Artificial Insemination." (editorial) *Fertility & Sterility* 35(4) (April 1981):395–6.

Slome, J. "Artificial Insemination by Donor." *British Medical Journal* 2 (1973):365.

Small, E. C., et al. "A View of Artificial Insemination." *Advances in Psychosomatic Medicine* 12 (1985):105–23.

Smith, G. P. "Artificial Insemination Redivius: Permutations Within a Penumbra." *Journal of Legal Medicine* (Chicago) 2 (June 2, 1981):113–30.

————. "For Unto Us a Child Is Born Legally," *American Bar Association Journal* 56 (1970):143.

————. "Great Expectations of Convoluted Realities: Artificial Insemination Influx." *Family Law Review* 1980 3:37–44.

Smith, K. D., et al. "The Influence of Ovulatory Dysfunction and Timing on the Success of Artificial Insemination with Fresh or Cryopreserved Semen." *Fertility & Sterility* 36(4) (Oct. 1981)496.

Smith, P. E. "Selection Against Genetic Defects in Donors." *Clinical Genetics* 26(2) (August 1984):87–108.

Sokoloff, B. "Alternative Methods of Reproduction: Effects on the Child." *Clinical Pediatrics* 26(1987)1:11.

Somerville, M. "Birth Technology, Parenting and Deviance." *International Journal of Law & Psychiatry,* 5 (1982):123–153.

Sorich, Carol, and R. Siebert. "Toward Humanizing AID." *Child Welfare* 16(4) (April 1982):207–16.

Spallanzi, L. "Osservazioni ed Esperienze Intorno ai Vermicelli Spermatici dell'Uomo e degle Animali." *Opuscoli di Fisica Animale e Vegetale,* Modena 1776.

Spann, W. "The Reproductive Process from the Legal Viewpoint." (German) *Munchener Medizinische Wochenschrift* 125(49) (Nov. 25, 1983):1091–2.

Steigrad, Stephen. "The AID Process." *Adoption and AID—Issues and Concerns* (seminar) Crown Street Hospital, Sydney, Australia, April 3, 1982.

Steinberg, E., and K. D. Smith. "Artificial Insemination with Fresh or Frozen Semen." *Journal of the American Medical Association* 233 (1973):778.

Stern, Susan. "Lesbian Insemination." *Co-Evolution Quarterly* 108 (Summer 1980):17.

Stewart, C. R., et al. "The Development of a Psychosocial Approach to Artificial Insemination of Donor Sperm." *New Zealand Medical Journal* 95(721) (Dec. 8, 1982):853–6.

Stewart, G. J., et al. "Transmission of Human T-Cell Lymphotrophic Virus Type III (HTLV-III) by Artificial Insemination Donor." *Lancet* 2 (1985):581–84.

Stewart, W. "What Should the Doctor Know about Exogamous Artificial Insemination?" *Journal of the American Medical Women's Association* 9(1) (1954):368–70.

Stone, C. "Sperm Bank." *U.S.* Oct. 26, 1982.

Stone, Olive. "Discussion: Legal Aspects." CIBA Foundation Symposium #17, *Excerpta Medica*. North Holland: Elsevier, 1973.

Stone, S. C. "Complications and Pitfalls of Artificial Insemination." *Clinical Obstetrics & Gynecology*. 23 (1980):667–82.

Strickler, R. C., et al. "Artificial Insemination with Fresh Donor Semen." *New England Journal of Medicine* 293 (1975):848.

Strong, C., et al. "The Single Woman and Artificial Insemination by Donor." *Journal of Reproductive Medicine* 29(5) (May 1984):293–9.

Sulewski, J. M., et al. "A Longitudinal Analysis of Artificial Insemination with Donor Semen." *Fertility & Sterility* 29 (1978):527.

Sullivan, J. "Families: Is This the End?" *The Age,* Melbourne, Australia, August 17, 1982.

Symonds, E. M. "Factors Influencing Successful AID with Frozen Semen." in *Frozen Human Semen,* D. Richardson, et al., eds. London: Royal College of Obstetricians and Gynaecologists, 1979.

Tagatz, G. E., et al. "AID Utilizing Donor Semen." *Minnesota Medicine* 63 (1980):539.

Tauber, P. I. "Insemination from the Physician's Viewpoint." *Munchener Medizinische Wochenschrift* (German) 125(47) (Nov. 25, 1983): 1086–9.

Tekavcic, B. "Are There Any Psychological Consequences in Husband,

Wife and Donor after AID?" *Fertility & Sterility* VII World Congress, in *Fertility & Sterility: Proceedings of the VII World Congress,* T. Hasegawa, et al., eds. Kyoto, Japan, Oct. 1973. New York: Elsevier, 1973.

Teper, S., et al. "Artificial Insemination by Donor: Problems and Perspectives." *Proceedings of the Annual Symposium of the Eugenics Society.* 19 (1983):19–52.

Thompson, W. "Counselling Patients for Artificial Insemination and Subsequent Pregnancy." *Clinical Obstetrics and Gynaecology* 9(1) (April 1982):211–25.

Thorneycroft, I. H., et al. "Donor Fertility in an Artificial Insemination Program." *Fertility & Sterility* 41(1) (Jan. 1984):144–5.

Timmons, M. C., et al. "Genetic Screening of Donors for Artificial Insemination." *Fertility & Sterility* 35(4) (April 1981):451–6.

Trounson, A. O., et al. "Artificial Insemination by Frozen Donor Semen: Results of a Multicentre Australian Experience." *International Journal of Andrology* 2 (April 4, 1981):227–34.

Tyler, E. T. "The Clinical Use of Frozen Semen Bank." *Fertility & Sterility,* 24(5)413–16.

Van der Ven, H. H., et al. "Effect of Heterologous Seminal Plasma on the Fertilizing Capacity of Human Spermatozoa as Assessed by the Zona-free Hamster Egg Test." *Fertility & Sterility* 13(5) (Oct. 1983):50.

Veevers, J. E. "Voluntarily Childless Wives: An Exploratory Study." *Sociology and Social Research* 57 (April 1975):356–66.

Vernon, G. A., and J. A. Broadway. "Attitudes Toward Artificial Insemination and Some Variables Associated Therewith." *Marriage & Family* 21 (1959):43.

Verp, M. S., et al. "The Necessity of Formal Genetic Screening in Artificial Insemination by Donor." *Obstetrics and Gynecology* 62(4) (Oct. 1983):474–9.

Virro, M. R., et al. "Pregnancy Outcome in 242 Conceptions after Artifical Insemination with Donor Sperm and Effects of Maternal Age on the Prognosis for Successful Pregnancy." *American Journal of Obstetrics and Gynecology* 148(5) (March 1, 1984):518–24.

Wadlington, Walter. "Artificial Insemination: the Dangers of a Poorly-kept Secret." *Northwestern University Law Review* 64 (Jan.-Feb. 1970):6.

Waltzer, H. "Psychological and Legal Aspects of Artificial Insemination (AID): An overview." *American Journal of Psychotherapy* 36(1) (Jan. 1982):91-102.

Warming, B. "Insemination Procedures—Cervical Cap." *Fertility & Sterility* 34(4) (Oct. 1980):407–8.

Warner, M. P. "Review of AID after 32 years Experience." *New York State Journal of Medicine* 13 (Dec. 1974):2358–61.

Waters, E. "The Baby Makers." *Family Circle* (Australia) Dec. 4, 1984.

Watters, W. W., and J. Sousa-Poza. "Psychiatric Aspects of AID." *Canadian Medical Association Journal* 95 (1966):106.

Weinstock, F. "Artificial Insemination—the Problem and the Solution." *Family Law Quarterly* 5 (1971):369.

Weisman, A. I. "Studies on Human Artificial Insemination." *Western Journal of Surgical Obstetrics & Gynecology* 55 (1947):348–51.

———. "Selection of Donors for Use in Artificial Insemination." *Western Journal of Surgical Obstetrics & Gynecology* 50 (1942):142.

Wellisch, E. "Children Without Genealogy: A Problem of Adoption." *Mental Health* 13:1(1952).

Whelan, D. "The Law and Artificial Insemination with Donor Semen (AID)." *Medical Journal of Australia* 1 (Jan. 14, 1978):56–8.

Whitelaw, M. J. "Use of the Cervical Cap to Increase Fertility in Case of Oligospermia." *Fertility & Sterility.* 1(1950)33.

Wieder, Herbert. "On Being Told of Adoption." *Psychoanalytical Quarterly* 46 (Jan. 1977):1.

Wimmer, H. "Sperm Trade Across the Atlantic?" (German) *MedWelt* 1983 34(1).

Wing, R., et al. "Artificial Donor Insemination: Analysis of 149 Cases at North Carolina Memorial Hospital." *Southern Medical Journal* 77(5) (May 1984):607–10.

Wolfers, H. "Psychological Aspects of Vasectomy." *British Medical Journal* 4 (1970):297–300.

Wong, P. C., et al. "Sperm Washing and Swimming Technique Using Antibodies Removes Microbes from Human Semen." *Fertility & Sterility* (45)1 (Jan. 1986):97–100.

Wood, C., et al. (letter) "Artificial Insemination by Donor Clinics." *Medical Journal of Australia* 2(8) (Oct. 18, 1980):462.

Worsnop, D., et al. "Human Artificial Insemination Donors in Melbourne from our Medical Schools." *Australian Family Physician* 3(218) (1982):20–4.

Younger, J. B. et al. "The Use of One-day Lutenizing Hormone Assay for Timing of Artificial Insemination in Infertility Patients." *Fertility & Sterility* 30(1978)648.

Zacur, H., and J. Rock. "Diagnosis and Treatment of Infertility." *Female Patient* Feb. 8, 1983.

Ziporyn, T. "Artificial Human Reproduction Poses Medical, Social Concern." *Journal of the American Medical Association* 255 (1986):13–15.

Index

Abortion
   availability of, 23, 31, 43
   and IVF, 67
   public discussion of, 72
   See also Miscarriage
Access to DI, 32, 94, 157, 202,
   232, 277, 300
Achilles, Rona, 49, 62, 73, 85,
   140, 152, 155, 217, 292,
   319–20, 323, 352
Adoptees, 73
   access to origins by, 221
   numbers of, 293
   psychological disturbances
   of, 339–40
   rights of, 320
   searching by, 340–42
   as victims of system, 1, 21,
   81, 225, 325
Adoption, 10, 12, 21, 23, 40,
   43–46, 51, 66, 81
   American Congress on, 352
   closed, 166
   cooperative, 350
   after DI, 12, 66
   failed, 300

legislation on, 245–46
open, 164–69, 346–47
in other cultures, 165–66
reform of, 1, 10, 51, 327
See also Search for biological
   parent in adoption
Adultery
   court rulings in DI cases,
   260–62, 264
   and DI, 56, 63, 68, 247–48
   DI seen as, 176, 202
   religious view of DI as, 52,
   210
   secrecy and, 82
   because of sterility, 200
Age
   of DI recipients, 94, 100–101
   of donors, 133, 173, 259
AIDS
   from DI, 64, 109, 125, 134,
   202, 230
   quarantining for, 102–3
   screening by law, 255–56,
   267, 278
American Academy of Pediatrics, 81

American Association of Tissue Banks (AATB), 64, 108–10

Andrews, Lori, 146, 180, 257, 258

Animal breeding, 207, 232, 234, 267

Annas, George, xiv–xvi, 239, 246, 279, 280

Anonymity, xiii, xiv, 9, 12, 133
  donors and, 126–59
  donors' feelings about, 149–50, 153, 154, 174, 184, 309
  frozen semen and, 107
  legal reform and, 290
  need to end, 81
  problems of, 155
  as protection against paternity suit, 46
  record keeping and, 110, 276
  significance of social ties and, 49
  See also Records, Secrecy

Ariel, Suzanne, 298–300, 321–22, 346

Attitudes toward DI, *See* Social attitudes

Azoospermia, 3, 4, 8, 23, 25, 78, 101, 361, 363

Baran, Annette, 77, 81, 164, 296, 301

Basal body temperature charts, 19, 62, 64, 65, 123, 368–70

Berger, D., 28, 55, 59, 60, 65, 70, 89, 296, 314

Biological ties. *See* Achilles, Rona; Blood lineage

Biopsy
  endometrial, 98
  ovarian, 98
  sperm for DI through, 364–65
  testicular, 4, 5, 93

Birth, 45, 50, 72

Birth certificate, 45, 50, 72
  donor's name on, 194
  falsification of, 213, 214, 222–25, 293, 313, 336
  legislation about, 247
  truthful, 354

Blended families, 199–200, 239, 240, 352

Blizzard, Joseph, 59, 71, 82, 208, 240, 311, 312, 335

Blood donors, 139–41, 152, 226, 264

Blood group matching, 134, 200, 253, 280

Blood lineage, 11, 35, 49–50, 60–61, 73
  anxiety about, 239, 300, 323, 352
  false strain in, 260, 275
  loss of, 239, 286–87, 289
  single women and lesbians, 171, 190
  See also Genealogical bewilderment, Genetic contamination

Blood tests for paternity, 200, 204, 224, 230, 244, 253, 275

Bok, Sissela, 282–85. *See also*

Secrecy bond
Caesarean section, 72, 101, 235
Case law, 260–66
Catholicism, 52, 210–11, 262
Cellular consciousness, 26, 78, 176, 181, 351
Center for Reproductive Alternatives, 159, 171
Cervical cap, 14, 15, 93, 95, 182, 375
Cervical cup, 15, 67, 93, 95
Cervical mucus, 12, 14
  evaluation of, 18, 96, 123
  hostile, 86, 91
  as indicator of fertility, 370–74
  infected, 17
  role of, 368, 371
Chemotherapy, 29, 108, 203, 363
Child
  best interests of, xv, 36, 169, 211, 239, 352
  right to know of DI, 11, 21, 288, 309, 352, 355
  right to know paternal origins, 2, 10, 215, 288, 309
Chromosomal abnormalities
  from frozen semen, 116
  from ovulation induction, 97, 103
Church of England, 211–13
Clomid (clomiphene citrate), 96–97, 363, 368
Conflicts, 28, 79, 178, 324, 350
  Oedipal, 64–66, 73, 78

See also Deception, Incest, Psychological reactions, Secrecy
Congenital malformations, 103, 115
Consent, 257
  of donor, 136, 140, 148, 158–59, 251
  of donor's wife, 151, 250
  implied, 265, 285
  of recipients, 248–53, 265
  See also Contracts
Contracts, 12, 175
  against making, 218–19
  Church of England, 212
  with couple, 198, 250–53
  with donor, 186, 187–89
  lesbians, 189, 192, 195
  single women, 187
  validity of, 13, 249
Corea, Gena, 88, 232–33
Counseling
  DI couple, 57, 68, 278, 281, 328
  donor, 159, 187, 281
  infertility, 37, 203
  single women and lesbians, 228, 379
  See also Support groups
Custody of DI child
  battle between couple for, 81
  in divorce, 261
  donor's protection from, 356
  and illegitimacy, 242

Deception, xiii, 10, 21, 45,

Deception (*Cont.*)
58, 70, 71, 80
and blood groups, 129
of child, 284–87
Church of England's posi-
tion on, 212–13
of extended family, 213,
216, 252, 285, 287, 296,
309
of husband, 311
inheritance, custody, and
support, and, 223
by physicians, 290–91,
213–24
of siblings, 344
of wife, 88
See also Secrecy

Decision making, 37, 42, 59
Denial
of DI, 78, 348
of donor, 213, 216, 307
of infertility, 31
of problems, 328
Depersonalization of donor,
53–54, 61, 73, 78, 155–56
See also Stranger/donor
Depression
postpartum, 308
prenatal, 307
See also Emotional aspects,
Psychological reactions
Disabled women, 202, 225,
229
Disclosure
in adoption, 315
arguments against, 332–34
art of, 336–39

to child, 120, 124, 196,
326–32
counseling for, 33
couple's responsibility for,
326–32
destructiveness of, 81, 287,
299, 301–2, 303–4, 336,
344
to family, 37, 59–60, 216,
329
language of, 334, 338
medical students' opinions
on, 331
nonidentifying information,
273, 276
reactions by offspring to,
336–39
timing of, 334–36
Divorce, 33, 41, 42, 67, 72, 77,
226
child's rights, 267
and DI child, 355
and stored semen, 158
See also Custody, Support
obligations
Donors
altruism of, 137–38, 154,
155, 158
anonymity of, 139, 174, 184
attitudes of, 191–92, 216,
280
characteristics of, 148–49
commitment of, 175–76
extent of use of, 91, 124–25,
145–46
family of, 21, 149–50, 151,
185
feelings about contact with
child, 150

feelings about recipients,
149, 170
fertility of, 173
known to offspring, 309
legal rights of, 157–58,
186–89
litigation and, 258, 307, 309
matching characteristics of
husband, 129, 134, 398
moral responsibility of, 161
motivations of, 134, 137,
142, 155
number of offspring by, 140,
145, 171, 309
as patients, 217, 249
personal profiles of, 119–20,
152–55, 190–92
recruitment of, 128, 173–74,
200, 328
selection of, 129, 134, 148,
169
sources of, 127–28, 200
questionnaire, 193
visitation rights of, 254
See also Depersonalization,
Known donors, Payment,
Responsibilities, Rights,
Selection, Stranger/donor
Donors' Offspring, 77, 303–6
Drugs, fertility. *See* Clomid

Emotional aspects of DI, 19,
51, 56–57, 58, 60, 78
of DI procedure, 61–68,
100–101
fear of error as, 71, 129
and pregancy, 45, 50, 51,
69–72, 170, 347
See also Fantasies, Genetic

contamination, Psycho-
logical reactions, Racism,
Stranger/donor
Epididymovasostomy,
364–65
Estoppel, 261–62
Eugenics, 116, 117, 120, 202,
255
Expense of DI, 64, 67, 182,
197
Extended family, 60, 83, 229
contact with, 347
DI concealed from, 185,
186
false bonds with, 312
sharing DI with, 314, 329,
330
through DI, 178–82
See also Blended families,
Deception, Secrecy

Fantasies, 133, 286–87
of adoptees, 167, 318, 345
of child, 293, 303, 319, 332
of donor, 139
of husband, 223
of mother in pregnancy, 65,
78, 302
of recipients, 324, 343
See also Emotional aspects
of DI, Psychological reactions, Secrecy,
Stranger/donor
Fathers, confused paternity,
319
Feminist Women's Health
Center, 122–25
Fertility, 129–30
Feversham Committee, 274

Follow-up, lack of, 75
See also Records, Secrecy
Foster children, 40, 46, 47
Frozen semen, 29, 102, 111,
125
advantages of, 106–8
coding, 105
disadvantages of, 115–16
effects of freezing on, 115,
116, 124
future use of, 123
history of, 106
inventory and coding of,
112
no control over, 104–5
posthumous use of, 203
safety of, 109
shipping of, 112, 115, 118
storage of, 102
success rates with, 115
thawing, 112, 375
use of, 102
See also Semen, Sperm
banks

Genealogical bewilderment,
xiii, 10, 51, 76, 316, 319
of adoptees, 192, 194
definition of, 292
in IVF, 213
Genetic contamination, 56,
74–75, 133, 207, 300,
301, 302, 332. See also
Racism
Genetic engineering, 206, 234.
See also Eugenics
Genetic heritage
denial of, 63, 304, 312, 424

identity formed by, 323
interest in, 319, 339
right to, 169, 180, 215,
246–47
See also Anonymity
Genetic indications for DI, 66,
202, 222
See also Physicians
Genetic screening of donors,
xiv, 135, 235–37, 281,
356. See also Eugenics
GIFT, 365
Go-between, 173, 189, 193,
194, 379
Grieving infertility, 7, 25,
30–36. See also Genea-
logical bewilderment
Guilt, 32–33, 52
searching for origins, 293
"survivor," 70, 76

Hereditary diseases, 66, 202,
308
fear of, 295, 312
Heredity
missing/confused, 320–23
psychology of, 292–95
See also Genealogical bewilderment
Homosexual men
attitudes toward DI, 199,
379
semen donations from,
132–33, 189, 192, 195
Huntington's chorea, 86, 222,
302, 382
Hysterosalpingogram, 16,
97–98

Illegitimacy, 242–43. *See also*
    Case law
Immunological reaction to
    sperm, 91, 108
    See also Cervical mucus,
    hostile
Inbreeding
    fear of, 145, 308–9, 312
    prevented by using frozen
    semen, 108, 111
    See also Incest
Incest
    cases of, 76, 146
    fear of, 65, 68, 145, 209,
    308
    taboo, 82
    unwitting, 155, 169
Infections
    in DI, 64, 130, 230, 255
    and infertility, 362
    screening donors for, 134,
    255, 280
    See also AIDS, Screening
Infertility
    confusion with virility, 25
    emotional aspects of, 23,
    24, 25, 26, 30–39, 85,
    97, 197
    female workup, 97–101
    insurance coverage for, 201
    rising incidence of, 237
    secondary, 29, 42
    male
    causes of, 361–63
    definition of, 360–61
    physiology of, 359–60
    psychosomatics, 361, 362
    workup, 363

See also Social attitudes
Inheritance, 243–44, 245,
    247
Insemination
    attempts per cycle, 90–93,
    98–99
    to conceal male infertility,
    50, 52
    definitions of, 90–93
    dropouts from, 99, 125
    duration of, 66, 98–99
    history of, 86–90
    husband and, 90–91, 108
    incidence of, 89–90
    indications for, 85–86
    multiple donors and, 99,
    156
    posthumous, 158, 203, 277
    same donor, 61, 106, 156
    statistical results of, 99–101
    techniques of, 93–94
    See also Deception, Donors,
    Genetic indications,
    Known donors, Screen-
    ing, Stranger/donor
Instincts, generative, 42, 53,
    178, 197–98, 200
International Soundex Re-
    union Registry, 349
In vitro fertilization (IVF), xii,
    xv, 67, 197, 201
    attitudes toward, 208
    known donors and, 163
    male infertility and, 365
    stored embryos from, 204

Judaism, 55, 209–10

Karma, 350
Karpel, M., 282, 287–89
Karyotyping, 110, 135, 278
Known donors, 51, 169
  anxiety with, 178
  case histories of, 13–18,
    180, 182–186
  commitment of, 175–77
  difficulties with, 177, 290
  disclosure of, 179
  lesbians' use of, 194, 195
  meeting, 178, 180
  role with child, 178–82,
    189, 191
  selection of, 177, 217
  sources of, 173–74, 217
  questionnaire for, 175

Laparoscopy, 98
Legal dilemmas, 206,
    240–44, 247–54
Legal history, 259. *See also*
    Case law
Legislation, 259, 260–71
  Australia, 272–74
  Canada, 27
  Europe, 277–79
  Great Britain, 274–76
  Sweden, 278
  U.S. proposed, 259, 267
Legitimacy, 244–46, 252,
    275, 354
Lesbians, 83, 92, 105, 122,
    188–96
  anonymity, 173
  case law, 266
  contracts, 192, 195
  custody by, 254, 266

discrimination in access to
    DI, 202, 208, 280
  donors for, 189
  fear of paternity suit, 223
  known donor and, 192–94
  open DI and, 170, 182
  relatives and gay men as do-
    nors, 379
  rights of, 155, 156, 157,
    225–32, 267, 288
  same donor for couple, 379
  self-insemination, 379–81
  studies of offspring, 231–32
Lifton, Betty Jean, 289, 293,
    297, 300, 317, 324, 325,
    328, 331, 345
Linde, Carey, 307–9
Liquid nitrogen. *See* Frozen
    sperm, Sperm banks
Lying. *See* Deception, Secrecy

Malpractice, 256
Marriage, exclusive union in,
    xiv, 47, 209, 212
Masturbating for DI, 93, 126,
    131, 141–45, 154–55,
    191
  emotional reactions to, 58,
    199
  religious objections to,
    210–11
Medicalization of DI, 9, 10,
    140, 155, 203, 206, 273
Medical profession's control
    of DI, xiv, 21, 33, 36, 45,
    54, 93, 140, 193, 214
  evaluating couples, 234

ignoring psychological dimension, 206, 234
lesbians, 193, 202–3, 263, 267
omnipotence, 317
secrecy, 214–15
semen brokers, 157
Medical students
attitudes toward disclosure to child, 331
as donors 121, 127, 130–32, 214, 258, 309
Menstrual cycle, 366–67. *See also* Ovulation
Microsurgery for male infertility, 5, 6, 7, 8, 365
Miscarriage, 103, 116, 130, 256

Naming of DI child, 71, 73
Negligence, 255–57

Offspring
concerns of, 304–6
feelings about DI, 291, 328–29
feelings about donor, 186, 304–6, 348–49
right to genetic past, 339–40
right to visit donor, 258
suit against parents, 231, 250
See also Deception, Genealogical bewilderment, Secrecy, Stranger/donor
Oligospermia, 90, 361
Open DI, 11, 21, 59, 154, 246

Open records, 315–17
Outcome
donors' knowledge of, 124, 146–48
informing donors of, 124, 146–48, 355
negative, 78–82
partner's attitude toward, 100–101
positive, 76–78
See also Emotional aspects of DI, Psychological reactions
Ovulation, 366–67
anovulation, 61, 96, 369
charting, 372–73
inducing, 61
measuring, 96
timing of, 93
See also Basal body temperature charts

Pannor, R., 77, 81, 164, 296, 301
Parenting, 27, 35, 41, 75, 82, 319
gay, 231
Paternity suit, 223, 253–54
by donor, 245
fear of, 146
single women and lesbians avoid, 223, 229
Patriarchy, 27, 156, 198, 216, 244
See also Legitimacy
Payment of donors, 135, 137, 138–39, 142, 154, 173, 211

Payment of donors (*Cont.*)
  prohibition of, 273, 281
  resentment of DI child, 295,
    321, 328
Perjury, 155
Physicians, poor knowlege of
    genetics, 130, 135, 234
Polygyny, 236
Postcoital test, 16, 97
Pratten, Alan and Shirley,
    307–8
Psychological reactions, 91,
    101, 157
  to child, 72–76, 79–82
  of donors, 133–34, 170
  to male infertility, 24–27,
    33, 51, 53, 69, 78
  See also Emotional aspects
    of DI, Genetic contami-
    nation, Racism,
    Stranger/donor
Public opinion. *See* Social atti-
    tudes

Racism, 69, 71, 129. *See also*
    Genetic contamination
Records, xiii, 188, 217–24
  central registries, 272, 273
  Church of England, 212
  destruction of, 342
  of donor as patient, 217
  falsification of, 258–59
  fight to maintain, 308,
    343–44
  of known donors, 187
  lack of, 304, 313
  no copy to couple of, 252
  permanent, 101–11, 121,
    179, 188, 258, 273,
    354–57
  physicians', 111, 113, 158,
    159, 258, 347
  reform of, 259, 281, 341
  sealed, 83, 280, 296, 315,
    344
  single women and lesbians,
    188–89
  of sperm banks, 110, 113,
    116, 121, 159
  updating, 304, 315–16, 356
Reform, 279
Reincarnation, 350
Relatives, use of for DI, 13,
    29, 171–72, 208, 277,
    304
Religious considerations,
    209–213. *See also* Ca-
    tholicism, Church of
    England, Judaism
Repository of Germinal
    Choice, 54, 152, 343
  donor questionnaire from,
    383–95
Reproductive technology, 41,
    50, 83
  commercialism of, 201
  as control over women,
    232–38
  doubletalk in, 232–33
  government regulation of,
    232
  impact on women, 232
  legal issues of, 240
  spiritual aspects of, 350–51
  unexpected outcomes of,
    204

Resemblance, physical
in adoption, 20
in DI, 20, 73, 297, 310, 325
disappointment with, 276
matching donor, 108
Resolve, Inc., 24, 30, 34, 36,
38, 39, 65, 182
Responsibilities
of DI parent, 355
of donor, 159, 161, 355–56
of offspring, 354–55
of practitioners, 356–57
Retrieval of sperm, 153, 176,
195
Retrograde ejaculation, 307
Rh blood factor, 66, 86, 134,
220
Rights
of donor, 157–58, 186–203
to reproduce, 198–200,
206, 225–38
of widow to DI, 203, 267,
277
See also Lesbians, Single
women
Risk factors in DI families, 81.
See also Deception, Emotional aspects, Psychological reactions, Secrecy

Screening of donor, 109, 135,
137, 355, 382–395. *See
also* Donors, Genetic
screening, Known donors
Scripts for disclosure,
examples, 336–37
lack of in DI, 313

Search for biological parent
in adoption, 339, 345–49
in DI, 32–33, 308,
325–26
effect on relationships of,
340–45, 347–48
guilt over, 293
as result of pregnancy, 342
support in, 355
Search organizations,
348–49, 356
Second DI child, 46, 71, 76,
81, 91, 108
Secrecy, xii, xv, 11, 49, 50,
58–59, 68, 70, 72, 76,
79, 81, 82–84, 213
anxiety of, 310–11
burden of, 21, 282–317
conflicts because of, 284,
314
dynamics of communication
in, 288–89
nature and context of,
286–88
philosophical dimensions
of, 282–286
and relatives, 172, 186,
326–34
violation of rights by,
289–92
See also Berger, D.; Deception
Secrecy bond
of donor and child, 180,
184, 191
of mother and donor, 21,
180, 195, 350
See also Known donors

Selection of donors, 255, 382–96
  questionnaire, 382–83
  See also Donors, Genetic screening, Known donors
Self-insemination, 182, 265, 266
  classes in, 123, 125
  difficulties with, 377–78
  with in-laws, 276
  legal aspects of, 249, 262, 267
  techniques of, 14, 67, 374–75
Semen analysis, 2, 3, 7, 23, 110, 130, 360
  done in adolescence, 237
Semen brokers, 237. *See also* Sperm banks
Semen freezing. *See* Frozen semen
Semen mixing, 92–93, 129, 156, 223, 253
  prohibition, 273
Semiadoption, 261
Sex ratio of offspring, 43, 103–4, 125
Sex selection, 108, 234–45, 375–77
Sexuality, 35, 36, 51, 78
  depersonalization of with DI, 20
  between donor and recipient, 170
  of donors, 141
  embarrassment with, 287, 294, 313
  illegitimacy of, 243, 316

Single Mothers by Choice, 227
Single women and DI, 79, 83, 105, 227, 288, 381
  custody case of, 254
  denial of donor by, 156
  discrimination in access to DI, 202, 208, 222, 280
  in Great Britain, 276
  openness of, 170, 182
  responsibilities of, 378
  rights of, 267
  secrecy of, 92
  visitation rights of donor, 254
  See also Feminist Women's Health Center
Social attitudes about DI, 205–8
  and lesbians, 378–81
  and single women, 82, 222
Speculum, 93, 373–74
Sperm banks
  commercial, 108–13
  consumer selection of, 119, 123
  disadvantages of, 115
  liabilities of, 117
  of Nobel Prize winners. *See* Respository for Germinal Choice
  profits of, 111–15
  regulation of, 109
Sperm Bank of Northern California, 122–25
Sperm filtering and concentration, 6

standards for sperm in, 109,
115, 134
sample catalog from,
400–401
sample contract with,
397–98
sample fee schedule of, 399
sample release from, 396
See also Frozen semen, Sex
selection
Sterilization. *See* Vasectomy
Stigma, 4, 50, 70, 316, 360
illegitimacy as, 243, 265
of lesbians and single
women, 170, 193
secrecy and, 296, 301, 310,
311, 335
Stranger/donor, 51, 65, 75,
82, 93, 127, 247, 252,
311, 324, 328
fear of, 10, 29, 51, 96, 190
See also Anonymity
Stress
of donors, 147–48, 155
of infertility 61, 66
of physicians, 214
waiting for DI pregnancy,
215, 277–78
Suicide, 81
Support groups, 37, 58, 312,
314, 332, 356
Support obligations, donor's
fear of, 257, 258, 309
Surrogate mothers, xii, 12, 47,
161–63
exploitation of, 233
legal aspects of, 245
openness of, 161–63, 310

relatives as, 161, 172, 274
remuneration of, 201
and sperm banking, 108
unexpected outcomes of,
204–5, 273
Sweden, 315, 327–28, 331

Testicles
biopsy of, 4
examination of, 364
temperature of, 359
Test-tube babies. *See* In vitro
fertilization
Triadoption Library, 348
Trust
in adoption, 10
in DI, 59, 62, 69, 188
guardian of, 192
in physician, 104–5, 140
violation of, 289
See also Deception, Disclosure, Secrecy
Tubal occlusion
evaluation of, 15
psychosomatic, 26
See also Hysterosalpingogram
Turner, Candace, 77, 303–6

Ultrasound, 96
Uniform Parentage Act, 245,
279–80

Variocele, 362
surgical removal of, 364
Vasectomy, 3, 9, 15, 42, 66,
77, 114

Vasectomy (*Cont.*)
  and remarriage, 86, 265,
    272, 358
  reversal of, 5, 201, 364
Vendor, 138–39, 188
Venereal disease. *See* AIDS,
  Infections
Visitation
  of donor, 254, 265
  by lesbian partner, 266

Waiting list
  for adoption, 8, 9, 217
  for DI, 58, 60, 68, 94
Waller Commission, 239
Warnock Commission, 145,
  201, 239, 290
Wrongful birth suit, 257
Wrongful life suit, 231,
  256–57